Sex, Gender and Substance Use

Sex, Gender and Substance Use

Editor

Lorraine Greaves

MDPI • Basel • Beijing • Wuhan • Barcelona • Belgrade • Manchester • Tokyo • Cluj • Tianjin

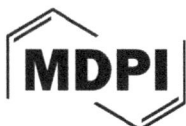

Editor
Lorraine Greaves
Centre of Excellence for Women's Health & University of British Columbia
Canada

Editorial Office
MDPI
St. Alban-Anlage 66
4052 Basel, Switzerland

This is a reprint of articles from the Special Issue published online in the open access journal *International Journal of Environmental Research and Public Health* (ISSN 1660-4601) (available at: https://www.mdpi.com/journal/ijerph/special_issues/sex_gender_substance_use).

For citation purposes, cite each article independently as indicated on the article page online and as indicated below:

LastName, A.A.; LastName, B.B.; LastName, C.C. Article Title. *Journal Name* **Year**, *Volume Number*, Page Range.

ISBN 978-3-0365-0200-7 (Hbk)
ISBN 978-3-0365-0201-4 (PDF)

© 2021 by the authors. Articles in this book are Open Access and distributed under the Creative Commons Attribution (CC BY) license, which allows users to download, copy and build upon published articles, as long as the author and publisher are properly credited, which ensures maximum dissemination and a wider impact of our publications.

The book as a whole is distributed by MDPI under the terms and conditions of the Creative Commons license CC BY-NC-ND.

Contents

About the Editor vii

Preface to "Sex, Gender and Substance Use" ix

Lorraine Greaves
Missing in Action: Sex and Gender in Substance Use Research
Reprinted from: *Int. J. Environ. Res. Public Health* **2020**, *17*, 2352, doi:10.3390/ijerph17072352 . . . 1

Lorraine Greaves and Natalie Hemsing
Sex and Gender Interactions on the Use and Impact of Recreational Cannabis
Reprinted from: *Int. J. Environ. Res. Public Health* **2020**, *17*, 509, doi:10.3390/ijerph17020509 . . . 9

Andreea C. Brabete, Lorraine Greaves, Natalie Hemsing and Julie Stinson
Sex- and Gender-Based Analysis in Cannabis Treatment Outcomes: A Systematic Review
Reprinted from: *Int. J. Environ. Res. Public Health* **2020**, *17*, 872, doi:10.3390/ijerph17030872 . . . 25

Natalie Hemsing and Lorraine Greaves
Gender Norms, Roles and Relations and Cannabis-Use Patterns: A Scoping Review
Reprinted from: *Int. J. Environ. Res. Public Health* **2020**, *17*, 947, doi:10.3390/ijerph17030947 . . . 41

Lindsay Wolfson, Julie Stinson and Nancy Poole
Gender Informed or Gender Ignored? Opportunities for Gender Transformative Approaches in Brief Alcohol Interventions on College Campuses
Reprinted from: *Int. J. Environ. Res. Public Health* **2020**, *17*, 396, doi:10.3390/ijerph17020396 . . . 73

Dian-Jeng Li, Shiou-Lan Chen and Cheng-Fang Yen
Multi-Dimensional Factors Associated with Illegal Substance Use Among Gay and Bisexual Men in Taiwan
Reprinted from: *Int. J. Environ. Res. Public Health* **2019**, *16*, 4476, doi:10.3390/ijerph16224476 . . . 91

Sílvia Font-Mayolas, Mark J. M. Sullman and Maria-Eugenia Gras
Sex and Polytobacco Use among Spanish and Turkish University Students
Reprinted from: *Int. J. Environ. Res. Public Health* **2019**, *16*, 5038, doi:10.3390/ijerph16245038 . . . 105

Isabel Corrales-Gutierrez, Ramon Mendoza, Diego Gomez-Baya and Fatima Leon-Larios
Understanding the Relationship between Predictors of Alcohol Consumption in Pregnancy: Towards Effective Prevention of FASD
Reprinted from: *Int. J. Environ. Res. Public Health* **2020**, *17*, 1388, doi:10.3390/ijerph17041388 . . . 119

Di Xiao, Lan Guo, Meijun Zhao, Sheng Zhang, Wenyan Li, Wei-Hong Zhang and Ciyong Lu
Effect of Sex on the Association Between Nonmedical Use of Opioids and Sleep Disturbance Among Chinese Adolescents: A Cross-Sectional Study
Reprinted from: *Int. J. Environ. Res. Public Health* **2019**, *16*, 4339, doi:10.3390/ijerph16224339 . . 135

Nadia Minian, Anna Ivanova, Sabrina Voci, Scott Veldhuizen, Laurie Zawertailo, Dolly Baliunas, Aliya Noormohamed, Norman Giesbrecht and Peter Selby
Computerized Clinical Decision Support System for Prompting Brief Alcohol Interventions with Treatment Seeking Smokers: A Sex-Based Secondary Analysis of a Cluster Randomized Trial
Reprinted from: *Int. J. Environ. Res. Public Health* **2020**, *17*, 1024, doi:10.3390/ijerph17031024 . . . 147

Carol Hubberstey, Deborah Rutman, Rose A. Schmidt, Marilyn Van Bibber and Nancy Poole
Multi-Service Programs for Pregnant and Parenting Women with Substance Use Concerns: Women's Perspectives on Why They Seek Help and Their Significant Changes
Reprinted from: *Int. J. Environ. Res. Public Health* **2019**, *16*, 3299, doi:10.3390/ijerph16183299 . . . 161

Julie Stinson, Lindsay Wolfson and Nancy Poole
Technology-Based Substance Use Interventions: Opportunities for Gender-Transformative Health Promotion
Reprinted from: *Int. J. Environ. Res. Public Health* **2020**, *17*, 992, doi:10.3390/ijerph17030992 . . . 179

Rachel O'Donnell, Kathryn Angus, Peter McCulloch, Amanda Amos, Lorraine Greaves and Sean Semple
Fathers' Views and Experiences of Creating a Smoke-Free Home: A Scoping Review
Reprinted from: *Int. J. Environ. Res. Public Health* **2019**, *16*, 5164, doi:10.3390/ijerph16245164 . . . 193

Naomi C. Z. Andrews, Mary Motz, Bianca C. Bondi, Margaret Leslie and Debra J. Pepler
Using a Developmental-Relational Approach to Understand the Impact of Interpersonal Violence in Women Who Struggle with Substance Use
Reprinted from: *Int. J. Environ. Res. Public Health* **2019**, *16*, 4861, doi:10.3390/ijerph16234861 . . 211

Mary Motz, Naomi C. Z. Andrews, Bianca C. Bondi, Margaret Leslie and Debra J. Pepler
Addressing the Impact of Interpersonal Violence in Women Who Struggle with Substance Use Through Developmental-Relational Strategies in a Community Program
Reprinted from: *Int. J. Environ. Res. Public Health* **2019**, *16*, 4197, doi:10.3390/ijerph16214197 . . . 225

Sarah C.M. Roberts
The Presence and Consequences of Abortion Aversion in Scientific Research Related to Alcohol Use during Pregnancy
Reprinted from: *Int. J. Environ. Res. Public Health* **2019**, *16*, 2888, doi:10.3390/ijerph16162888 . . 235

Katherine J. Karriker-Jaffe, Christina C. Tam, Won Kim Cook, Thomas K. Greenfield and Sarah C.M. Roberts
Gender Equality, Drinking Cultures and Second-Hand Harms from Alcohol in the 50 US States
Reprinted from: *Int. J. Environ. Res. Public Health* **2019**, *16*, 4619, doi:10.3390/ijerph16234619 . . 245

About the Editor

Lorraine Greaves, Ph.D. Senior Investigator, Centre of Excellence for Women's Health & Clinical Professor, University of British Columbia. Lorraine Greaves is a medical sociologist and founding director of the Centre of Excellence for Women's Health in Vancouver, Canada. She is a researcher on sex and gender influences on health, substance use, trauma and violence, cannabis and tobacco. She focuses on the translation of research evidence to practice and policy. She has published 12 books and numerous articles and reports on substance use, smoking, addictions, research methods and health promotion. She has been named on the Canadian Women in Global Health list and is the recipient of several awards including a Lifetime Achievement Award from the International Network of Women Against Tobacco and an honorary doctorate from the University of Ottawa. In Canada, she is a member of the Scientific Advisory Committee on Vaping Products, and Chair, Scientific Advisory Committee on Women's Health Products.

Preface to "Sex, Gender and Substance Use"

Welcome to this special collection of articles on Sex, Gender and Substance Use. While substance use research, prevention and treatment have been ongoing for decades, sex and gender science is in its relative infancy, with much work yet to be done on integrating sex and gender considerations into substance use research, practice and policy.

Substance use is a significant global public health issue. Its impact on individuals, families, communities, health and criminal justice systems, social cohesion, and governments is costly, sometimes deadly, and often experienced as intractable. Substance use is viewed through many different lenses, including moral, legal, social and psychological. It can also be viewed as a personal problem, a social or economic issue, a cultural practice and/or a criminal activity. Each of these lenses often leads to different social and legal responses, and very different understandings of the dynamics of substance use.

In all cases, however, substance use needs to be viewed with a sex and gender lens in order to fully understand and to respond to it most effectively. Sex-related factors affect how female and male bodies respond to substances, treatments and often differentially develop related diseases and conditions. These factors include hormones, anatomy, metabolism, reproductive systems, genetics and organ function. Such factors differentially affect safe levels of use, speed to intoxication or dependence, and responses to pharmaceuticals, therapeutics, etc. Recognizing such sex-related differences has led to sex-specific health advice regarding safe levels of alcohol consumption, for example. It is now established that females should drink less than males for these reasons.

Gender-related factors are somewhat more temporal and culturally driven, but no less impactful on substance use patterns, prevalence and responses to policy and treatment. Issues such as gender roles and norms, identities, and institutional gender regulations and laws affect the consumption practices of women and men, girls and boys, and gender diverse people. Such factors act on both men and women to differentially affect who takes up substance use, how they access substances and their subsequent patterns and trends. Noting these gender-related factors leads us to consider issues such as power and decision-making differences between men and women in relationships, high rates of substance use among gender minorities and the different impacts of gendered marketing of legal substances such as alcohol and tobacco on women and men. Such research has established, for example, that men use substances more than women and in higher quantities and may be affected by dominant masculinities that increase risk taking and decrease help seeking.

In this Special Issue Book, the authors address and report on sex, gender and sex-gender interactions in detail, and apply them to the analysis of prevalence and trends, interventions and programs, and substance use disorders. These papers consider legal and illegal drugs including alcohol, nicotine, cannabis, opioids and polydrug use, and draw on data from many different countries and cultures. They explore different gendered roles such as fathers, mothers, pregnant women and adolescents. The authors consider the interactions of substance use with other issues, such as intimate partner violence and abortion policy, as well as tailored treatment programs. In summary, the articles in this issue reflect just some of the many ways in which sex and gender affect substance use and responses to substance use.

Lorraine Greaves
Editor

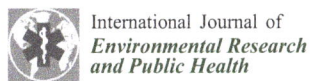

Editorial

Missing in Action: Sex and Gender in Substance Use Research

Lorraine Greaves [1,2]

1. Centre of Excellence for Women's Health, Vancouver, BC V6H 3N1, Canada; lgreaves@cw.bc.ca
2. School of Population and Public Health, Faculty of Medicine, University of British Columbia, 2206 East Mall, Vancouver, BC V6T 1Z3, Canada

Received: 27 March 2020; Accepted: 30 March 2020; Published: 31 March 2020

Abstract: Substance use and misuse is a significant global health issue that requires a sex- and gender-based analysis. Substance use patterns and trends are gendered: that is, women and men, girls and boys, and gender-diverse people often exhibit different rates of use of substances, reasons for use, modes of administration, and effects of use. Sex-specific effects and responses to substances are also important, with various substances affecting females and males differentially. Nevertheless, much research and practice in responding to substance use and misuse remains gender blind, ignoring the impacts of sex and gender on this important health issue. This special issue identifies how various aspects of sex and gender matter in substance use, illustrates the application of sex- and gender-based analyses to a range of substances, populations and settings, and assists in progressing sex and gender science in relation to substance use.

Keywords: sex factors; gender; substance abuse; drinking; alcohol; nicotine; research

---

1. Introduction

Substance use is a significant global health issue, with over 271 million people using illicit drugs each year [1], 2.3 billion using alcohol [2], and 1.4 billion using tobacco [3]. The consumption of substances, both licit and illicit, whether misused or not, can affect the mental and physical health and economic status of individuals, families, communities and bystanders, contribute to overall mortality and morbidity, and pose costs to health care and criminal justice systems. Substances can also be used to experience pleasure, respond to trauma, decrease pain, enhance social and cultural bonds, cope with stress, and adapt to problems in living. Hence, responding to substance use is complex, recognizing both health and social costs as well as patterns and motivations among those who use substances. There is a wide range of substances in use, including alcohol, nicotine, cannabis, opiates, and methamphetamines, as well as misuse of prescription drugs.

Sex and gender both affect substance use in critically important ways. Sex refers to biologically based factors characteristic of female and male bodies, such as hormones, genetics, anatomy, physiology, and organ function. These factors affect how particular bodies respond to the ingestion of substances such as alcohol, cannabis, opioids or nicotine, including the quantity required to create intoxication or effect, create harm or dependence, or cause damage to the body or brain. These factors also affect the range and frequency of resulting health conditions or diseases, such as cancer, heart disease, respiratory illnesses, or psychoses. Sex-specific factors also affect responses to therapeutics and other treatments. These aspects of understanding sex in its entirety are not new. The Institute of Medicine outlined the importance of sex in 2001 for all health researchers and made the fundamental point that "every cell has a sex" [4].

Gender refers to a host of socially and culturally determined factors that affect how men, women, boys, girls and gender-diverse people experience roles, relations, opportunities, customs and expectations. These factors affect individual and social understandings of femininity, masculinity, transgender identities and gender diversity, and are closely tied to cultural contexts. Gender roles and relations affect prevalence and consumption trends, access to substances, initiation into use, responses to advertising, marketing and promotion of legal substances, and how substance use functions in responding to gendered experiences of trauma, caregiving, poverty, social bonding, inequality or marginalization. Gender also affects responses to treatments, policies and health promotion or harm reduction messages. By its nature, gender reflects temporal and cultural interpretations of being men, women or gender diverse, and requires social science theorizing and conceptual development to hone the understanding, use and measurement of gender in its varied contexts.

Taken together, it is easy to see that both sex and gender comprise multiple elements that affect substance use and responses to substance use, such as policy, prevention, or practice. It is important to note that sex and gender also *interact* with each other to affect substance use, and its effects. Sex and gender also intersect with a range of other factors and characteristics such as sexual orientation, income, geography, age, ability, Indigenous status, religiosity, and culture, among others. The measurement challenges posed by these complexities have not been resolved, but these hurdles should not deter substance use researchers from pursuing the impact of sex, gender and sex-gender interactions in our work.

To assist with this process, I have suggested a breakdown of the elements comprising sex and gender for conceptual clarity in order to guide research, practice and policy making in health and in the substance use field. For diagrams, specific examples and to see its application in cannabis, see Greaves and Hemsing [5], in this issue. Sex, for example, includes the impact of hormones, genetics, physiology and anatomy, among many other biologically based aspects of human bodies. Identifying the element of interest in a study assists in sorting out research questions and agendas, clarifying use of terms and language, refining measurement and honing treatments and therapeutics.

It has been important, for example, to note that female and male responses to alcohol are different, and that females require less alcohol to become inebriated or to sustain damage. This is because female bodies typically have more fat, water and fewer enzymes for breaking down alcohol [6]. Hence, in 2012, Canada adopted sex-specific Low-Risk Alcohol Drinking Guidelines that encourage girls and women to drink less per day, week and sitting than men [7]. This not only had a direct impact on health promotion messaging, but also on clinical assessments of health behavior and on calculations of the rates of risky drinking in Canada. In fact, reducing the level of safe drinking for women immediately created a much wider risky drinking problem than had previously been considered [8]. Clearly, precision about such sex-specific effects also needs to be incorporated into all research designs, measures and analyses, to better inform programming and policy development.

Gender also breaks down into a wide range of aspects, but of primary interest are gender relations, gender roles and gender norms as they affect experiential opportunities in any given social context. The experiences of females and males are impacted by gendered attitudes and the assignment of gender roles and norms resulting in stereotypes deemed congruent with that particular sex. This has global ramifications that include more income inequality for women, less decision-making power in relationships, families and state apparatus, more unpaid work, and more subjugation via intimate partner violence, female genital mutilation (FGM), forced marriage and related concerns. The experiences of men include more familial and political authority, paid work and income, along with more subjection to criminal violence, injury and war experiences. Also of interest is the impact of gender identity. One's adherence and identification with dominant interpretations of masculinity, femininity, or gender-diverse identities, such as transgender, non-binary or other culturally specific gender-diverse groups, has an effect on how one performs gender, and is directly related to the patterns and prevalence of substance use. For example, gender minority status is often aligned with higher prevalence of substance use.

Sexual orientation is not to be confused with gender identity. Sexual orientation refers to the romantic and sexual preferences of individuals, and all gender identities can experience a range of sexual orientations including gay, lesbian, bisexual and pansexual. Of interest to the substance use field, though, is that sexual minority status is also a clear risk factor for higher prevalence of substance use.

Ultimately, applying sex and gender to substance use will facilitate the development of tailored treatment, personalized medicine, targeted policies and more precise health promotion and harm reduction. While the past twenty years has seen a rise in interest and application of sex and gender science in health, the substance use field has been slow to insist on the inclusion of these concepts. This special issue [5,9–23] is aimed at providing a remedy for this lack, and more importantly, to provide examples of the impact of sex and gender in a range of substances, cultures, populations and contexts.

These articles address concepts [5], different substances such as alcohol [12,19,23], cannabis [5,17,18], illegal drugs [13], nicotine [11,12], opioids [14], and multi drug use [10], populations such as gay and bisexual men [13], fathers [20], mothers [15], pregnant women [9,23], patients [9,17] and adolescents [14]. They address interactions with interpersonal violence [22], treatment responses [21], abortion policy [23], other harms [12] in a range of settings in countries including Spain, Scotland, Turkey, Canada, China, Taiwan, and the USA. All of the articles address some aspect of sex or gender, interactions between sex and gender, or gender-transformative responses [19] and all contextualize the discussion in a range of cultures and settings. Taken together, they provide a wide range of illustrations of how sex and gender affect both substance use and our responses to it, as well as how research can better address these concepts to derive important and meaningful evidence on which to build treatment and policy.

2. Issues with Language and Conceptual Clarity

The research literature has consistently demonstrated that sex and gender are often conflated both linguistically and conceptually, avoided altogether in research design or policy, or measured, but not reported upon or analyzed. In all cases, important understandings are missed or lost that could assist consumers, researchers, practitioners and policy makers in responding to substance use in more useful, accurate and ethical ways. This theoretical and conceptual "muddle" [24,25] is evident in the substance use literature.

For example, in preparing for the systematic review described in detail in Hemsing and Greaves [18] in this issue, aimed at identifying relevant evidence on four drugs (alcohol, cannabis, nicotine and opioids) that reflected on sex and/or gender, a team of researchers at the Centre of Excellence for Women's Health encountered several issues. We had intended to do a quality appraisal of each selected study and to use Morgan et al. Feminist Appraisal Tool to assist with the appraising of gender, as an additional filter prior to drawing conclusions [26]. However, as described, the response to our search was over 20,000 articles. Once we sifted through these, we found that the muddy conceptual use of sex and/or gender prevented us from confidently carrying out our intended overarching systematic review. Instead, based on this material, we developed several scoping reviews [5,16,18,19] and one small systematic review [17] because terms were either misused or imprecise, or in some cases conflated or used in contradictory ways in a single article. Our intention for systematically surveying the current evidence on sex, gender and substance use was undermined because precise engagement with sex and gender in research was, in essence, missing in action. Some examples of the issues we found include:

1. Using gender to refer to sex or using sex to refer to gender or using both interchangeably.
2. Collecting sex-specific or gender-specific data in the research design, but not reporting it.
3. Collecting sex- and/or gender-related data and reporting but not interpreting or analyzing them.
4. Collecting, reporting and analyzing sex/gender-specific data, but not discussing the impact on practice or policy.

These problems were so ubiquitous that the objective of appropriate analysis was undermined. But these issues are not unique to the literature we searched on substance use. Indeed, these issues are present in much of the extant health literature. While sex and gender science is growing, and more training and resources are available to guide researchers, peer reviewers and students [27], policy makers [28], and practitioners [29,30], there is considerable room for improvement and precision.

3. Implications for Substance Use Research, Practice and Policy

Clearly, it is time to raise the bar on integrating sex and gender more precisely and consistently in substance use research. The articles in this special issue illustrate investigations and analyses on various aspects of sex and gender and substance use in a variety of populations and settings. All of them address sex and/or gender in some way. In addition, one addresses a sexual minority. While not all of the authors identify exactly which aspect of sex or gender is being addressed, readers can, after reviewing the definitions and diagrams [5], and the detailed gender-based analysis addressing cannabis use [18], begin to place the various studies in more precise groups.

Hubberstey et al. [15] consider the gendered social determinants of substance use among disadvantaged women in order to analyze the nature of help required, focusing on the gendered roles, norms and relations affecting women with children who use substances. Andrews et al. [21] offer an elegant description of the links between early intimate partner violence(IPV) and hypothalamic-pituitary-adrenal axis (HPA) dysfunction, relational deficits and pathways to substance use among women with substance use issues. Essentially, this is a study of sex and gender interactions, focused on a high-risk population of women and children. Motz et al. [22] build on this by demonstrating how the *Breaking the Cycle* program in Toronto, Canada, is constructed to repair these effects of early IPV on women who use substances and their children.

O'Donnell et al. [20] consider the gendered aspects of creating smoke-free homes for children through a scoping review on the nascent area of engaging fathers in such activity, and highlights the barriers and facilitators that fathers might face. Focusing on fathers and caregiving is a step toward more gender-transformative approaches to smoke-free home initiatives that have traditionally focused on mothers. Wolfson et al. [19] directly assess the gender-transformative impact of brief interventions on alcohol, via a cogent sex and gender analysis of existing literature in that area. Similarly Stinson et al. [16] address the gendered use of technology to respond to substance use treatment and interventions.

Minian et al. [10] examine a treatment intervention assessing the impact of an online treatment for alcohol use in smokers, and then analyze these results by sex and gender to check for differential outcomes. Similarly, Brabete et al. [17] examine the paucity of evidence on sex-related factors affecting treatment for Cannabis Use Disorder, highlighting the need for research attention on this issue. Font-Mayolas et al. [11] perform a sex disaggregation of descriptive prevalence data on various routes of nicotine administration comparing Turkish and Spanish university students. Their preliminary descriptions and survey questions regarding reasons for use establish basic descriptions of behavior by sex category and invite a two-country comparison. Li et al., from Taiwan [13], address illicit substance use among sexual minority men and the interaction with dynamics such as homophobic bullying and cyberviolence.

The journey towards more precise usage of sex and gender concepts and terminology is ongoing. However, it is not a frill or an option when designing, doing and reporting on research that is intended to influence policy and practice in the field. Knowing the sex-specific tolerance limits and effects of various substances such as alcohol or cannabis on male and female bodies, is essential to designing accurate and relevant prevention, harm reduction, health promotion, and treatment. Understanding the differential health impacts and diseases that result for males and females from using substances is critical for improving diagnoses, medical care and for refining treatment protocols and programs.

Understanding that gender roles, norms and identities have a direct impact on how and why substances are used, how often, how they are accessed, and what their consumption might mean to users is critically important to designing treatment, policy or prevention. Gender also affects all of our responses to the marketing and promotion of legal substances, and what meanings we associate with substances such as cigarettes, e-cigarettes, alcohol and, in some jurisdictions, cannabis. Further, our gender identity affects how health care practitioners respond to us, diagnose and treat us, often based on stereotypes about masculinity and femininity. Knowing that gender minorities experience above average rates of substance use alerts us to the impact of both gendered and transphobic stigma and discrimination.

Taken together, sex and gender contribute to explaining the generally lower prevalence of substance use among women, and the higher rates and amounts of use by men. They may also explain the different subjective effects reported by men and women, and boys and girls, of substances such as cannabis or nicotine. Knowing that men experience higher rates of substance use in general alerts us to the impacts of masculinities.

Knowing that those in sexual minorities are consistently at higher risk for use alerts us to the overarching effects of minority stress, homophobia and discrimination. Knowing that these patterns are also gendered, in that bisexual girls and women are the group at highest risk for substance use is a clue as to how important it is to modify our substance use response systems to improve both gender and health equity.

In short, the field of sex and gender science has a lot to offer to the field of substance use. This special issue is an attempt to fill the gaps in the field, where all too often researchers ignore these concepts and factors in designing, doing and reporting on research. These gaps have a direct and negative impact on the health of individuals and groups, and on the ability to be effective practitioners in substance use treatment and prevention.

4. Conclusions

Integrating sex and gender analyses into research design not only improves science [31], and increases reproducibility, efficiency and accuracy [32], but also advances social justice and gender equity [26,33]. There are numerous issues of design and measurement that are yet to be resolved [34] and there are considerable challenges in designing methods and measures to address sex and gender and interactions with health determinants [35,36]. Nonetheless, it is heartening to see more research funders in several countries ask for sex and gender concepts to be included in research proposals and offer training for researchers and peer reviewers. It is important that some governments insist on sex- and gender-based analyses of policy and programming (see, for example, Sweden [37], and New Zealand [38]), and offer resources and examples to educate. It is critically important that some journals have adopted sex and gender equity in research (SAGER) [39] guidelines to uphold basic requirements for reporting sex and gender in the research articles that they publish. And, it is critical that implementation and knowledge transfer of evidence includes sex and gender [40]. All of these measures blend together to advance sex and gender science, and to raise the bar on the quality of health research. It is my hope that this special issue will do the same for the field of substance use.

Funding: The work described in this article and several other articles in this special issue [5,16–19] was supported by a grant from the Canadian Institutes of Health Research, Institute of Gender and Health. Grant # 384548.

Conflicts of Interest: The author declares no conflict of interest.

References

1. The United Nations Office on Drugs and Crime (UNODC). *World Drug Report*; United Nations: Vienna, Austria, 2019.
2. World Health Organization. *Global Status Report on Alcohol and Health 2018*; World Health Organization: Geneva, Switzerland, 2019.
3. World Health Organization. *WHO Global Report on Trends in Prevalence of Tobacco Use 2000–2025*; World Health Organization: Geneva, Switzerland, 2019.
4. Institute of Medicine. *Exploring the Biological Contributions to Human Health: Does Sex Matter?* National Academy Press: Washington, DC, USA, 2001.
5. Greaves, L.; Hemsing, N. Sex and Gender Interactions on the Use and Impact of Recreational Cannabis. *Int. J. Environ. Res. Public Health* **2020**, *17*, 509. [CrossRef] [PubMed]

6. Mancinelli, R.; Binetti, R.; Ceccanti, M. Woman, alcohol and environment: Emerging risks for health. *Neurosci. Biobehav. Rev.* **2007**, *31*, 246–253. [CrossRef] [PubMed]
7. Stockwell, T. Canada's low-risk drinking guidelines. *CMAJ* **2012**, *184*, 75. [CrossRef] [PubMed]
8. Bialystok, L. Recalculating risk: An opportunity for gender transformative alcohol education for girls and women. In *Making it better: Gender-Transformative Health Promotion*; Greaves, L., Pederson, A., Poole, N., Eds.; Canadian Scholars' Press: Toronto, ON, Canada, 2014; pp. 93–110.
9. Corrales-Gutierrez, I. Understanding the Relationship between Predictors of Alcohol Consumption in Pregnancy: Towards Effective Prevention of FASD. *Int. J. Environ. Res. Public Health* **2020**, *17*, 1388. [CrossRef]
10. Minian, N. Computerized Clinical Decision Support System for Prompting Brief Alcohol Interventions with Treatment Seeking Smokers: A Sex-Based Secondary Analysis of a Cluster Randomized Trial. *Int. J. Environ. Res. Public Health* **2020**, *17*, 1024. [CrossRef]
11. Font-Mayolas, S.; Sullman, M.J.; Gras, M.-E. Sex and Polytobacco Use among Spanish and Turkish University Students. *Int. J. Environ. Res. Public Health* **2019**, *16*, 5038. [CrossRef]
12. Karriker-Jaffe, K.J. Gender equality, drinking cultures and second-hand harms from alcohol in the 50 US states. *Int. J. Environ. Res. Public Health* **2019**, *16*, 4619. [CrossRef]
13. Li, D.-J.; Chen, S.-L.; Yen, C.-F. Multi-dimensional factors associated with illegal substance use among gay and bisexual men in Taiwan. *Int. J. Environ. Res. Public Health* **2019**, *16*, 4476. [CrossRef]
14. Xiao, D. Effect of sex on the association between nonmedical use of opioids and sleep disturbance among Chinese adolescents: A cross-sectional study. *Int. J. Environ. Res. Public Health* **2019**, *16*, 4339. [CrossRef]
15. Hubberstey, C. Multi-Service Programs for Pregnant and Parenting Women with Substance Use Concerns: Women's Perspectives on Why They Seek Help and Their Significant Changes. *Int. J. Environ. Res. Public Health* **2019**, *16*, 3299. [CrossRef]
16. Stinson, J.; Wolfson, L.; Poole, N. Technology-Based Substance Use Interventions: Opportunities for Gender-Transformative Health Promotion. *Int. J. Environ. Res. Public Health* **2020**, *17*, 992. [CrossRef] [PubMed]
17. Brabete, A.C. Sex-and Gender-Based Analysis in Cannabis Treatment Outcomes: A Systematic Review. *Int. J. Environ. Res. Public Health* **2020**, *17*, 872. [CrossRef] [PubMed]
18. Hemsing, N.; Greaves, L. Gender Norms, Roles and Relations and Cannabis-Use Patterns: A Scoping Review. *Int. J. Environ. Res. Public Health* **2020**, *17*, 947. [CrossRef] [PubMed]
19. Wolfson, L.; Stinson, J.; Poole, N. Gender Informed or Gender Ignored? Opportunities for Gender Transformative Approaches in Brief Alcohol Interventions on College Campuses. *Int. J. Environ. Res. Public Health* **2020**, *17*, 396. [CrossRef] [PubMed]
20. O'Donnell, R. Fathers' Views and Experiences of Creating a Smoke-Free Home: A Scoping Review. *Int. J. Environ. Res. Public Health* **2019**, *16*, 5164. [CrossRef]
21. Andrews, N.C. Using a developmental-relational approach to understand the impact of interpersonal violence in women who struggle with substance use. *Int. J. Environ. Res. Public Health* **2019**, *16*, 4861. [CrossRef]
22. Motz, M. Addressing the impact of interpersonal violence in women who struggle with substance use through developmental-relational strategies in a community program. *Int. J. Environ. Res. Public Health* **2019**, *16*, 4197. [CrossRef]
23. Roberts, S. The Presence and Consequences of Abortion Aversion in Scientific Research Related to Alcohol Use during Pregnancy. *Int. J. Environ. Res. Public Health* **2019**, *16*, 2888. [CrossRef]
24. Hammarström, A. Central gender theoretical concepts in health research: The state of the art. *J. Epidemiol. Community Health* **2014**, *68*, 185–190. [CrossRef]
25. Hammarström, A.; Hensing, G. How gender theories are used in contemporary public health research. *Int. J. Equity Health* **2018**, *17*, 34. [CrossRef]
26. Morgan, T.; Williams, L.A.; Gott, M. A feminist quality appraisal tool: Exposing gender bias and gender inequities in health research. *Crit. Public Health* **2017**, *27*, 263–274. [CrossRef]
27. CIHR Institute of Gender and Health. *Science is Better with Sex and Gender*; CIHR Institute of Gender and Health: Ottawa, ON, Canada, 2018.
28. Status of Women Canada. What is Sex and Gender Based Analysis Plus (SGBA+)? 2018. Available online: https://cfc-swc.gc.ca/gba-acs/index-en.html (accessed on 25 March 2020).

29. Schmidt, R. *New Terrain Tools to Integrate Trauma and Gender Informed Responses into Substance Use Practice and Policy*; Centre of Excellence for Women's Health: Vancouver, BC, Canada, 2018.
30. Greaves, L.; Poole, N. *Integrating Sex and Gender Informed Evidence into Your Practices: Ten Key Questions on Sex, Gender & Substance Use*; Centre of Excellence for Women's Health: Vancouver, BC, Canada, 2020.
31. Johnson, J.L.; Greaves, L.; Repta, R. Better science with sex and gender: Facilitating the use of a sex and gender-based analysis in health research. *Int. J. Equity Health* **2009**, *8*, 14. [CrossRef]
32. Tannenbaum, C. Sex and gender analysis improves science and engineering. *Nature* **2019**, *575*, 137–146. [CrossRef] [PubMed]
33. Greaves, L. *CIHR 2000: Sex, Gender and Women's Health*; Centre of Excellence for Women's Health: Vancouver, BC, Canada, 1999.
34. Oliffe, J.L.; Greaves, L. *Designing and Conducting Gender, Sex, and Health Research*; SAGE: Thousand Oaks, CA, USA, 2011.
35. Austin, S. Gender-based analysis, women's health surveillance and women's health indicators—Working together to promote equity in health in Canada. *Int. J. Public Health* **2007**, *52*, S41–S48. [CrossRef]
36. Hankivsky, O. The odd couple: Using biomedical and intersectional approaches to address health inequities. *Glob. Health Action* **2017**, *10* (Suppl. S2), 1326686. [CrossRef] [PubMed]
37. European Institute for Gender Equality. Sweden. 2020. Available online: https://eige.europa.eu/gender-mainstreaming/countries/sweden (accessed on 25 March 2020).
38. New Zealand Ministry for Women. Bringng Gender In. Available online: https://women.govt.nz/gender-tool (accessed on 25 March 2020).
39. Heidari, S. Sex and gender equity in research: Rationale for the SAGER guidelines and recommended use. *Res. Integr. Peer Rev.* **2016**, *1*, 2. [CrossRef]
40. Tannenbaum, C.; Greaves, L.; Graham, I.D. Why sex and gender matter in implementation research. *BMC Med. Res. Methodol.* **2016**, *16*, 145. [CrossRef]

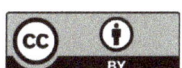

© 2020 by the author. Licensee MDPI, Basel, Switzerland. This article is an open access article distributed under the terms and conditions of the Creative Commons Attribution (CC BY) license (http://creativecommons.org/licenses/by/4.0/).

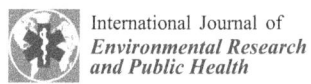

Review

Sex and Gender Interactions on the Use and Impact of Recreational Cannabis

Lorraine Greaves [1,2] and Natalie Hemsing [1,*]

1. Centre of Excellence for Women's Health, Vancouver, BC V6H 3N1, Canada; lgreaves@cw.bc.ca
2. School of Population and Public Health, University of British Columbia, Vancouver, BC V6T 1Z4, Canada
* Correspondence: nhemsing@cw.bc.ca; Tel.: +604-875-2633

Received: 1 January 2020; Accepted: 9 January 2020; Published: 14 January 2020

Abstract: Cannabis is the second most frequently used substance in the world and regulated or legalized for recreational use in Canada and fourteen US states and territories. As with all substances, a wide range of sex and gender related factors have an influence on how substances are consumed, their physical, mental and social impacts, and how men and women respond to treatment, health promotion, and policies. Given the widespread use of cannabis, and in the context of its increasing regulation, it is important to better understand the sex and gender related factors associated with recreational cannabis use in order to make more precise clinical, programming, and policy decisions. However, sex and gender related factors include a wide variety of processes, features and influences that are rarely fully considered in research. This article explores myriad features of both sex and gender as concepts, illustrates their impact on cannabis use, and focuses on the interactions of sex and gender that affect three main areas of public interest: the development of cannabis use dependence, the impact on various routes of administration (ROA), and the impact on impaired driving. We draw on two separate scoping reviews to examine available evidence in regard to these issues. These three examples are described and illustrate the need for more comprehensive and precise integration of sex and gender in substance use research, as well as serious consideration of the results of doing so, when addressing a major public health issue such as recreational cannabis use.

Keywords: sex; gender; cannabis

1. Introduction

Cannabis is the second most frequently used substance in the world, after alcohol [1]. It is an illegal substance in most countries, but increasingly becoming regarded as a controlled substance in various states in the USA and, as of 2018, all of Canada [2]. In 2018, recreational cannabis was legalized in Canada, 17 years after the regulation of medical use. Recreational cannabis use is also legal in Uruguay–for personal use since 1974, and for cultivation and sale since 2013 [3]. Eleven US states plus Washington, D.C. and two US territories (Guam, Northern Mariana Islands) have also introduced legal recreational cannabis use among adults and fifteen US states have decriminalized cannabis. Cannabis is semi-legal in several other countries. For example, Argentina, South Africa, and Mexico have identified punishment for possession of cannabis for personal consumption as unconstitutional; the Netherlands tolerates public consumption and sale of cannabis in licensed coffee-shops; and in Spain personal consumption and cultivation of cannabis is tolerated [3].

When legalization of recreational cannabis occurred in Canada in October 2018, efforts to research the impacts of legalization and use were accelerated and numerous key clinical and public policy issues emerged. In Canada, 17.1% of the population report using recreational cannabis in the past three months, with 20.3% of males and 14% of females reporting such use [4].

While it is unclear how cannabis policies will evolve in other countries, there will undoubtedly be a rapidly evolving legal and social environment in various countries and jurisdictions, as cannabis use increasingly comes to the attention of regulators. However, its widespread use globally indicates that developing evidence of its impacts is already a critical global health issue. Hence, it is important to actively monitor recreational cannabis use patterns and trends, in particular in Canada and other jurisdictions where legalization has occurred, in order to understand the implications of such regulation and legalization.

It is clear from the wider substance use research field that sex- and gender-related factors (fully defined below) have a profound effect on substance use, the effects of use, and the response to interventions, approaches to treatment and overall policies [5]. As cannabis use trends evolve, it is therefore essential to collect and analyze evidence on sex and gender related factors and the effects on the benefits and risks of cannabis use. In the past, however, the integration of sex and gender concepts in substance use research and policy has often been overlooked [5], thereby preventing the building of evidence for effective programming for all sub populations and individuals. Integrating sex and gender in a disciplined manner within all future cannabis research will inform tailored harm reduction messaging, health information, and prevention and treatment responses for all genders.

1.1. How Do Sex and Gender Matter in Substance Use?

Sex related factors include the biological factors and mechanisms that are affected by, or affect, substance use in male and female bodies, while gender related factors include the effects on all people of gender norms, relations, identity and gendered institutional factors including customs, laws and regulations. Further, sex and gender related factors interact to influence patterns of substance use, effects of use, and responses to treatment. For example, Becker et al. argue that "gender and sex differences in addiction are a complicated interaction between sociocultural factors and neurobiological sex differences" [6]. It is also essential to take a transdisciplinary approach to addictions research in order to capture the myriad conceptual and theoretical perspectives that impact use and responses to substance use [7], including both sex and gender [8]. More specifically, investigating and analyzing interactions between aspects of sex and gender in cannabis research is an important step in understanding the full impact of cannabis use and legalization, as well as developing the required evidence for effective policy, programming, messaging and treatment.

Sex related factors include a number of aspects of human biology, physiology, anatomy and genetics (see Figure 1). Bodily characteristics at birth are either male or female, with a small percentage of individuals who are labelled as intersex due to ambiguous characteristics [9]. These male or female characteristics contribute to a lifetime of developmental milestones, processes and stages, and determine reproductive capacity. In addition, a range of processes are affected by sex-based factors such as rates of metabolism, production of sex hormones, organ function, and development and distribution of adipose tissue, among others. These factors affect the ingestion of substances, including cannabis, and their rate of absorption, effects and impacts on the body and brain. These sex-based factors can also affect the response to therapeutic and treatment regimes, such as pharmaceutical treatments.

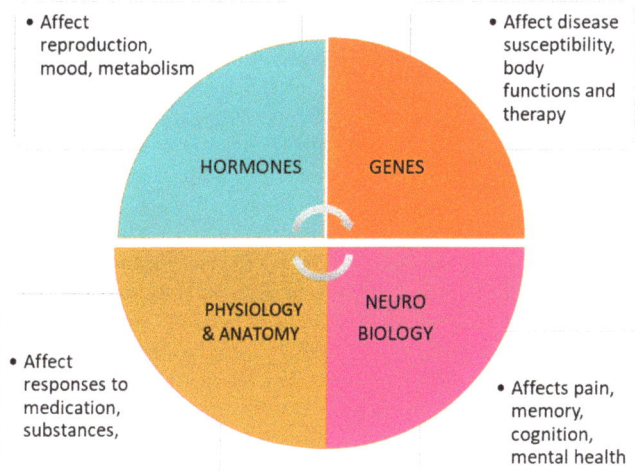

Figure 1. Sex related factors. These factors include reproductive characteristics, physiological processes, susceptibility to substances, and impacts on all body systems.

Gender is often assumed or ascribed, based on our sex. Gender related factors are those connected to the gender relations we experience, the gender roles and norms to which we are exposed and influenced by, our gender identities (such as feminine, masculine, or gender diverse) and the gendered regulations and rules embedded in institutions such as education, politics and religion (see Figure 2). These factors are often temporal and culturally dependent and can change over time.

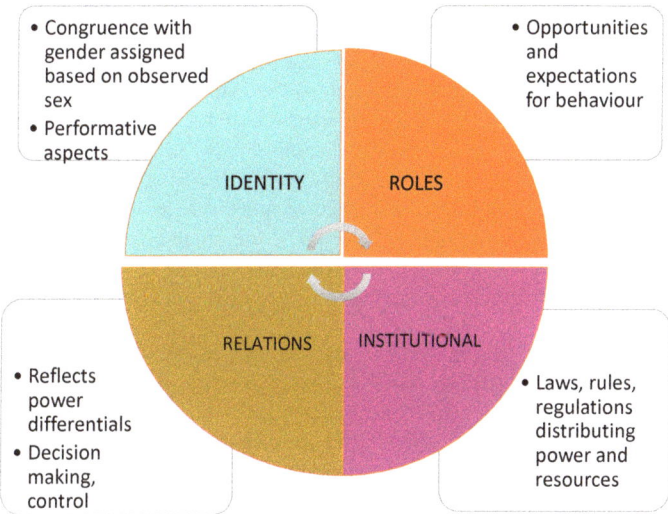

Figure 2. Gender related factors. These factors include culturally driven influences on relationships, opportunities, access to power, resources, decision making, autonomy, and identity.

For example, substance use initiation patterns can be influenced by gendered relationships with partners or household members or friends, affecting our access and usage of cannabis. These influences can heighten dominant understandings of masculinity or femininity, and be expressed in intimate partnerships, peer groups, friendships, or families. Gendered roles such mothering or fathering are often impacted by substance use, in that caregiving is often seen as anathema to substance use, particularly for mothers for whom the stigma associated with substance use is acute. Gender identities and the 'performance' of our identities; whether feminine, masculine, or gender diverse (transgender, non-binary, or queer) have an impact on how and why substances such as cannabis are used, ingested, and in what contexts, not to mention how they are marketed and advertised when legal. Finally, large institutions affect substance use by imposing standards, moral teachings, or public education that implies restrictions, rules or opportunities based on gender, all of which can restrict or encourage substance use in gendered ways.

This wide range of gender related factors combine to create social and cultural contexts for substance use that in turn interact and intersect with the sex-based factors, along with a range of other characteristics such as sexual orientation, age, income, ethno/racial characteristics, Indigenous status, ability, rural and remote life, occupation, etc., to create both clinical and public health impacts.

In short, both sex and gender are of relevance and importance to any researcher or clinician investigating any substance use, including recreational cannabis. If such concepts are introduced (in disciplined and precise ways) into research designs, measured, analyzed, and reported, the resulting evidence will contribute to improved public education and health information for the population. This will enable the promotion of safe cannabis use, which is especially important in a rapidly changing policy environment. Further, including sex and gender in the analysis of the impact of policy can lead to more tailored and sharpened regulations, standards and public policy.

1.2. Gendered Trends of Use

Similar to most substances, more men than women use cannabis. According to data from the 2019 National Cannabis Survey in Canada, more men than women reported cannabis use in the past three months (20.3% vs. 14%). Further, men are more likely to report greater frequency of use and are twice as likely as women to report daily or almost daily use (8% of men vs. 4% of women). Indeed, after alcohol, cannabis is the most commonly used substance in Canada. These national statistics on cannabis use in Canada mirror evidence from the US and Europe where boys and men also report greater prevalence of cannabis use. Indeed, the prevalence of cannabis use among boys and men is higher compared to girls and women for past year [10–12], lifetime [13,14], and past 90 day use [15]. However, again, similar to historical trends of other substances there is evidence of a narrowing in the gender gap [14,16]. Some researchers suggest that the diffusion of cannabis use and experimentation appears similar to that observed with tobacco, with use beginning among men and more educated and higher income groups first, with later diffusion to women and lower socioeconomic status groups [16]. While population based data on prevalence of cannabis use among transgender populations are limited, a study conducted in the USA with $n = 1210$ transgender adults identified cannabis use among 24.4% of the sample; and cannabis use was significantly greater among transgender men compared to transgender women [17].

The majority of available studies and surveys have focused on gendered patterns and preferences for cannabis use. These forms of data are instrumental in offering insight into modes of use and trends of use. For example, there is evidence of gendered preferences for cannabis routes of administration [18], and that dominant gender norms may be reinforced or resisted through cannabis use behaviors [19]. With respect to sex related factors, some recent reviews have examined preclinical and clinical research on sex differences in the therapeutic effects of cannabis and potential for abuse [20] and on the sex-specific neurobiological mechanisms of cannabis use and dependence and associations with psychiatric symptoms [21]. Early evidence of sex differences from animal studies and (to a lesser extent) human studies suggests that females may be more sensitive to cannabis or cannabinoids in general [21], may transition to problematic cannabis use faster than males, and exhibit more intense withdrawal symptoms during abstinence [20].

Clearly, sex and gender related factors both matter in the context of cannabis use and there is much yet to explore in research and clinical practice. Overall, evidence on either sex or gender and cannabis use is lacking and nascent [22]. However, there is also a clear lack of research examining the interactions of sex and gender based factors on cannabis use and its effects. Hence, this paper draws on evidence from two scoping reviews to explore sex and gender based factors, and the potential interactions of these factors in the context of three key and current cannabis use practice and policy issues: cannabis use dependence, cannabis routes of administration (ROA), and driving under the influence of cannabis. These three exemplars comprise: a key clinical issue, a key health promotion/harm reduction issue, and key public policy issue. These are all important issues in early phases of legalized cannabis regimes, and all currently under scrutiny in Canada.

2. Materials and Methods

This article draws on evidence from two scoping reviews examining sex and gender related factors in the context of cannabis use, including: (1) a scoping review on sex, gender and substance use which identified $n = 784$ papers on cannabis; and (2) a more specific scoping review on sex, gender and cannabis routes of administration. The methods for the former are described in full in Hemsing and Greaves [23]. The methods for the latter review are described below.

Scoping Review on Routes of Administration

We conducted a second scoping review of the academic and grey literature to identify literature on cannabis routes of administration (ROA). Specifically, we searched the literature for evidence on sex, gender and cannabis smoking or cannabis vaping, and health promotion, harm reduction and policy approaches to ROA.

The research questions were:

(Q1) How do sex and gender related factors impact:

    (a)   The mode of cannabis or tobacco/nicotine use (ROA)?
    (b)   The health effects of various cannabis routes of administration?

(Q2) What existing health promotion, harm reduction and policy approaches to cannabis ROA are available? Do these approaches include a sex/gender/equity lens?

The following academic databases were searched:
Medline, Embase (including Ovid), Cochrane; CINAHL, PsycINFO, Social Work Abstracts, Women's Studies International, and Social Science Citation Index via Clarivate Analytics

The search covered studies published in the past 10 years (2009 to 2019) combining the following search terms on sex/gender and ROAs:

women; man; women; men; girl; boy; girls; boys; trans; transgender; female; male; sex; gender AND cigar*; e-cigar*; tobacco; nicotine; smoking; vaping; "heat not burn"; marijuana; cannabis; cannabinoid.

In total, $n = 2332$ studies were identified after duplicates were removed. One researcher screened abstracts and full papers, including studies that measured and analyzed some aspect of sex or gender, and that examined cannabis or tobacco routes of administration. Following abstract screening and full paper screening, $n = 122$ studies were included. In addition, we conducted a targeted search on the co-use of cannabis and tobacco and identified an additional 80 studies; after abstract and full paper screening, 19 of these studies were identified as relevant. In total, $n = 131$ papers were included in the scoping review.

This paper draws on some of the key findings from these two scoping reviews to consider the interplay of sex and gender in the context of cannabis use on three topic areas: cannabis use dependence, driving under the influence and cannabis routes of administration. Given the paucity of evidence on the interaction of sex and gender in cannabis use, relevant findings on sex, gender and substance use are included to explore biological and social interactions.

3. Results

3.1. Cannabis Use Dependence

Cannabis use disorder (CUD) affects approximately 10% of cannabis users [1]. It results in a range of symptoms, such as using cannabis in larger amounts or greater frequency than intended, challenges with cutting down, and withdrawal symptoms including anxiety and insomnia [24]. Despite the minority of users developing CUD, it is a high priority public health issue as dependency can interfere with social and economic activities, as well as negatively impact health and wellbeing. Monitoring the potential CUD effects post cannabis legalization is a key aspect of assessing the clinical impact of such legislation.

Sex and gender related factors both affect the development and impact of cannabis use disorder. Similar to other substance use, there is emerging evidence that females transition more quickly to cannabis use dependence compared to males, a process often called "telescoping" [25,26]. Cross-sectional studies analyzing US national data reported no differences between females and males in the age at first or heavy cannabis use, age at onset of CUD, total number of episodes of cannabis abuse or dependence, or in the number of criteria met for cannabis dependence [25]. However, the time from age at first use of cannabis to the age at onset of the CUD was longer among males (mean = 2.64 years vs. 2.24 years, $F = 5.20$, $p < 0.05$), providing support for telescoping among females who use cannabis [25].

Similarly, a second study found that while prevalence of CUD was greater among males, females reported a shorter duration from onset of cannabis use to onset of CUD compared to men (mean of 5.8 vs. 4.7 years) [26]. Clinical research also indicates greater abuse liability among females, such that females reported greater subjective effects at lower doses of oral THC (5 mg), while males reported greater subjective effects at higher doses (15 mg) [27]. The authors suggest these sex differences in subjective effects may contribute to the more rapid progression to dependence (telescoping) observed in females [27]. Clearly, more robust research on cannabis telescoping is needed to inform tailored prevention and harm reduction approaches for women and girls, in particular.

There is also emerging evidence that females may experience greater severity of cannabis dependence. In animal studies (mostly rodents) females have demonstrated slightly greater withdrawal symptoms compared to males, which is one component of dependence [28,29]. However, there are clear challenges in translating findings from animal to human studies including: more controlled experimental conditions, different methods of administration, the tendency to use synthetic forms of cannabinoids, and translational challenges due to the differences between animal and human bodies. Unfortunately, females tend to be underrepresented in human studies despite evidence of a telescoping effect [30].

However, there is some evidence based on self-reports of more severe CUD symptoms among women. Analysis of the US National Epidemiological Survey of Alcohol and Related Conditions (n = 43,093) found that both women and men who used cannabis reported a lower quality of life compared to those who did not use cannabis, and women and men with CUD reported a lower quality of life compared to those without CUD [31]. However, the negative effect of cannabis use on mental quality of life scores was more pronounced for women. Each daily joint smoked was associated with a greater decrease in mental quality of life summary scores in women compared to men [31]. This effect does not appear to be due to higher prevalence of depression among women who used cannabis, as there was no difference in the prevalence of mood and anxiety disorders between women and men in the sample who used cannabis. In our review, another study also reported greater CUD severity in women. In a sample of treatment-seeking adults with CUD, women reported greater withdrawal intensity, more co-occurring mental health issues (including lifetime panic disorder and current agoraphobia), and more days of poor physical health [32].

Both the telescoping effect and differences between women and men in the severity of CUD, may reflect the influence of sex hormones, the endocannabinoid system, and pharmacodynamics and pharmacokinetics. Neurobiological differences have been identified in the endogenous cannabinoid system of females and males. Studies examining the neural regions of rats have reported greater CB1 receptor desensitization and downregulation in females, which may in part explain cannabis telescoping among females [33]. In addition, sex hormones may modulate cannabinoid sensitivity [34–36]. However, studies on the influence of sex hormones on responses to cannabinoids in humans are lacking [21]. Cannabis pharmacodynamics and pharmacokinetics may also be implicated in the development of dependence. While sex differences in the metabolism of cannabinoids have been demonstrated in animal studies, these findings have not, to date, been found in human studies. For example, female rats metabolize THC more quickly than males [37,38], although this effect was reversed when CBD was provided to the rats before injection with THC [38]. Female rats also produce more 11-OH-Δ^9-THC, the primary active metabolite of THC, while males metabolize THC to 11-OH-Δ^9-THC and other inactive metabolites [21]. Further research is required to investigate the biological mechanisms underpinning sex differences in the progression to cannabis use dependence and the severity of cannabis use dependence.

While it has not yet been investigated, there may also be a gendered dimension to the greater severity of CUD reported by women. Women experience greater stigma and discrimination when they use substances of any kind, and this may partially explain the greater severity of CUD observed among women in some observational studies. For example, women may experience and report more shame and blame regarding their substance use, particularly if they are pregnant or parenting [39]. In general, women with substance use issues tend to experience more isolation and less social support compared to men [6]. The experience of stigma creates additional barriers to accessing substance use services and supports for substance use dependence and related health and social services, which may exacerbate the negative effects of women's cannabis use dependence. Identifying the specific sex and gender factors associated with greater CUD severity among women, and tailoring treatment responses to ameliorate these risks is an important consideration for intervention development.

However, despite evidence of a telescoping effect and greater severity of CUD for females, males are more likely to be diagnosed with CUD [13] and tend to report a younger age of onset of CUD [40]. If there is evidence of a more rapid progression to dependence among females, and emerging evidence that females with CUD may be more severely impacted, why are men more likely to be diagnosed with CUD? As argued by Becker and colleagues, biological vulnerability does not equate to greater prevalence of dependence [6]. While biological factors impact the reinforcing effects of cannabis, social and environmental factors also influence the development of CUD [41]. Specifically, gender roles and norms may impact the risk of developing CUD. Men and boys tend to have greater prevalence of cannabis use, initiate earlier and use cannabis more frequently; and being male has been identified as one of the greatest risk factors for developing CUD [41].

Gender differences in the prevalence of substance use are in part due to men's greater access to substances relative to women [42]. Substance use is more socially acceptable among boys and men relative to girls and women, and therefore men tend to have greater opportunities and access to substances in their social environments. In addition, adherence to dominant masculine norms boys has been associated with increased risk taking and substance use behaviors in general [43]. This is also reflected in the cannabis research literature suggesting that men tend to engage in riskier patterns of use, thereby increasing their risk of cannabis use dependence. For example, boys and men tend to report using a greater variety of cannabis routes of administration [18], and use higher potency cannabis products including cannabis concentrates [44] both of which increase the risk of dependence. With expanding cannabis legalization and increasing normalization of use, it will be crucial to monitor changes in gendered patterns of use and risks of dependence, particularly given the emerging evidence on greater biological vulnerability to dependence among females.

3.2. Routes of Administration

Routes of administration (ROA) refer to the various methods of using, inhaling or ingesting cannabis. These include: smoking, vaporizing, heating, ingesting oils or edibles, or using topical versions of cannabis such as creams. It is often assumed that smoking cannabis is the standard approach, both in popular culture and often implicitly, in policy and health promotion. However, examining and comparing the effects of ROAs using sex and gender related factors is essential to creating more precise and harm reducing health information and advice. The majority of the studies on cannabis ROAs that include an analysis of sex or gender have simply described prevalence and patterns of use. Men and boys tend to report higher rates of inhalation ROAs (smoking and vaping), including: joints, blunts, vaporizers, and concentrates [15,45], and water pipes/bongs [46]. There is some evidence that young women [47] and girls [48] may prefer edible cannabis products.

Several human studies have examined the pharmacokinetics of smoked cannabis. Some have demonstrated higher concentrations of THC and THC-COOH levels among females compared to males after administration of smoked [49,50] or vaporized cannabis [50], and greater subjective ratings of cannabis intoxication among females [49]. In contrast, a study with young adults aged 19–25 years who regularly used cannabis (1–4 days per week) found that females smoked less of the cannabis cigarette compared to males to reach their desired effect, but that blood THC and THC-COOH (a metabolite of THC) levels were lower among females compared to males even after adjusting for differences in the dose of THC inhaled [51]. The authors suggest that the similar subjective effects experienced by females at lower doses may reflect sex differences in the endocannabinoid system, as some animal studies have demonstrated greater cannabinoid type-1 (CB1) receptor availability and binding affinity with cannabinoids in females [51]. Ovarian hormones may also influence the subjective effects of cannabis in females; studies with other substances have revealed differences in subjective effects depending on menstrual cycle phase, though similar research on cannabis is currently lacking [51].

Further, Matheson et al. (2019) suggest that there may be sex differences in cannabis smoking topography [51]. In their experiment, females and males smoked for the same duration yet females smoked less of the cannabis cigarette suggesting they took smaller puffs, inhaled less deeply or held the smoke in the lungs for a shorter duration [51]. This finding may be influenced by neuro-biological factors, such as greater cannabinoid sensitivity among females [21], causing females to titrate their dose via their smoking behaviors. There could also be gender related influences; for example, a qualitative study with cannabis using women and men found that women often reported only smoking part of a joint, and typically avoided more "intense" ROAs such as water pipes/bongs, instead preferring a more gradual high [52]. The authors suggest these patterns of cannabis use align with feminine norms regarding the avoidance of excessive substance use and intoxication [52].

Recently, the emergence of e-cigarette or vaping associated lung injury (EVALI), highlights how gendered cannabis ROA preferences may shape health risks. EVALI has primarily affected young men (70%) in the USA and the majority of the reported cases have involved vaping THC products [53]. In the context of an unregulated market, young men may be more likely to access counterfeit cannabis vaping cartridges that are contaminated, increasing their risk of EVALI. Combined with broad improvements in the regulation of vaping products, tailored prevention and harm reduction responses are needed.

The preferences of women and girls for edible cannabis may reflect gender roles and norms regarding the social acceptability of substance use. Inhalation methods are more visible, while edible use can be easily concealed. This may be a more desirable option for girls and women, to avoid experiencing discrimination and stigma related to their cannabis use. This was reflected in a focus group study which found that girls reported a preference for edible cannabis because these products are more discreet [54]. However, given the challenges of titrating edible cannabis dosage, these trends and preferences signal the need for gender informed harm reduction messaging.

There is also evidence of differences in preferred ROA within groups of women and men. For example, women who are pregnant may prefer inhalation methods, because of the difficulty ingesting due to nausea [55]. This is an example of how biological factors—hormonal changes and/or pregnancy-related nausea, may underpin preferences for cannabis ROAs.

Culture can also intersect with gender roles to influence preferred routes of administration. Mixing cannabis with tobacco, often called "spliffs" is a common practice in some countries, particularly in the UK, European countries, and Australia [56]. In a qualitative study with Australian men who "mulled" (smoked a mixture of cannabis and tobacco), men described the effects of mixing tobacco and cannabis as producing a milder, more manageable "high" [56]. They described feeling more "grounded" than if they smoked only cannabis, and they preferred this effect as they were able to continue to participate in family and work responsibilities. In addition, blunt use–hollowed out cigars filled with cannabis, have been promoted through hip-hop culture [57], and are particularly popular among young Black males in the USA [58–62]. However, cannabis use ROAs that combine cannabis and tobacco, such as spliff and blunt use, confer greater risk of dependence [57] as well as adverse respiratory health effects. Gendered and/or culturally sensitive harm reduction messaging that addresses the risks associated with co-use of cannabis and tobacco is warranted.

In short, the sex and gender interactivity affecting ROA choices and effects should be areas of key concern to clinicians, researchers, and health promotion and harm reduction specialists. Currently precise and gendered health information aimed at the general public about ROA choices is lacking, along with tailored information that includes basic evidence on sex and gender.

3.3. Driving Under the Influence of Cannabis

Driving under the influence of cannabis is a key public policy issue in jurisdictions that have legalized recreational cannabis. Discussions about legalization of cannabis often focus on estimating risks associated with possible impaired driving. Not surprisingly, after the legalization of cannabis in Canada in 2018 there has been increased interest in understanding cannabis related impairment and preventing and responding to driving under the influence of cannabis. This emphasis formed one of the key focal areas of health promotion and messaging campaigns aimed at young people in particular [63].

Impaired driving is a gendered activity, with the prevalence of driving after cannabis use higher among men. In a Swedish study, a greater proportion of men were apprehended with THC concentrations detected in their blood (94% vs. 6%), and among those with detected THC, blood concentrations were higher in men than in women (mean 2.1 ng/mL vs. mean 1.4 ng/mL) when cannabis was the only substance detected [64]. In a US study, among college students who reported past month cannabis use, 43.9% of males and 8.7% of females reported driving after cannabis use [65]. In addition, males were more likely to report riding as a passenger with someone who had recently used cannabis (51.2% vs. 34.8%). O'Malley and colleagues' analysis of US high school seniors also found that male students were more likely to report driving after smoking cannabis; however, there was no gender difference in riding as a passenger after cannabis use [66].

Gendered patterns of cannabis use likely influence the risk of driving under the influence of cannabis. In one study, males were more likely to both vape and use cannabis edibles; and more frequent vaping was associated with driving under the influence [67]. As discussed above, in general, boys and young men tend to engage in riskier substance use behaviors. Boys and men are also more likely to co-use cannabis and alcohol, which significantly increases impairment, driving errors and accidents [68]. Further, compared to women, men tend to perceive lower harm with driving under the influence of cannabis, are less likely to believe that cannabis negatively affects their driving ability, are more likely to perceive their friends as approving of driving under the influence of cannabis, and are more likely to report an intention to drive after cannabis use in the future [69]. These gendered patterns of cannabis use and beliefs and perceptions are clear and critically important targets for gender specific harm reduction and health promotion efforts. Specifically, gender informed harm reduction messaging is needed that addresses both driving after cannabis use and riding as a passenger with a driver who has recently consumed cannabis.

Sex differences in the subjective effects of cannabis may impact impairment. As noted above, the greater subjective effects that females tend to experience at lower doses and with a lower blood level of THC may suggest the potential for greater impairment with a lower dose of cannabis among females [51]. It is possible that females may require more time to achieve sobriety before driving, though further research is required to investigate sex differences in the metabolism of cannabinoids and the effects on intoxication and impaired driving. This evidence can be used to inform more precise and refined harm reduction and health promotion responses, messages, and recommendations. Sex specific measures of impairment are lacking; further research is needed to understand sex differences in cannabis impairment and effects on attention and driving to inform measures of impairment and enforcement of impaired driving laws.

It is clear that more research is needed to examine sex differences in driving related impairment. In simulated studies by Anderson et al., they found no evidence of any sex differences. They studied the effects of inhaled THC on attention impairment among people who used cannabis occasionally (participants reported using cannabis at least once per month, but no more than 10 times per month), while driving in a simulator [70], and found no sex differences in the impact of cannabis use. In another study, participants reduced their overall driving speed and performed more poorly on a neuropsychological test following the driving simulation, but no sex differences were observed [71]. In short, this vital area of public policy is still lacking in research that would enable health promoters and enforcement officials to better target their messaging and policy using comprehensive sex and gender related evidence.

4. Discussion

Research on sex and gender related factors and cannabis use and its effects is in its infancy. This area needs considerable attention and growth in light of the high level of cannabis use globally, as well as the legalization of cannabis in various jurisdictions. We have reported elsewhere on known sex and gender related factors that appear to affect use, impact and effect of cannabis use [22]. In this article we have elucidated the various components of sex and gender that are relevant to the study of recreational cannabis use (and other substances) and illustrated how sex and gender interact and combine their effects. We illustrated these interactions in three examples relevant to health outcomes, health promotion and public policy: the development of CUD, the differential choices and impacts of ROA, and cannabis impaired driving.

Aside from one review that acknowledges the influence of both social and biological factors on cannabis use [41], most of the literature we found in our searches for sex and gender influences on cannabis use and ROA has examined either sex related or gender related factors. Going forward, a framework may be useful for examining the interactions of sex and gender, along with other social dimensions of health and equity. There have been calls for understanding intersectional factors affecting health, including the intersection of sex and gender [72]. While intersectional frameworks have been criticized for not adequately attending to biological factors, some proponents have identified opportunities for integrating biological and social dimensions of health within this framework, and begun to consider how biological factors intersect with other factors including gender, class, and ethnicity to address health inequities [73].

Physiological aspects of sex are increasingly understood as being influenced by gender-related social dynamics [74]. Yet, most of the evidence on gender and cannabis to date has focused on noting simple differences between women and men and boys and girls in patterns and prevalence of use. The evidence on sex differences in cannabis use is largely confined to animal studies, and studies on humans have not consistently included female participants and/or integrated a full sex-based analysis. More research is needed to understand how male and female bodies respond to cannabis use and the respective health consequences of use, and the influence of social factors on biological mechanisms. This evidence can then be used to inform more precise harm reduction and health promotion messaging, similar to the sex specific Canadian Lower Risk Drinking Guidelines [75]. Overall, the development of precise, sex, and gender tailored responses to cannabis use are needed to reduce harms, maximize benefits, and improve clinical treatment and health promotion.

Despite these current limitations and insufficiencies, these early findings on cannabis use dependence, cannabis routes of administration, and driving while under the influence have important implications for prevention, health literacy, public education, and treatment. For example, tailored messaging is needed to address risky patterns and consequences of use among boys and men, including greater and more frequent cannabis use, inhaling high potency/high THC products, co-use with alcohol and tobacco, and driving or riding with drivers under the influence of cannabis. For women, emerging evidence on female vulnerabilities to developing dependence and severity of CUD could inform prevention and treatment responses. If telescoping occurs more quickly in females, compounded by increased social stigma directed at women, treatment options should be more readily available for women at the earliest stage possible.

In addition, gender specific efforts can be made to address and reduce discrimination and stigma for all groups, via public education and in the design and delivery of substance use services. Further, considering sex and gender together in cannabis use, can pave the way for gender transformative initiatives in health promotion and messaging. Such approaches simultaneously reduce risky use and work toward gender and health equity in cannabis prevention, harm reduction and treatment responses, thereby alleviating inequities associated with cannabis use [76,77].

It will be critical to continue to monitor and collect data on gendered cannabis use patterns. Patterns of use may change as recreational cannabis becomes increasingly normalized, and producers and advertisers tailor product promotions to target specific groups. As discussed, the gender gap appears to be narrowing [16] and there are indications that cannabis vapour product producers are marketing specific devices to girls and women [78]. If the gender gap in cannabis use continues to narrow, and girls and women begin to use different cannabis ROAs, this will likely affect their health and social consequences of cannabis use including cannabis dependence and driving under its influence.

5. Conclusions

While research on recreational cannabis use is rapidly expanding in response to a shifting policy landscape, research specifically focussed on the impact of sex and gender on its use is in its infancy. More adherence and precision is required in applying sex and gender related concepts to the study of substance use in general, and cannabis use in particular. Robust studies are needed to investigate a full spectrum of sex related factors in the effects of cannabis use; and to explore how gender norms, roles, relations and identities all impact cannabis use and health and social consequences. Further, as illustrated using the examples of CUD, ROA and impaired driving, research is needed that examines the interactions of sex with gender related factors and other social determinants of health including class, age, income, and ethnicity to address and prevent inequities in health related to cannabis use. Advancing knowledge on the interaction of sex, gender and equity based factors will inform more responsive health promotion, effective harm reduction, and precise treatment approaches for all genders.

Author Contributions: Both authors contributed to the analysis of literature review findings and manuscript preparation. All authors have read and agreed to the published version of the manuscript.

Funding: This research was supported by funding from the Canadian Institutes of Health Research Institute of Gender and Health (CIHR-IGH) Knowledge Translation Team Grant, and the Health Canada Substance Use and Addictions Program.

Conflicts of Interest: The authors declare no conflict of interest.

References

1. World Health Organization. *The Health and Social Effects of Nonmedical Cannabis Use*; World Health Organization: Geneva, Switzerland, 2016.
2. Health Canada. *Cannabis Laws and Regulations*; Government of Canada: Ottawa, ON, Canada, 2019.
3. Adinoff, B.; Reiman, A. Implementing social justice in the transition from illicit to legal cannabis. *Am. J. Drug Alcohol Abus.* **2019**, *45*, 673–688. [CrossRef] [PubMed]
4. Statistics Canada. *Prevalence of Cannabis Use in the Past Three Months, Self-Reported*; Statistics Canada: Ottawa, ON, Canada, 2019.
5. Schmidt, R.; Poole, N.; Greaves, L.; Hemsing, N. *New Terrain: Tools to Integrate Trauma and Gender Informed Responses into Substance Use Practice and Policy*; Centre of Excellence for Women's Health: Vancouver, BC, Canada, 2018.
6. Becker, J.B.; McClellan, M.L.; Reed, B.G. Sex differences, gender and addiction. *J. Neurosci. Res.* **2017**, *95*, 136–147. [CrossRef] [PubMed]
7. Greaves, L.; Poole, N.; Boyle, E. *Transforming Addiction: Gender, Trauma, Transdisciplinarity*; Routledge: New York, NY, USA, 2015.
8. Einstein, G. Bridging the biological and social in neuroscience. In *Transforming Addiction: Gender, Trauma, Transdisciplinarity*; Greaves, L., Poole, N., Boyle, E., Eds.; Routledge: New York, NY, USA, 2015.
9. Meyer-Bahlburg, H.F.L. Intersex care development: Current priorities. *LGBT Health* **2017**, *4*, 77–80. [CrossRef] [PubMed]
10. Cranford, J.A.; Eisenberg, D.; Serras, A.M. Substance use behaviors, mental health problems, and use of mental health services in a probability sample of college students. *Addict. Behav.* **2009**, *34*, 134–145. [CrossRef]
11. Carliner, H.; Mauro, P.M.; Brown, Q.L.; Shmulewitz, D.; Rahim-Juwel, R.; Sarvet, A.L.; Wall, M.M.; Martins, S.S.; Carliner, G.; Hasin, D.S. The widening gender gap in marijuana use prevalence in the U.S. During a period of economic change, 2002–2014. *Drug Alcohol Depend.* **2017**, *170*, 51–58. [CrossRef]
12. Felton, J.W.; Collado, A.; Shadur, J.M.; Lejuez, C.W.; MacPherson, L. Sex differences in self-report and behavioral measures of disinhibition predicting marijuana use across adolescence. *Exp. Clin. Psychopharmacol.* **2015**, *23*, 265–274. [CrossRef]
13. Farmer, R.F.; Kosty, D.B.; Seeley, J.R.; Duncan, S.C.; Lynskey, M.T.; Rohde, P.; Klein, D.N.; Lewinsohn, P.M. Natural course of cannabis use disorders. *Psychol. Med.* **2015**, *45*, 63–72. [CrossRef]
14. Johnson, R.M.; Fairman, B.; Gilreath, T.; Xuan, Z.M.; Rothman, E.F.; Parnham, T.; Furr-Holden, C.D.M. Past 15-year trends in adolescent marijuana use: Differences by race/ethnicity and sex. *Drug Alcohol Depend.* **2015**, *155*, 8–15. [CrossRef]
15. Cuttler, C.; Mischley, L.K.; Sexton, M. Sex differences in cannabis use and effects: A cross-sectional survey of cannabis users. *Cannabis Cannabinoid Res.* **2016**, *1*, 166–175. [CrossRef]
16. Legleye, S.; Piontek, D.; Pampel, F.; Goffette, C.; Khlat, M.; Kraus, L. Is there a cannabis epidemic model? Evidence from France, Germany and USA. *Int. J. Drug Policy* **2014**, *25*, 1103–1112. [CrossRef]
17. Gonzalez, C.A.; Gallego, J.D.; Bockting, W.O. Demographic characteristics, components of sexuality and gender, and minority stress and their associations to excessive alcohol, cannabis, and illicit (noncannabis) drug use among a large sample of transgender people in the united states. *J. Prim. Prev.* **2017**, *38*, 419–445. [CrossRef] [PubMed]
18. Baggio, S.; Deline, S.; Studer, J.; Mohler-Kuo, M.; Daeppen, J.B.; Gmel, G. Routes of administration of cannabis used for nonmedical purposes and associations with patterns of drug use. *J. Adolesc. Health* **2014**, *54*, 235–240. [CrossRef] [PubMed]
19. Haines, R.J.; Johnson, J.L.; Carter, C.I.; Arora, K. "I couldn't say, I'm not a girl"—Adolescents talk about gender and marijuana use. *Soc. Sci. Med.* **2009**, *68*, 2029–2036. [CrossRef] [PubMed]
20. Cooper, Z.D.; Craft, R.M. Sex-dependent effects of cannabis and cannabinoids: A translational perspective. *Neuropsychopharmacology* **2018**, *43*, 34. [CrossRef]
21. Nia, A.B.; Mann, C.; Kaur, H.; Ranganathan, M. Cannabis use: Neurobiological, behavioral, and sex/gender considerations. *Curr. Behav. Neurosci. Rep.* **2018**, *5*, 271–280.
22. Greaves, L.; Hemsing, N.; Brabete, A.C.; Poole, N. *Sex, Gender and Cannabis*; Centre of Excellence for Women's Health: Vancouver, BC, Canada, 2019.

23. Hemsing, N.; Greaves, L. Gender norms, roles and relations and cannabis use patterns: A scoping review. *Int. J. Environ. Res. Public Health.* [Electronic Resource] in review.
24. Jafari, S.; Tang, T. Diagnosis and treatment of marijuana dependence. *Br. Columbia Med. J.* **2016**, *58*, 315–317.
25. Khan, S.S.; Secades-Villa, R.; Okuda, M.; Wang, S.; Perez-Fuentes, G.; Kerridge, B.T.; Blanco, C. Gender differences in cannabis use disorders: Results from the national epidemiologic survey of alcohol and related conditions. *Drug Alcohol Depend.* **2013**, *130*, 101–108. [CrossRef]
26. Kerridge, B.T.; Pickering, R.; Chou, P.; Saha, T.D.; Hasin, D.S. DSM-5 cannabis use disorder in the national epidemiologic survey on alcohol and related conditions-III: Gender-specific profiles. *Addict. Behav.* **2018**, *76*, 52–60. [CrossRef]
27. Fogel, J.S.; Kelly, T.H.; Westgate, P.M.; Lile, J.A. Sex differences in the subjective effects of oral delta-thc in cannabis users. *Pharmacol. Biochem. Behav.* **2017**, *152*, 44–51. [CrossRef]
28. Marusich, J.A.; Lefever, T.W.; Antonazzo, K.R.; Craft, R.M.; Wiley, J.L. Evaluation of sex differences in cannabinoid dependence. *Drug Alcohol Depend.* **2014**, *137*, 20–28. [CrossRef] [PubMed]
29. Harte-Hargrove, L.C.; Dow-Edwards, D.L. Withdrawal from thc during adolescence: Sex differences in locomotor activity and anxiety. *Behav. Brain Res.* **2012**, *231*, 48–59. [CrossRef] [PubMed]
30. Schlienz, N.J.; Budney, A.J.; Lee, D.C.; Vandrey, R. Cannabis withdrawal: A review of neurobiological mechanisms and sex differences. *Curr. Addict. Rep.* **2017**, *4*, 75–81. [CrossRef] [PubMed]
31. Lev-Ran, S.; Imtiaz, S.; Taylor, B.J.; Shield, K.D.; Rehm, J.; Le Foll, B. Gender differences in health-related quality of life among cannabis users: Results from the national epidemiologic survey on alcohol and related conditions. *Drug Alcohol Depend.* **2012**, *123*, 190–200. [CrossRef] [PubMed]
32. Sherman, B.J.; McRae-Clark, A.L.; Baker, N.L.; Sonne, S.C.; Killeen, T.K.; Cloud, K.; Gray, K.M. Gender differences among treatment-seeking adults with cannabis use disorder: Clinical profiles of women and men enrolled in the achieving cannabis cessation-evaluating n-acetylcysteine treatment (accent) study. *Am. J. Addict.* **2017**, *26*, 136–144. [CrossRef] [PubMed]
33. Farquhar, C.E.; Breivogel, C.S.; Gamage, T.F.; Gay, E.A.; Thomas, B.F.; Craft, R.M.; Wiley, J.L. Sex, thc, and hormones: Effects on density and sensitivity of cb1 cannabinoid receptors in rats. *Drug Alcohol Depend.* **2019**, *194*, 20–27. [CrossRef]
34. Marusich, J.A.; Craft, R.M.; Lefever, T.W.; Wiley, J.L. The impact of gonadal hormones on cannabinoid dependence. *Exp. Clin. Psychopharmacol.* **2015**, *23*, 206–216. [CrossRef]
35. Struik, D.; Sanna, F.; Fattore, L. The modulating role of sex and anabolic-androgenic steroid hormones in cannabinoid sensitivity. *Front. Behav. Neurosci.* **2018**, *12*, 249. [CrossRef]
36. Craft, R.M.; Marusich, J.A.; Wiley, J.L. Sex differences in cannabinoid pharmacology: A reflection of differences in the endocannabinoid system? *Life Sci.* **2013**, *92*, 476–481. [CrossRef]
37. Wiley, J.L.; Burston, J.J. Sex differences in Δ^9-tetrahydrocannabinol metabolism and in vivo pharmacology following acute and repeated dosing in adolescent rats. *Neurosci. Lett.* **2014**, *576*, 51–55. [CrossRef]
38. Britch, S.C.; Wiley, J.L.; Yu, Z.; Clowers, B.H.; Craft, R.M. Cannabidiol-δ9-tetrahydrocannabinol interactions on acute pain and locomotor activity. *Drug Alcohol Depend.* **2017**, *175*, 187–197. [CrossRef] [PubMed]
39. Cleveland, L.M.; Bonugli, R.J.; McGlothen, K.S. The mothering experiences of women with substance use disorders. *Adv. Nurs. Sci.* **2016**, *39*, 119–129. [CrossRef] [PubMed]
40. Foster, K.T.; Li, N.; McClure, E.A.; Sonne, S.C.; Gray, K.M. Gender differences in internalizing symptoms and suicide risk among men and women seeking treatment for cannabis use disorder from late adolescence to middle adulthood. *J. Subst. Abus. Treat.* **2016**, *66*, 16–22. [CrossRef] [PubMed]
41. Courtney, K.E.; Mejia, M.H.; Jacobus, J. Longitudinal studies on the etiology of cannabis use disorder: A review. *Curr. Addict. Rep.* **2017**, *4*, 43–52. [CrossRef] [PubMed]
42. McHugh, R.K.; Votaw, V.R.; Sugarman, D.E.; Greenfield, S.F. Sex and gender differences in substance use disorders. *Clin. Psychol. Rev.* **2018**, *66*, 12–23. [CrossRef]
43. Wilkinson, A.L.; Fleming, P.J.; Halpern, C.T.; Herring, A.H.; Harris, K.M. Adherence to gender-typical behavior and high frequency substance use from adolescence into young adulthood. *Psychol. Men Masc.* **2018**, *19*, 145–155. [CrossRef]
44. Daniulaityte, R.; Zatreh, M.Y.; Lamy, F.R.; Nahhas, R.W.; Martins, S.S.; Sheth, A.; Carlson, R.G. A twitter-based survey on marijuana concentrate use. *Drug Alcohol Depend.* **2018**, *187*, 155–159. [CrossRef]
45. Lee, D.C.; Crosier, B.S.; Borodovsky, J.T.; Sargent, J.D.; Budney, A.J. Online survey characterizing vaporizer use among cannabis users. *Drug Alcohol Depend.* **2016**, *159*, 227–233. [CrossRef]

46. Noack, R.; Hofler, M.; Lueken, U. Cannabis use patterns and their association with DSM-iv cannabis dependence and gender. *Eur. Addict. Res.* **2011**, *17*, 321–328. [CrossRef]
47. Doran, N.; Papadopoulos, A. Cannabis edibles: Behaviours, attitudes, and reasons for use. *Environ. Health Rev.* **2019**, *62*, 44–52. [CrossRef]
48. Friese, B.; Slater, M.D.; Battle, R.S. Use of marijuana edibles by adolescents in california. *J. Prim. Prev.* **2017**, *38*, 279–294. [CrossRef] [PubMed]
49. Cooper, Z.D.; Haney, M. Comparison of subjective, pharmacokinetic, and physiological effects of marijuana smoked as joints and blunts. *Drug Alcohol Depend.* **2009**, *103*, 107–113. [CrossRef] [PubMed]
50. Spindle, T.R.; Cone, E.J.; Schlienz, N.J.; Mitchell, J.M.; Bigelow, G.E.; Flegel, R.; Hayes, E.; Vandrey, R. Acute pharmacokinetic profile of smoked and vaporized cannabis in human blood and oral fluid. *J. Anal. Toxicol.* **2019**, *43*, 233–258. [CrossRef] [PubMed]
51. Matheson, J.; Sproule, B.; Di Ciano, P.; Fares, A.; Le Foll, B.; Mann, R.E.; Brands, B. Sex differences in the acute effects of smoked cannabis: Evidence from a human laboratory study of young adults. *Psychopharmacology* **2019**, 1–12. [CrossRef]
52. Dahl, S.L.; Sandberg, S. Female cannabis users and new masculinities: The gendering of cannabis use. *Sociology* **2015**, *49*, 696–711. [CrossRef]
53. Perrine, C.G.; Pickens, C.M.; Boehmer, T.K. *Characteristics of a Multistate Outbreak of Lung Injury Associated with E-Cigarette Use, or Vaping—United States*; Centre for Disease Control and Prevention: Atlanta, GA, USA, 2019.
54. Friese, B.; Slater, M.D.; Annechino, R.; Battle, R.S. Teen use of marijuana edibles: A focus group study of an emerging issue. *J. Prim. Prev.* **2016**, *37*, 303–309. [CrossRef]
55. Westfall, R.E.; Janssen, P.A.; Lucas, P.; Capler, R. Survey of medicinal cannabis use among childbearing women: Patterns of its use in pregnancy and retroactive self-assessment of its efficacy against 'morning sickness'. *Complementary Ther. Clin. Pract.* **2006**, *12*, 27–33. [CrossRef]
56. Banbury, A.; Zask, A.; Carter, S.M.; Van Beurden, E.; Tokley, R.; Passey, M.; Copeland, J. Smoking mull: A grounded theory model on the dynamics of combined tobacco and cannabis use among adult men. *Health Promot. J. Aust.* **2013**, *24*, 143–150. [CrossRef]
57. Montgomery, L.; Bagot, K. Let's be blunt: Consumption methods matter among black marijuana smokers. *J. Stud. Alcohol Drugs* **2016**, *77*, 451–456. [CrossRef]
58. Timberlake, D.S. Characterizing blunt smokers by their acquisition of cannabis. *Subst. Use Misuse* **2018**, *53*, 1419–1423. [CrossRef]
59. Schauer, G.L.; Berg, C.J.; Kegler, M.C.; Donovan, D.M.; Windle, M. Assessing the overlap between tobacco and marijuana: Trends in patterns of co-use of tobacco and marijuana in adults from 2003–2012. *Addict. Behav.* **2015**, *49*, 26–32. [CrossRef] [PubMed]
60. Koopman Gonzalez, S.J.; Cofie, L.E.; Trapl, E.S. "I just use it for weed": The modification of little cigars and cigarillos by young adult African American male users. *J. Ethn. Subst. Abus.* **2017**, *16*, 66–79. [CrossRef] [PubMed]
61. Timberlake, D.S. The changing demographic of blunt smokers across birth cohorts. *Drug Alcohol Depend.* **2013**, *130*, 129–134. [CrossRef] [PubMed]
62. Macleod, J.; Robertson, R.; Copeland, L.; McKenzie, J.; Elton, R.; Reid, P. Cannabis, tobacco smoking, and lung function: A cross-sectional observational study in a general practice population. *Br. J. Gen. Pract.* **2015**, *65*, e89–e95. [CrossRef]
63. Health Canada. *Drug-Impaired Driving*; Health Canada: Ottawa, ON, Canada, 2018.
64. Jones, A.W.; Holmgren, A.; Kugelberg, F.C. Driving under the influence of cannabis: A 10-year study of age and gender differences in the concentrations of tetrahydrocannabinol in blood. *Addiction* **2008**, *103*, 452–461. [CrossRef]
65. Whitehill, J.M.; Rivara, F.P.; Moreno, M.A. Marijuana-using drivers, alcohol-using drivers, and their passengers: Prevalence and risk factors among underage college students. *JAMA Pediatr.* **2014**, *168*, 618–624. [CrossRef]
66. O'Malley, P.M.; Johnston, L.D. Driving after drug or alcohol use by U.S. High school seniors, 2001–2011. *Am. J. Public Health* **2013**, *103*, 2027–2034.
67. Jones, C.B.; Hill, M.L.; Pardini, D.A.; Meier, M.H. Prevalence and correlates of vaping cannabis in a sample of young adults. *Psychol. Addict. Behav.* **2016**, *30*, 915. [CrossRef]

68. Dubois, S.; Mullen, N.; Weaver, B.; Bédard, M. The combined effects of alcohol and cannabis on driving: Impact on crash risk. *Forensic Sci. Int.* **2015**, *248*, 94–100. [CrossRef]
69. Earle, A.M.; Napper, L.E.; LaBrie, J.W.; Brooks-Russell, A.; Smith, D.J.; de Rutte, J. Examining interactions within the theory of planned behavior in the prediction of intentions to engage in cannabis-related driving behaviors. *J. Am. Coll. Health* **2019**, 1–7. [CrossRef]
70. Anderson, B.M.; Rizzo, M.; Block, R.I.; Pearlson, G.D.; O'Leary, D.S. Sex differences in the effects of marijuana on simulated driving performance. *J. Psychoact. Drugs* **2010**, *42*, 19–30. [CrossRef] [PubMed]
71. Anderson, B.M.; Rizzo, M.; Block, R.I.; Pearlson, G.D.; O'Leary, D.S. Sex, drugs, and cognition: Effects of marijuana. *J. Psychoact. Drugs* **2010**, *42*, 413–424. [CrossRef] [PubMed]
72. Bauer, G.R. Incorporating intersectionality theory into population health research methodology: Challenges and the potential to advance health equity. *Soc. Sci. Med.* **2014**, *110*, 10–17. [CrossRef]
73. Hankivsky, O.; Doyal, L.; Einstein, G.; Kelly, U.; Shim, J.; Weber, L.; Repta, R. The odd couple: Using biomedical and intersectional approaches to address health inequities. *Glob. Health Action* **2017**, *10*, 1326686. [CrossRef]
74. Van Anders, S.M.; Steiger, J.; Goldey, K.L. Effects of gendered behavior on testosterone in women and men. *Proc. Natl. Acad. Sci. USA* **2015**, *112*, 13805. [CrossRef] [PubMed]
75. Canadian Centre on Substance Use and Addiction. *Canada's Low-Risk Alcohol Drinking Guidelines*; CCSA: Ottawa, ON, Canada, 2018.
76. Greaves, L. Raising the bar on women's health promotion. In *Making It Better: Gender Transformative Health Promotion*; Greaves, L., Pederson, A., Poole, N., Eds.; CSPI: Toronto, ON, Canada, 2014; pp. 1–16.
77. Pederson, A.; Poole, N.; Greaves, L.; Gerbrandt, J.; Fang, M.L. Envisioning gender-transformative health promotion. In *Making It Better: Gender Transformative Health Promotion*; Greaves, L., Pederson, A., Poole, N., Eds.; CSPI: Toronto, ON, Canada, 2014; pp. 17–41.
78. Hakkarainen, P. Vaporizing the pot world—Easy, healthy, and cool. *Drugs Alcohol Today* **2016**, *16*, 185–193. [CrossRef]

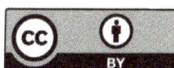 © 2020 by the authors. Licensee MDPI, Basel, Switzerland. This article is an open access article distributed under the terms and conditions of the Creative Commons Attribution (CC BY) license (http://creativecommons.org/licenses/by/4.0/).

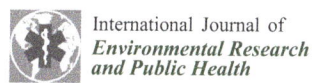 International Journal of
*Environmental Research
and Public Health*

Review

Sex- and Gender-Based Analysis in Cannabis Treatment Outcomes: A Systematic Review

Andreea C. Brabete [1,*], Lorraine Greaves [1,2], Natalie Hemsing [1] and Julie Stinson [1]

1. Centre of Excellence for Women's Health, E311-4500 Oak Street, Vancouver, BC V6H 3N1, Canada; lgreaves@cw.bc.ca (L.G.); nhemsing@cw.bc.ca (N.H.); juliestinson7@gmail.com (J.S.)
2. School of Population and Public Health, University of British Columbia, Vancouver, BC V6T 1Z4, Canada
* Correspondence: andreea.c.brabete@gmail.com; Tel.: +1-514-621-8601

Received: 31 December 2019; Accepted: 28 January 2020; Published: 30 January 2020

Abstract: There is evidence that sex- and gender-related factors are involved in cannabis patterns of use, health effects and biological mechanisms. Women and men report different cannabis use disorder (CUD) symptoms, with women reporting worse withdrawal symptoms than men. The objective of this systematic review was to examine the effectiveness of cannabis pharmacological interventions for women and men and the uptake of sex- and gender-based analysis in the included studies. Two reviewers performed the full-paper screening, and data was extracted by one researcher. The search yielded 6098 unique records—of which, 68 were full-paper screened. Four articles met the eligibility criteria for inclusion. From the randomized clinical studies of pharmacological interventions, few studies report sex-disaggregated outcomes for women and men. Despite emergent evidence showing the influence of sex and gender factors in cannabis research, sex-disaggregated outcomes in pharmacological interventions is lacking. Sex- and gender-based analysis is incipient in the included articles. Future research should explore more comprehensive inclusion of sex- and gender-related aspects in pharmacological treatments for CUD.

Keywords: sex- and gender-based analysis; SGBA; cannabis use disorder; randomized controlled trial

1. Introduction

Growing evidence related to the importance of sex- and gender-based factors within health research has led to increased interest among researchers, funding agencies, scientific journals and database creators to find innovative ways of examining these factors in previously unexplored areas [1–3]. The integration of sex- and gender-related factors into research, policy, or health programs revisits or identifies the influence of components such as anatomy, physiology, genetics and other bodily characteristics biological (sex-based) and the social and cultural milieu affecting humans socio-cultural (gender-based) is known as sex- and gender-based analysis (SGBA) [4]. Sex and gender are not independent of other social characteristics and they might interact with each other and other characteristics to influence health outcomes [5].

Randomized controlled trials (RCT) provide the strongest research evidence and are often used to test the efficacy of new pharmacological interventions. However, sex- and gender-based analysis in RCTs is very scarce. For example, in a study that analyzed 100 Canadian-led or funded RCTs, Welch et al. found that 98% of studies included sex in the description of sociodemographic characteristics of the participants, while only 6% conducted a subgroup analysis across sex, and only 4% reported sex-disaggregated data. None of the examined articles included a definition of "sex" or "gender" nor a comprehensive sex- and gender-based analysis [6]. Failing to include a sex- and gender-based analysis of the outcomes might have important and serious clinical consequences for individuals or subgroups of patients.

There are differences between women and men in referrals and pathways to substance use treatment in general. For example, women are less likely to be referred to residential treatment than men [7]; women are more likely to be referred to outpatient treatment vs. residential treatment [7,8]. Women tend to access substance use services via primary health care or mental health services vs. specialty substance use treatment services [8,9], while men are more likely to enter treatment via the criminal justice system [10]. Lack of awareness of options, stigma, confrontational treatment models, and lack of childcare are some of the common barriers encountered by women when accessing treatments for substance use [9]. Women tend to enter treatment with a more severe clinical profile and more problems related to mental health, family, interpersonal relationships, and physical health [9–12]; while men have more legal, criminal, and financial problems [13].

There are also differences in response to treatment for other substance use. For example, evidence derived using a sex- and gender-based analysis reveals that women have additional difficulties in tobacco smoking cessation. Women have poorer smoking cessation outcomes with some pharmacological supports, including nicotine replacement therapy, regardless of whether combined with counselling [14]; and buproprion [15]. In contrast, treatment with varenicline has shown similar, or better, outcomes for women compared to men [16–18]. Women tend to require more smoking quit attempts before achieving cessation. While women report lower quit rates, the use of any medication increases women's likelihood of cessation [19].

Women and men receiving treatment for alcohol use disorder (AUD) report similar rates in reductions and/or abstinence from alcohol, including medical management and behavioral counselling for AUD [20]; treatment with the medication acamprosate (based on a meta-analysis) [21]; and residential treatment [22]. Studies on the effectiveness of naltrexone treatment for AUD treatment are mixed, with some studies reporting similar outcomes for women and men [22,23], and others reporting a greater reduction in craving scores for women [24], or greater reductions in alcohol use (and other substance use) in men [25]. The limited evidence examining sex differences in treatment outcomes for opioid use disorder (OUD) have reported similar improvements in opioid use outcomes for women and men following a medical management intervention (tapering with buprenorphine–naloxone) either alone or combined with counselling [26].

2. Sex- and Gender-Based Analysis in Cannabis Research

There is growing evidence that sex- and gender-related factors are involved in cannabis patterns of use, health effects and biological mechanisms. Men and boys are more likely to initiate cannabis use earlier, and use more frequently and in greater quantities, compared to women and girls. However, the gender gap has been narrowing over time [27,28]. For example, an analysis of US trends in adolescent cannabis use from 1999 to 2009 revealed that in 1999, 51% of boys and 43.4% of girls reported lifetime cannabis use, while in 2013, this decreased to 42.1% for boys and 39.2% for girls [27]. Furthermore, sex and gender factors also intersect with factors such as education and cultural context. Evidence suggests that the diffusion of cannabis experimentation among men appears similar to that observed with tobacco, with use beginning among men and the most educated groups first, in countries such as USA and Germany. In France, cannabis experimentation continues to be more prevalent among women with higher education [28].

Not everyone who uses cannabis transitions to cannabis use disorder (CUD). It is estimated that approximately 9% of those who initiate cannabis use will meet the criteria for cannabis use dependence. Those who initiate during adolescence have an increased likelihood (16.6%) of developing CUD [29,30]. Multiple factors have been associated with cannabis use disorder in women and men. Specifically, both frequency of use and form of cannabis used have been associated with CUD. Among females, cannabis use with strangers was more strongly related to being diagnosed with CUD according to the Diagnostic and Statistical Manual of Mental Disorders (DSM-IV) compared to males [31]. Compared to women, men have a younger age of onset for CUD [32]. Polysubstance use, trauma and violence may also be risk factors for CUD. In a US study, sexual abuse and history of alcohol use disorder were more strongly associated with 12 month CUD among females, compared to males [33]. Men with lifetime CUD were more likely than women to be diagnosed with any psychiatric disorder, any substance use disorder and antisocial personality disorder, whereas women with CUD had more mood and anxiety disorders [34].

Similar to other substance use, there is some evidence that females transition more quickly to cannabis use dependence compared to males. Studies found that women demonstrate a "telescoping effect", meaning a shorter duration from onset of cannabis use to onset of CUD [34–36]. In a nationally representative sample of the U.S. population, there were no gender differences in the age at first or heavy cannabis use, age at onset of CUD, total number of episodes of cannabis abuse or dependence, or in the number of criteria met for cannabis dependence. However, the time from age at first use of cannabis to the age at onset of the CUD was shorter among women [34].

The results of studies on the subjective effects of cannabis are mixed, and seem to depend on the dose, route of administration (oral vs. smoked) and population (e.g., user vs. non user) [37]. After inhaling tetrahydrocannabinol (THC), women rated themselves as "higher" than men [38]; and reported higher ratings of cannabis as "good" and desire to "take again" compared to men [39]. Another study demonstrated women were more likely to describe cannabis as "good" at low doses, while men more likely to report the same at high doses [40]. In animal studies, female rats exhibit greater drug seeking behavior. In one study that primed rats for drug use and cues before a period of absence, females exhibited higher baseline cannabis intake during training, and reinstate responding for the cannabinoid at higher levels than males [41].

Finally, women and men report different CUD symptoms. For example, several studies report that women have worse withdrawal symptoms compared to men mostly related to gastrointestinal and mood symptoms [42–45]. Men are more likely than women to report experiencing insomnia and vivid dreams as withdrawal symptoms [45]. These findings have important implications since withdrawal symptoms correlate with relapse [46]. Moreover, in a sample of treatment-seeking adults with cannabis use disorder, women reported more co-occurring mental health issues (including lifetime panic disorder and current agoraphobia), and more days of poor physical health [45]. Although CUD is associated with poorer mental health and quality of life in both women and men, this pattern is more pronounced in women with CUD [47]. Animal studies also illustrate the impact of sex-related factors on withdrawal symptoms. Several studies show that females have slightly greater withdrawal symptoms than males [48]. After a week of daily THC treatment in Sprague–Dawley rats, Harte-Hargrove et al. observed the presence of locomotor depression in females but not males during the abstinence period [49].

3. Objective of the Present Study

This systematic review draws on a much broader scoping review on sex- and gender-related factors in substance use (initiation/uptake, patterns of use), effects, and prevention, treatment or harm reduction outcomes for four substances (opioids, alcohol, tobacco/nicotine and cannabis use). It also examined harm reduction, health promotion/prevention and treatment interventions and programs that include sex, gender and gender transformative elements to address each of the four substances. The methodology of the scoping review is described in full elsewhere [50].

Despite the evidence regarding sex and gender differences in, and impacts of cannabis use, little is known about sex- and gender-related factors in pharmacological interventions for cannabis dependence. Pharmacological interventions for cannabis dependence have been recently reviewed [51,52], but sex and gender factors have not been closely examined. Therefore, the purpose of this systematic review was to evaluate the effects of sex and gender factors in cannabis pharmacological interventions.

Our initial research question was:

What cannabis pharmacological interventions are available that include sex, gender and gender transformative elements and how effective are these in addressing cannabis use?

After examining the results of the original scoping review and realizing that there is a lack of examination of sex and gender factors in substance use interventions, and more specifically in cannabis pharmacological interventions, we decided to analyze the studies on cannabis pharmacological interventions that included women and men and sex-disaggregated the outcomes of the interventions for both sexes. In addition, we assessed the role of sex- and gender-based analysis in the included studies.

The research question was then updated to:

What cannabis pharmacological interventions are available that include both sexes and how effective are these in addressing cannabis use for women and men?

4. Methods

This systematic review was conducted in accordance with the Preferred Reporting Items for Systematic Reviews and Meta-Analyses (PRISMA) [53].

4.1. Search Strategy

A systematic search of the literature was undertaken to identify relevant studies published in English between 2007 and 2019 (up to fourth week of October). The following databases were used: PubMed, CINAHL, PsycINFO, and Embase. The search strategy was developed based on keywords and Medical Subject Headings (MeSH) terms. We based our search strategy on the search strategy developed for the scoping review [50] and, in addition, we also included more keywords relevant to pharmacological interventions such as "drug therapy", "pharmacotherapy", "pharmacology", "cessation", "addiction treatment" that were not included in the previous scoping review. An additional search was also completed from a recent systematic review on cannabis pharmacological interventions. Thirty-eight articles were included for the screening in this systematic review.

4.2. Literature Screening

Searches in four databases resulted in $n = 6098$ unique returns. Firstly, titles and abstracts were screened by a single reviewer for relevance. Then, the full-text of the articles were obtained and reviewed by two reviewers according to the inclusion criteria. These inclusion criteria were: (a) English language articles from a selection of Organization for Economic Cooperation and Development (OECD) member countries such as Australia, Austria, Belgium, Canada, Denmark, Finland, France, Germany, Greece, Iceland, Ireland, Italy, Luxembourg, Netherlands, New Zealand, Norway, Portugal, Spain, Sweden, Switzerland, United Kingdom, United States; (b) the population of interest included: women, girls, men, boys of all ages and sociodemographic characteristics; (c) studies including pharmacotherapies that targeted cannabis use (in addition to other comorbid conditions) and presented sex-disaggregated data; (d) studies that analyzed outcomes such as cannabis abstinence or cannabis reduction; (e) randomized clinical trials. Articles were excluded if: (a) although both women and men were included in the study, outcomes of the interventions were not sex-disaggregated; (b) the study did not examine a pharmacological intervention aiming to modify cannabis use; (c) studies were conducted in a non-OECD country; (d) studies analyzed baseline characteristics of the population but the analyses are not done in relationship to the pharmacological treatment. Figure 1 provides an overview of the literature search returns, the number of articles included and excluded at each level of screening, and the final number of included articles.

4.3. Study Selection

The abstract screening was conducted by a single reviewer. Full papers of the included studies at this stage ($n = 68$) were then retrieved and assessed by two independent reviewers. Inter-rater reliability was calculated, and the overall kappa was 0.78. Differences between the reviewers in the inclusion of articles were resolved through discussion and consensus was reached.

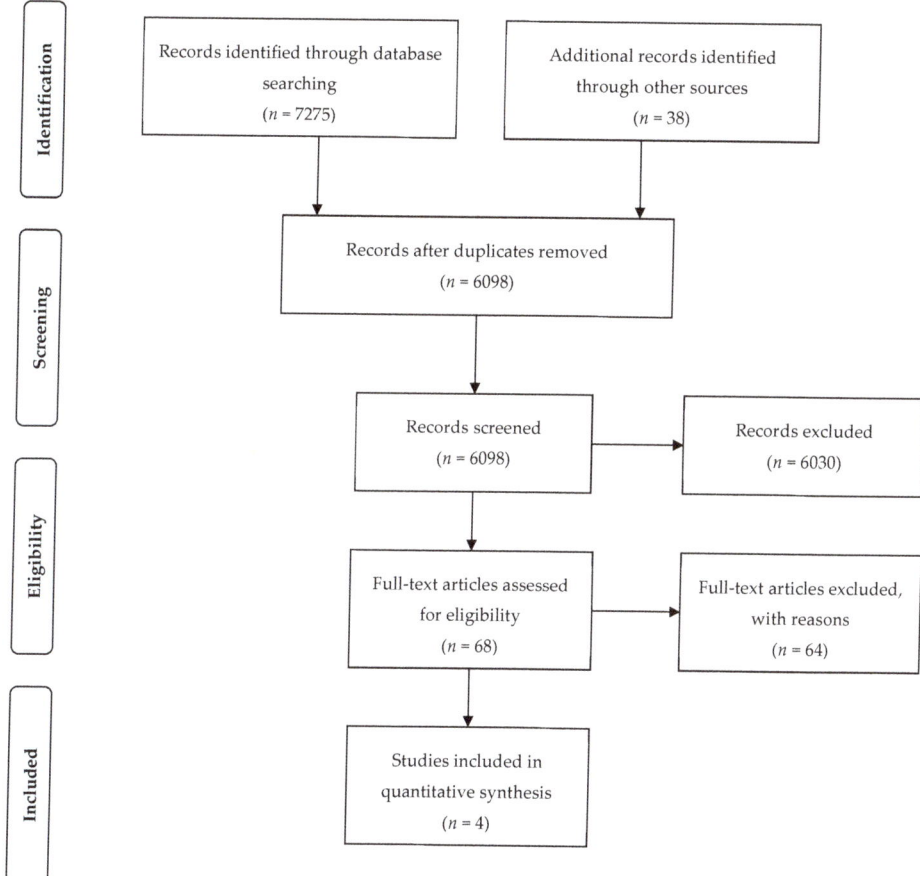

Figure 1. Preferred Reporting Items for Systematic Reviews and Meta-Analyses (PRISMA) diagram of study selection.

4.4. Data Extraction

Data regarding the following information was extracted by one reviewer from the four papers included in this systematic review: (1) study details (authors and year of publication); (2) aim of the study; (3) study design; (4) country of study; (5) setting of the study; (6) details on recruitment; (7) inclusion and exclusion criteria; (8) method of allocation to intervention/control; (9) details regarding the intervention; (10) sample size and demographics; (11) baseline comparisons; (12) outcomes; (13) details on the sex, gender or diversity analysis; (14) follow up periods; (15) methods of analysis; (16) results; (17) results regarding the sex, gender or diversity based factors in findings; (18) attrition details; (19) study limitations; (20) evidence gaps and/or recommendations for future research.

4.5. Sex- and Gender-Based Analysis in the Included Studies

Research can incorporate sex- and gender-based analysis in several ways. Hammarström presented a tool that researchers might use when developing gender research [54]. Although Hammarström [54] does not employ the term "sex- and gender-based analysis", in this paper we used the concept sex- and gender-based analysis as in the scoping review conducted by McCarthy et al. [55]. The authors reviewed 458 articles on pharmacy practice research and found that only six studies mention any information related to sex and gender considerations and only three were classified as SGBA according to Hammarström's model [55]. Table 1 presents the classification based on Hammarström's typology [54]. For the sex- and gender-based analysis of the included articles, we examined the following characteristics:

1. *Use of sex and gender in the aim and research questions*: were sex and gender included in the aim of the study or explicitly mentioned in the research question and the study design?
2. *Study design and reporting results*: how were the outcomes analyzed and reported in relation to sex and gender?
3. *Interpretation of sex/gender findings*: how were findings related to sex and gender included in the interpretation of the data?
4. *Intentional and accurate use of language*: were the terms sex and gender used intentionally and appropriately by the authors of the study?

Table 1. Sex- and gender-based analysis in health research.

Research Phase	Model 1: Sex/Gender Differences	Model 2: Sex and Gender-Based Analysis (SGBA)	Model 2(a): SGBA+	Model 3: Intersectional Approach
Research question	Sex/gender included, but not primary focus of study. Sex/gender included in the study design or the reporting but are not specifically stated in the research question or aim of the study.	Specific questions related to sex/gender. Looking for sex/gender differences, or the impact of sex/gender an explicit aim of the study or stated research question.	Specific questions related to sex/gender, and additional subgroups/identities included. Research question includes sex/gender and other factors such as race, age, sexual orientation, etc.	Specific questions related to sex/gender, and additional subgroups/identities included. Research question includes sex/gender and other factors such as race, age, sexual orientation, etc.
Data analysis and reporting of findings	Disaggregation by sex/gender; sex as confounder/controlled for (e.g., included in a model). Data related to the outcomes is reported for different sex/gender groups or sex/gender is controlled for in the analysis.	Sex/gender as analysis category Beyond reporting results by different sex/gender group, there is testing of significance between gender groups in relation to the outcomes of the study.	Sex/gender as analysis category; other factors included (e.g., race, SES). There is testing of significance between sex/gender groups in relation to the outcomes of the study and related to other factors such as race, ethnicity, age, etc. But as seperate analysis, not combined into one analysis. Must be beyond reporting demographic characteristics of a sample.	Multi-faceted analysis of multiple factors. More than one factor is included in the same analysis (e.g., comparing young and old white and Hispanic men, to the same 4 groups of women).
Interpretation of sex/gender findings	Findings related to sex and gender are not necessarily included in the interpretation of the data. Differences reported are not necessarily explained.	Findings related to sex and/or gender are reported in the discussion/conclusion. The differences reported in the results section are interpreted and explained.	Findings related to sex and/or gender are reported in the discussion/conclusion in relationship to at least another factor.	Findings related to sex and/or gender are reported in the discussion/conclusion in relationship to other factors such as race, age, etc. The differences reported in the results section are interpreted and explained.
Use of language	Not dependent on specific aim, design/results and interpretation.	Not dependent on specific interpretation and use of language.	Not dependent on specific interpretation and use of language.	Not dependent on specific interpretation and use of language.

Adapted from: Hammarstrom (2007) [54]; McCarthy et al. (2017) [55].

5. Results

5.1. Included Studies

Four randomized controlled trials involving 623 participants met the inclusion criteria for this review [56–59]. Characteristics of the studies are described in Table 2. In total, 316 participants received the intervention while 307 participants received placebo. The number of women included in the studies oscillated between 16 [58] and 86 [57]. Disaggregating by sex, 170 women and 453 men were included in the randomized controlled trials and 82 women and 234 men received the pharmacological intervention.

In the placebo group there were 88 women and 219 men. In addition to the pharmacological intervention and placebo, some form of psychological intervention was offered in all included studies.

Table 2. Characteristics and findings of included studies.

Cornelius et al. (2010) [56]	Characteristics and Findings of Included Studies
Study design	Randomized controlled trial
Participants	Recruitment: Through referrals from the Western Psychiatric Institute and Clinic (WPIC) treatment programs and by responding to newspaper, radio, and bus advertisements. Setting: Outpatient clinic, Pittsburgh, USA. Scheduled for 12 weeks. Participants: In total, 70 participants between 14 and 25 years of age at baseline and comorbid presence of both a current CUD (using DSM-IV) and a current major depressive disorder (MDD). Exclusion criteria: Diagnosis of bipolar disorder, schizoaffective disorder, or schizophrenia; subjects with hyper- or hypothyroidism, significant cardiac, neurological, or renal impairment, and significant liver disease; substance abuse or dependence other than alcohol abuse or dependence, nicotine dependence, or cannabis abuse; any history of intravenous drug use; pregnancy, inability or unwillingness to use contraceptive methods, and an inability to read or understand study forms. Sample size: Intervention, 34; placebo, 36. Demographics: Mean age 21.1 years ±2.4 years; 61% male; 56% Caucasian, 37% African-American. In total, 94% cannabis dependent, using on average of 76% of days in prior month; 20 participants met diagnostic criteria for alcohol dependence; seven for alcohol abuse and 16 reported a history of an antidepressant medication in the moth prior to recruitment.
Interventions	Intervention: In total, one capsule of 10 mg of fluoxetine for 2 weeks and increased to two capsules of 10 mg of fluoxetine. Placebo: In total, one capsule of 10 mg of placebo and after 2 weeks, two capsules of 10 mg of placebo. The low dose was used to maximize the safety and minimize the risk of medication side effects. In total, nine sessions of cognitive behavior therapy (CBT) for depression and CUD, and motivation enhancement therapy (MET) for CUD.
Outcomes	Severity of abuse or dependence (cannabis and alcohol), number of days of cannabis use, quantity and frequency, number completing the treatment Timeline follow-back method (TLFB) for the cannabis use behaviors and other substance use behaviors; Hamilton Rating Scale for Depression (HAM-D-27) for observer-rated depressive symptoms; Beck Depression Inventory (BDI) for participant-rated depressive symptoms; Number of drinks per drinking day, the number of drinking days, number of heavy drinking days (defined as greater than or equal to four drinks per day for women and five for men); Side Effects Questionnaire for Children and Adolescent for the side effects during each assessment throughout the course of the clinical trial.
Findings	The group that received fluoxetine did not have better cannabis or depressive than the group that received placebo. The improvement of the depressive symptoms and decrease of number of days of cannabis use may have resulted either from the psychosocial therapy or the natural course of the disorders.
Gray et al. (2017) [57]	
Study design	Randomized controlled trial
Participants	Recruitment: Community media advertisements. Setting: Outpatient, six sites within the National Drug Abuse Treatment Clinical Trials Network, USA. Scheduled duration 12 weeks. Participants: In total, 302 treatment-seeking adults ages 18–50 with CUD and submitting a positive Urine cannabinoid testing UCT during the initial screening visit. Exclusion criteria: Individuals with acutely unstable medical or psychiatric disorders, DSM-IV-TR substance dependence aside from cannabis or tobacco, contraindications for N-acetylcysteine (NAC) treatment, or recent synthetic cannabinoid use. Sample size: Intervention, 153; placebo, 149. Demographics: Mean age 29.8 years ±8.74 years; 71.5% male; 58.3% White; 27.8% Black or African-American. Mean cannabis use 26.0/30 days at baseline.
Interventions	Intervention: In total, two capsules of 600 mg of United States Pharmacopeia grade NAC powder (twice daily dose). Placebo: In total, two capsules of 600 mg of placebo (twice per day). Riboflavin 25 mg was added to all capsules (100 mg/day total) as a biomarker for medication adherence. All participants received contingence management twice weekly during treatment. Medical management.
Outcomes	Urine specimens were collected at baseline, twice weekly throughout treatment, at end-of-treatment. UCT at post-treatment follow-up. Medication adherence included taking ≥80% of prescribed study medication per study week, confirmed by urine riboflavin level >1500 ng/mL. Adverse effects at each study visit.
Findings	No statistically significant differences between the NAC and placebo groups in cannabis abstinence. In the NAC group, 22.3% of urine cannabinoid tests were negative compared to 22.4% in the placebo group. Exploratory analysis within medication-adherent subgroups revealed no significant differential abstinence outcomes by treatment group.

Table 2. *Cont.*

McRae-Clark et al. (2015) [59]	
Study design	Randomized controlled trial.
Participants	Recruitment: Media and internet advertisements. Setting: Outpatient. Scheduled duration 12 weeks. Participants: In total, 175 participants between 18 and 65 years of age and met DSM-IV criteria for current cannabis dependence. Exclusion criteria: current dependence on any other substance (with the exception of caffeine and nicotine), history of psychotic, bipolar or eating disorder, current suicidal or homicidal risk, current major depression, current treatment with psychoactive medication (with the exception of stimulants and non-benzodiazepine sedative/hypnotics), major medical illness or disease, significant cognitive impairment, hypersensitivity to buspirone or other product component, current consumption of substances that inhibit or induce CYP3A4, and pregnancy, lactation or inadequate birth control. Sample size: intervention, 88; placebo, 87. Demographics: Mean age 24.00 years (23.1-25 years); 76.6% male; 64% Caucasian.
Interventions	Intervention: Dosage initiated at 5 mg buspirone or placebo twice daily and increased by 5–10 mg every three to four days as tolerated, to a maximum dose of 60 mg daily for 12 weeks. Placebo: Up to 60 mg of placebo. Adjunctive motivational enhancement therapy sessions (MET) during the first four weeks of the treatment period.
Outcomes	Semi-quantitative urine cannabinoid tests (UCTs) for cannabinoids administered at screening and weekly throughout the study. Proportion of negative urine test during treatment. Point prevalence of abstinence by urine test at the end of the treatment Number of reporting adverse events.
Findings	No differences of UCTs and the weekly creatinine adjusted cannabinoid levels between the two groups. Although participants in both groups reduced their cannabis craving over the course of the study, there were no differences between the buspirone and placebo groups. However, participants who attained abstinence from cannabis reported less cannabis craving.
McRae-Clark et al. (2016) [58]	
Study design	Randomized controlled trial
Participants	Recruitment: Media and internet advertisements. Setting: Outpatient, 8 weeks. Participants: In total, 76 participants between 18 and 65 years of age and CUD. Exclusion criteria: current dependence on any other substance (exception caffeine and nicotine), history of psychotic, bipolar, or eating disorder, current suicidal or homicidal risk, current treatment with psychoactive medication (exception stimulants and non-benzodiazepine sedative/hypnotics) or CYP3A4 inhibitors, major medical illness or disease, pregnancy, lactation, or inadequate birth control, patients that would be unable to comply with study procedures or assessments. Sample size: Intervention, 41; placebo, 35. Demographics: Mean age 22.2 (21.3–23.1) years; 79% male; 54.8% Caucasian.
Interventions	Intervention: In total, 10 mg daily dose of Vilazodone tablets provided by Forest Pharmaceuticals for 7 days, increased to 20 mg daily for 7 days, followed by 40 mg daily as tolerated. Placebo: In total, 10 mg daily dose of placebo tablets for 7 days, increased to 20 mg daily for 7 days, followed by 40 mg daily. Both groups received three adjunctive motivational enhancement therapy sessions (MET). First session, prior to medication initiation. Second session, approximately 1 week later. Third session, week 4.
Outcomes	Quantitative urine cannabinoid tests (UCTs) for cannabinoids administered at screening and weekly throughout the study. Self-report cannabis use measured by TLFB (Time-Line Follow-Back). Marijuana Craving Questionnaire (MCQ) for levels of cannabis craving. Adverse effects assessed weekly. Medication compliance by weekly patient report. Proportion of scheduled visits attended.
Findings	The vilazodone group did not show greater efficacy when compared to the placebo group on cannabis use outcomes. Participants in both groups reported lower cannabis use with no differences between the two groups.

Several medications with different mechanisms of action were applied in the studies included in this review. Cornelius et al. [57] examined the role of fluoxetine while McRae-Clark et al. [58] used vilazodone. Both medications are selective serotonin reuptake inhibitors. The effect of buspirone, a serotonin 5-HT1A partial agonist, was explored by McRae-Clark et al. [59]. Lastly, Gray et al. [57] examined the effect of N-acetylcysteine, a supplement promoting glutamate release and modulating N-methyl-D-aspartate (NMDA).

All studies were undertaken in outpatient settings. In one study, the scheduled duration for the clinical trial was 8 weeks [58] while in the three other studies, it was 12 weeks [56,57,59]. The four selected studies were all conducted in the USA. The mean age of participants was between 16.64 [56] and 29.8 years [57]. Three studies included young adults [57–59] and one study targeted adolescents [56]. In one study, participants had comorbid major depression and cannabis use disorders [56]. The other three studies excluded people with psychiatric conditions.

5.2. Sex-Disaggregated Outcomes

In one of the included articles, sex was not a significant predictor of cannabis abstinence, and there was no sex-by-treatment interaction [57]. Females showed a greater improvement with time on depressive symptoms ($F = 5.01$, $p = 0.028$) and DSM cannabis abuse criteria count than males ($F = 4.22$, $p = 0.044$) [56]. In a study using buspirone McRae-Clark et al. (2015) [59] found that UCTs were negative in 8.7% of buspirone and 4.5% of placebo of male participants. In females, 2.4% of buspirone participant UCTs were negative and 12.9% of placebo; although the difference was not statistically significant ($p = 0.007$). Regarding the creatinine adjusted cannabinoid levels, there was a sex by treatment interaction indicating that for males, those randomized to buspirone treatment had significantly lower creatinine adjusted cannabinoid levels as compared to those randomized to placebo. For females, those randomized to placebo had lower creatinine adjusted cannabinoid levels compared to those randomized to buspirone [59]. Examining the effect of vilazodone, McRae-Clark (2016) found that males had significantly lower creatinine-adjusted cannabinoid levels and a trend for increased negative urine cannabinoid tests compared to females [58].

5.3. Sex- and Gender-Based Analysis of the Included Studies

The assessments of the role of sex- and gender-based analysis in the included studies is presented in Table 3. While Cornelius et al. and Gray et al.'s studies were classified in the sex/gender differences category, McRae-Clark et al. (2015) [59] and McRae-Clark et al. (2016) [58] were categorized as SGBA (see Table 3). Based on the categories that were analyzed, the results are as follows:

1. *Aim and research questions*: The four studies included sex/gender in the study design or the reporting. However, none of the studies included sex or gender in their major research question.

2. *Reporting sex/gender in the results*: In Cornelius et al.'s study [56] on the effects of fluoxetine in adolescents and young adults with comorbid depression and cannabis use dependence, sex by time was analyzed for the outcomes of the study (number of days participants used cannabis in past month; DSM cannabis dependence count; DSM CUD total count - DSM dependence + abuse symptoms). The authors also examined whether abstinence rates differed across sex [56]. Although Gray et al. did not find statistically significant results, they examined whether sex was a predictor of cannabis abstinence, and whether there was a sex-by-treatment interaction [57]. McRae-Clark (2016) used sex as one of the randomization variables in addition to the presence or absence of anxiety or depressive disorders [58]. Sex and sex by treatment group interactions were added to examine the effect of gender on the primary and secondary efficacy outcomes in a randomized clinical trial that tested the efficacy of vilazodone, a selective serotonin receptor inhibitor and partial 5-HT1A agonist, for treatment of cannabis dependence [58]. McRae-Clark et al. also conducted a sex- and gender-based analysis since they used sex as a stratified randomization variable [59]. Sex was analyzed in relationship to the negative UCTs and cannabinoid levels in this study that examined the efficacy of buspirone for participants with cannabis use dependence [59].

3. *Interpretation of Sex/Gender findings*: Cornelius et al. did not report their findings related to sex and/or gender in the discussion section [56]. Gray et al. did not discuss any aspects of sex or gender, likely because their results were not statistically significant [57]. The differences reported in the results section are interpreted and explained in McRae-Clark et al. (2015) [59] and McRae-Clark et al. (2016) [58]. McRae-Clark et al.'s study, which featured sex or gender in their research question, provided a comprehensive discussion of their interpretation of the impact of sex and gender in their findings [59].

In this study, the authors acknowledged that this is the first study to demonstrate a sex difference in response to a pharmacological treatment for cannabis dependence. The authors highlighted the importance of including gender in the development and evaluation of new treatments for addictive disorders [59]. However, they did not specify what sex or gender-related factors could be considered for the development and evaluation of new treatments for addictive disorders. McRae-Clark et al.'s (2016) study suggests that women with CUD might have more problems in achieving cannabis cessation compared to men with CUD [58]. Their findings are related to sex and gender in the discussion. They also note that their analyses of sex differences might have been underpowered, and they mention that women are underrepresented in pharmacological trials calling for higher representativity of women in future studies.

4. *Intentional and accurate use of terminology*: None of the included studies define sex and gender. Cornelius et al. use only the term sex and they do not mention gender [56], while Gray et al. used sex and gender interchangeably [57]. For example, in the sociodemographic table the authors use "gender" and throughout the paper they mentioned "sex". McRae-Clark et al. and McRae-Clark et al. used "gender" throughout the article though the study is in fact measuring sex although they also employ the terms females and males and women and men at the same time [58,59]. All four articles included in this systematic review lacked accuracy in the application of the concepts of sex and gender. Not even the articles that were categorized as applying a sex- and gender-based analysis in their studies used intentional and accurate terminology throughout the articles.

Table 3. SGBA applied to cannabis pharmacological interventions.

Authors	Publication Date	SGBA Categorization	Sex/Gender in the Research Question	Results	Interpretation of Sex/Gender Findings	Use of Terminology	Findings Related to Sex and Gender
[56]	2010	Sex/Gender Differences	No	Sex by time was analyzed in relation to the outcomes.	No	Use only sex	Females showed a greater improvement with time on the depressive symptoms and DSM cannabis abuse criteria count than males.
[57]	2017	Sex/Gender Differences	No	Examined whether sex was a predictor of cannabis abstinence, and whether there was a sex-by-treatment interaction.	No	Sex and gender used interchangeably	Sex was not a significant predictor of cannabis abstinence, and there was no sex-by-treatment interaction.
[59]	2015	SGBA	No	Sex was used as a randomized stratification variable. Sex was analyzed in relationship to the negative UCTs and cannabinoid levels.	Yes	Sex and gender used interchangeably	In males, 8.7% of buspirone participant UCTs were negative and 4.5% of placebo UCTs were negative. In females, 2.4% of buspirone participant UCTs were negative and 12.9% of placebo; although the difference was not statistically significant ($p = 0.007$). There was a sex by treatment interaction for the creatinine adjusted cannabinoid levels: for males, those randomized to buspirone treatment had significantly lower creatinine adjusted cannabinoid levels as compared to those randomized to placebo; for females, those randomized to placebo had lower creatinine adjusted cannabinoid levels compared to those randomized to buspirone.
[58]	2016	SGBA	No	Sex was used as a variable for randomization. Sex and sex by treatment group interactions were analyzed.	Yes	Sex and gender used interchangeably	Men had significantly lower creatinine-adjusted cannabinoid levels and a trend for increased negative urine cannabinoid tests than women. There were no sex differences regarding the self-reported frequency and amount of cannabis use; nor significant interactions between sex and treatment. Male participants randomized to vilazodone showed a reduction in the Purposefulness subscale of the MCQ; it did not happen for females.

6. Discussion

In this systematic review on sex- and gender-related factors in cannabis pharmacological interventions, there was a paucity of studies that sex-disaggregated outcomes for women and men or analyzed the sex- or gender-related factors in the interventions. Although overall the findings showed that the pharmacological interventions analyzed in the studies (fluoxetine, vilazodone, buspirone, N-acetylcysteine) are not effective for treating CUD, three of the four included studies found different results for women and men. Of the three studies, one showed that females demonstrated a greater improvement with time on the depressive symptoms and DSM cannabis abuse criteria count than males [56]. The other two studies suggest that women have worse results than men in cannabis pharmacological interventions [58,59].

The lack of reported sex-disaggregated results does not mean that there are no differences or similarities between women and men. However, it is not possible to accurately interpret these results. Given the emergent evidence of sex- and gender-related factors in cannabis research [42,43], sex- and gender-related factors may intervene in the efficacy of cannabis pharmacological interventions. As in the case of smoking cessation treatment, demonstrating that women have more difficulty maintaining long-term abstinence than men [60], two of the four included studies showed that women have worse outcomes when examining the efficacy of buspirone [59] and vilazodone [58].

Even though the included studies did not find a greater efficacy of the pharmacological intervention, two of the four studies found that women had better results in the placebo group while men had better results in the pharmacological intervention group [58,59]. The different mechanisms generating the placebo effect between women and men are not well understood. However, preliminary findings suggest that sex- and gender-related factors might also be intervening in the placebo effect [61].

Although two of the included studies described the integration of aspects of sex into research questions, analysis, reporting of findings and discussion, there is an overall lack of comprehensive integration and analysis of sex and gender in these randomized controlled trials. These findings are consistent with those found by Welch et al. (2017) examining the use of sex and gender considerations in 100 Canadian-led or funded RCTs [6]. This study showed that 98% of studies included sex in the description of sociodemographic characteristics of the participants and only 6% conducted a subgroup analysis across sex and 4% reported sex-disaggregated data. Even in those RCTs that included females, most of the studies did not sex-disaggregate the outcomes [6].

Studying the effect of sex- and gender-related factors in cannabis pharmacological interventions is challenging and there is still an overall lack of research on sex, gender and cannabis. To determine sex- and gender-related factors in pharmacological interventions for cannabis use, researchers urgently need to fill this void. The preliminary findings show that women might not benefit from certain pharmacological interventions. Including and reporting sex- and gender-related factors might contribute to better determine the effectiveness of pharmacological interventions for both women and men and tailor treatment for all individuals.

In the included studies, the terms "sex" and "gender" were used in an inconsistent way and there were no definitions provided for these terms. Three of the included studies used "sex" and "gender" interchangeably. Throughout the studies, authors used "male/female" and "women/men" and the use of "gender" was inaccurate. These findings are consistent with results from a study on Campbell and Cochrane systematic reviews [62]. Petkovic et al. (2018) found that reporting in systematic reviews is inadequate [62]. None of the studies in our systematic review included gender diverse populations or other gender considerations. Findings from a scoping review on how gender norms, roles and relations impact cannabis use patterns showed that there is a complex relationship between substance use and gender norms. While certain feminine and masculine norms might be protective, there are others that might be linked with greater risk of developing cannabis use dependence [50].

This systematic review has limitations. Since sex and gender are not often examined in pharmacological interventions for cannabis use, our results are limited. This is reflected in the small number of studies that met the inclusion criteria, and therefore, what we could draw from for interpretation. Our search strategy was designed taking into account that there is a growing body of literature that focuses on sex- and gender-related factors and we conducted searches using sex- and gender-related keywords [63]. However, since the use of sex and gender terms are not used in pharmacological interventions for cannabis use, we reviewed references from a recent systematic review [52] and screened those that were not captured by our search strategy. Sex and gender factors might have been tested in many other studies but not reported. We did not contact authors for further details on sex- and gender-based analysis, methods or results. Although we intended to apply the Feminist Quality Appraisal Tool [64] to analyze the ways in which gender is addressed in the included studies, the lack of deeper gender analysis did not support it. We did not perform a quality assessment of the studies since our aim was to examine the role of sex- and gender-related factors and the uptake of sex- and gender-based analysis. The included articles were assessed in two previous systematic reviews that examined the effectiveness of pharmacotherapies for cannabis dependence [51,52].

7. Conclusions

This systematic review aimed to examine the treatment outcomes in cannabis pharmacological interventions for women and men. In addition, it analyzed the uptake of sex- and gender-based analysis in pharmacological interventions for cannabis use. Despite the increasing evidence showing that sex and gender factors intervene in patterns of cannabis use, health effects and biological mechanisms, we found only four articles that sex-disaggregated the outcomes for both sexes on CUD treatment. Taking into account the poor uptake of sex- and gender-based analysis, future research should consider more consistent and disciplined integration of sex and gender in cannabis pharmacological interventions in order to improve outcomes for all individuals experiencing CUD.

Author Contributions: Conceptualization, A.C.B. and L.G.; methodology, A.C.B., N.H. and J.S.; data curation, A.C.B. and N.H.; writing—original draft preparation, A.C.B.; writing—review and editing, A.C.B., L.G., N.H. and J.S.; funding acquisition, L.G. All authors have read and agreed to the published version of the manuscript.

Funding: This research was funded by Canadian Institutes of Health Research, Team Grant: Impact of Gender on Knowledge Translation Interventions (Evaluating the Effectiveness of Sex- and Gender-Based Analysis on Knowledge Translation Interventions).

Conflicts of Interest: The authors declare no conflict of interest. The funders had no role in the design of the study; in the collection, analyses, or interpretation of data; in the writing of the manuscript, or in the decision to publish the results.

References

1. Tannenbaum, C.; Greaves, L.; Graham, I.D. Why sex and gender matter in implementation research. *Med. Res. Methodol.* **2016**, *16*, 145. [CrossRef]
2. Johnson, J.; Sharman, Z.; Vissandjée, B.; Stewart, E.D. Does a Change in Health Research Funding Policy Related to the Integration of Sex and Gender Have an Impact? *PloS ONE* **2014**, *9*, e99900. [CrossRef] [PubMed]
3. Institute of Gender and Health. *Science is Better with Sex and Gender, Strategic Plan*; Canadian Institutes of Health Research: Ottawa, ON, Canada, 2019.
4. Johnson, J.L.; Greaves, L.; Repta, R. *Better Science with Sex and Gender: A Primer for Health Research*; Women's Health Research Network: Vancouver, BC, Canada, 2007.
5. Krieger, N. Genders, sexes, and health: What are the connections—And why does it matter? *Int. J. Epidemiol.* **2003**, *32*, 652–657. [CrossRef] [PubMed]
6. Welch, V.; Doull, M.; Yoganathan, M.; Jull, J.; Boscoe, M.; Coen, S.E.; Marshall, Z.; Pardo Pardo, J.; Pederson, A.; Petkovic, J.; et al. Reporting of sex and gender in randomized controlled trials in Canada: A cross-sectional methods study. *Res. Integr. Peer Rev.* **2017**, *2*, 15. [CrossRef] [PubMed]
7. Bazargan-Hejazi, S.; Doull, M.; Yoganathan, M.; Jull, J.; Boscoe, M.; Coen, S.E.; Marshall, Z.; Pardo, P.J.; Pederson, A.; Petkovic, J.; et al. Gender comparison in referrals and treatment completion to residential and outpatient alcohol treatment. *Subst. Abuse* **2016**, *10*, S39943. [CrossRef] [PubMed]

8. Greenfield, S.F. Substance abuse treatment entry, retention, and outcome in women: A review of the literature. *Drug Alcohol Depend.* **2007**, *86*, 1–21. [CrossRef]
9. Grella, C.E.; Mitchell, P.K.; Alison, A.M. Gender and comorbidity among individuals with opioid use disorders in the NESARC study. *Addict. Behav.* **2009**, *34*, 498–504. [CrossRef]
10. Greenfield, S.F.; Rosa, C.; Putnins, S.I.; Green, C.A.; Brooks, A.J.; Calsyn, D.A.; Cohen, L.R.; Erickson, S.; Gordon, S.M. Gender research in the National Institute on Drug Abuse National Treatment Clinical Trials Network: A summary of findings. *Am. J. Drug Alcohol Abuse* **2011**, *37*, 301–312. [CrossRef]
11. Small, J.; Curran, G.M.; Booth, B. Barriers and facilitators for alcohol treatment for women: Are there more or less for rural women? *J. Subst. Abuse* **2010**, *39*, 1–13. [CrossRef]
12. Bold, K.W.; Epstein, E.E.; McCrady, B.S. Baseline health status and quality of life after alcohol treatment for women with alcohol dependence. *Addict. Behav.* **2017**, *64*, 35–41. [CrossRef]
13. Storbjörk, J. Gender differences in substance use, problems, social situation and treatment experiences among clients entering addiction treatment in Stockholm. *Nordisk. Alkohol. Nark.* **2011**, *28*, 185–209. [CrossRef]
14. Perkins, K.A.; Scott, J. Sex differences in long-term smoking cessation rates due to nicotine patch. *Nicotine Tob. Res.* **2008**, *10*, 1245–1250. [CrossRef] [PubMed]
15. Smith, P.H.; Andrea, H.W.; Zhang, J.; Erin, E. Sex Differences in Smoking Cessation Pharmacotherapy Comparative Efficacy: A Network Meta-analysis. *Nicotine Tob. Res.* **2017**, *19*, 273–281. [CrossRef] [PubMed]
16. Smith, P.H.; Zhang, J.; Weinberger, A.H.; Mazure, C.M.; McKee, S.A. Gender differences in the real-world effectiveness of smoking cessation medications: Findings from the 2010–2011 Tobacco Use Supplement to the Current Population Survey. *Drug Alcohol Depend.* **2017**, *178*, 485–491. [CrossRef] [PubMed]
17. Glatard, A.; Dobrinas, M.; Gholamrezaee, M.; Lubomirov, R.; Cornuz, J.; Csajka, C.; Eap, C.B. Association of nicotine metabolism and sex with relapse following varenicline and nicotine replacement therapy. *Exp. Clin. Psychopharmacol.* **2017**, *25*, 353–362. [CrossRef] [PubMed]
18. McKee, S.A.; Smith, P.H.; Kaufman, M.; Mazure, C.M.; Weinberger, A.H. Sex Differences in Varenicline Efficacy for Smoking Cessation: A Meta-Analysis. *Nicotine Tob. Res.* **2016**, *18*, 1002–1011. [CrossRef]
19. Smith, P.H.; Karin, A.K.; Sherry, A.M. Gender differences in medication use and cigarette smoking cessation: Results from the International Tobacco Control Four Country Survey. *Nicotine Tob. Res.* **2015**, *17*, 463–472. [CrossRef]
20. Greenfield, S.F.; Pettinati, H.M.; O'Malley, S.; Randall, P.K.; Randall, C.L. Gender differences in alcohol treatment: An analysis of outcome from the COMBINE study. *Alcohol Clin. Exp. Res.* **2010**, *34*, 1803–1812. [CrossRef]
21. Mason, B.J.; Lehert, P. Acamprosate for alcohol dependence: A sex-specific meta-analysis based on individual patient data. *Alcohol Clin. Exp. Res.* **2012**, *36*, 497–508. [CrossRef]
22. Hitschfeld, M.J.; Schneekloth, T.D.; Ebbert, J.O.; Hall-Flavin, D.K.; Karpyak, V.M.; Abulseoud, O.A.; Patten, C.A.; Geske, J.R.; Frye, M.A. Female smokers have the highest alcohol craving in a residential alcoholism treatment cohort. *Drug Alcohol Depend.* **2015**, *150*, 179–182. [CrossRef]
23. Baros, A.M.; Latham, P.K.; Anton, R.F. Naltrexone and cognitive behavioral therapy for the treatment of alcohol dependence: Do sex differences exist? *Alcohol Clin. Exp. Res.* **2008**, *32*, 771–776. [CrossRef] [PubMed]
24. Herbeck, D.M.; Schneekloth, T.D.; Ebbert, J.O.; Hall-Flavin, D.K.; Karpyak, V.M.; Abulseoud, O.A.; Patten, C.A.; Geske, J.R.; Frye, M.A. Gender differences in treatment and clinical characteristics among patients receiving extended release naltrexone. *J. Addict. Dis.* **2016**, *35*, 305–314. [CrossRef] [PubMed]
25. Pettinati, H.M.; Kampman, K.M.; Lynch, K.G.; Suh, J.J.; Dackis, C.A.; Oslin, D.W.; O'Brien, C.P. Gender differences with high-dose naltrexone in patients with co-occurring cocaine and alcohol dependence. *J. Subst. Abuse Treat.* **2008**, *34*, 378–390. [CrossRef] [PubMed]
26. McHugh, R.K.; Devito, E.E.; Dodd, D.; Carroll, K.M.; Potter, J.S.; Greenfield, S.F.; Connery, H.S.; Weiss, R.D. Gender differences in a clinical trial for prescription opioid dependence. *J. Subst. Abuse Treat.* **2013**, *45*, 38–43. [CrossRef]
27. Johnson, R.M.; Fairman, B.; Gilreath, T.; Xuan, Z.; Rothman, E.F.; Parnham, T.; Furr-Holden, C.D. Past 15-year trends in adolescent marijuana use: Differences by race/ethnicity and sex. *Drug Alcohol Depend.* **2015**, *155*, 8–15. [CrossRef]
28. Legleye, S.; Daniela, P.; Fred, P.; Céline, G.; Myriam, K.; Ludwig, K. Is there a cannabis epidemic model? Evidence from France, Germany and USA. *Int. J. Drug Policy* **2014**, *25*, 1103–1112. [CrossRef]

29. Hall, W.; Louisa, D. Adverse health effects of non-medical cannabis use. *Lancet* **2009**, *374*, 1383–1391. [CrossRef]
30. Lopez-Quintero, C.; Pérez, C.J.; Hasin, D.S.; Okuda, M.; Wang, S.; Grant, B.F.; Blanco, C. Probability and predictors of transition from first use to dependence on nicotine, alcohol, cannabis, and cocaine: Results of the National Epidemiologic Survey on Alcohol and Related Conditions (NESARC). *Drug Alcohol Depend.* **2011**, *115*, 120–130. [CrossRef]
31. Noack, R.; Hofler, M.; Lueken, U. Cannabis use patterns and their association with DSM-IV cannabis dependence and gender. *Eur. Addict. Res.* **2011**, *17*, 321–328. [CrossRef]
32. Foster, K.T.; Li, N.; McClure, E.A.; Sonne, S.C.; Gray, K.M. Gender Differences in Internalizing Symptoms and Suicide Risk Among Men and Women Seeking Treatment for Cannabis Use Disorder from Late Adolescence to Middle Adulthood. *J. Subst. Abuse Treat.* **2016**, *66*, 16–22. [CrossRef]
33. Blanco, C.; Rafful, C.; Wall, M.M.; Ridenour, T.A.; Wang, S.; Kendler, K.S. Towards a comprehensive developmental model of cannabis use disorders. *Addiction* **2014**, *109*, 284–294. [CrossRef] [PubMed]
34. Khan, S.S.; Secades-Villa, R.; Okuda, M.; Wang, S.; Pérez-Fuentes, G.; Kerridge, B.T.; Blanco, C. Gender differences in cannabis use disorders: Results from the National Epidemiologic Survey of Alcohol and Related Conditions. *Drug Alcohol Depend.* **2013**, *130*, 101–108. [CrossRef] [PubMed]
35. Schepis, T.S.; Desai, R.A.; Cavallo, D.A.; Smith, A.E.; McFetridge, A.; Liss, T.B.; Potenza, M.N.; Krishnan-Sarin, S. Gender differences in adolescent marijuana use and associated psychosocial characteristics. *J. Addict. Med.* **2011**, *5*, 65–73. [CrossRef] [PubMed]
36. Kerridge, B.T.; Desai, R.A.; Cavallo, D.A.; Smith, A.E.; McFetridge, A.; Liss, T.B.; Potenza, M.N.; Krishnan-Sarin, S. DSM-5 cannabis use disorder in the National Epidemiologic Survey on Alcohol and Related Conditions-III: Gender-specific profiles. *Addict. Behav.* **2018**, *76*, 52–60. [CrossRef]
37. Cooper, Z.D.; Craft, R.M. Sex-Dependent Effects of Cannabis and Cannabinoids: A Translational Perspective. *Neuropsychopharmacology* **2017**, *43*, 34–35. [CrossRef]
38. Anderson, B.M.; Matthew, R.; Robert, I.B.; Godfrey, P. Sex, drugs, and cognition: Effects of marijuana. *J. Psychoact. Drugs* **2010**, *42*, 413–424. [CrossRef]
39. Cooper, Z.D.; Haney, M. Investigation of sex-dependent effects of cannabis in daily cannabis smokers. *Drug Alcohol Depend.* **2014**, *136*, 85–91. [CrossRef]
40. Fogel, J.S.; Kelly, T.H.; Westgate, P.M.; Lile, J.A. Sex differences in the subjective effects of oral DELTA^9-THC in cannabis users. *Pharmacol. Biochem. Behav.* **2017**, *152*, 44–51. [CrossRef]
41. Fattore, L.; Fratta, W. How important are sex differences in cannabinoid action? *Br. J. Pharmacol.* **2010**, *160*, 544–548. [CrossRef]
42. Copersino, M.L.; Boyd, S.J.; Tashkin, D.P.; Huestis, M.A.; Heishman, S.J.; Dermand, J.C.; Simmons, M.S.; Gorelick, D.A. Sociodemographic characteristics of cannabis smokers and the experience of cannabis withdrawal. *Am. J. Drug Alcohol Abuse* **2010**, *36*, 311–319. [CrossRef]
43. Herrmann, E.; Weerts, E.; Vandrey, R. Sex Differences in Cannabis Withdrawal Symptoms Among Treatment-Seeking Cannabis Users. *Exp. Clin. Psychopharmacol.* **2015**, *156*, 415–421. [CrossRef]
44. Sherman, B.J.; McRae-Clark, A.L.; Baker, N.L.; Sonne, S.C.; Killeen, T.K.; Cloud, K.; Gray, K.M. Gender differences among treatment-seeking adults with cannabis use disorder: Clinical profiles of women and men enrolled in the achieving cannabis cessation-evaluating N-acetylcysteine treatment (ACCENT) study. *Am. J. Addict.* **2017**, *26*, 136–144. [CrossRef]
45. Cuttler, C.; Mischley, L.K.; Sexton, M. Sex Differences in Cannabis Use and Effects: A Cross-Sectional Survey of Cannabis Users. *Cannabis Cannabinoid Res.* **2016**, *1*, 166–175. [CrossRef] [PubMed]
46. Davis, J.P.; Smith, D.C.; Morphew, J.W.; Lei, X.; Zhang, S. Cannabis Withdrawal, Posttreatment Abstinence, and Days to First Cannabis Use Among Emerging Adults in Substance Use Treatment: A Prospective Study. *J. Drug Issues* **2016**, *46*, 64–83. [CrossRef] [PubMed]
47. Lev-Ran, S.; Imtiaz, S.; Taylor, B.J.; Shield, K.D.; Rehm, J.; Foll, B. Gender differences in health-related quality of life among cannabis users: Results from the National Epidemiologic Survey on Alcohol and Related Conditions. *Drug Alcohol Depend.* **2012**, *123*, 190–200. [CrossRef]
48. Marusich, J.A.; Lefever, T.W.; Antonazzo, K.R.; Craft, R.M.; Wiley, J.L. Evaluation of sex differences in cannabinoid dependence. *Drug Alcohol Depend.* **2014**, *137*, 20–28. [CrossRef]
49. Harte-Hargrove, L.C.; Dow-Edwards, D.L. Withdrawal from THC during adolescence: Sex differences in locomotor activity and anxiety. *Behav. Brain Res.* **2012**, *231*, 48–59. [CrossRef]

50. Hemsing, N.; Greaves, L. Gender norms, roles and relations and cannabis use patterns: A scoping review. *Int. J. Environ. Res. Public Health.* Forthcoming. [CrossRef]
51. Marshall, K.; Gowing, L.; Ali, R.; Le Foll, B. Pharmacotherapies for cannabis dependence. *Cochrane Database Syst. Rev.* **2014**, *12*. [CrossRef]
52. Nielsen, S.; Gowing, L.; Sabioni, P.; Le Foll, B. Pharmacotherapies for cannabis dependence. *Cochrane Database Syst. Rev.* **2019**, *1*. [CrossRef]
53. Moher, D.; Iberati, A.; Tetzlaff, J.; Altman, D.G.; PRISMA Group. Preferred reporting items for systematic reviews and meta-analyses: The PRISMA statement. *PLoS Med.* **2009**, *6*, e1000097. [CrossRef] [PubMed]
54. Hammarström, A. A tool for developing gender research in medicine: Examples from the medical literature on work life. *Gender Med.* **2007**, *4*, S123–S132. [CrossRef]
55. McCarthy, L.; Milne, E.; Waite, N.; Cooke, M.; Cook, K.; Chang, F.; Sproule, B.A. Sex and gender-based analysis in pharmacy practice research: A scoping review. *Res. Soc. Adm. Pharm.* **2017**, *13*, 1045–1054. [CrossRef] [PubMed]
56. Cornelius, J.R.; Bukstein, O.G.; Douaihy, A.B.; Clark, D.B.; Chung, T.A.; Daley, D.C.; Wood, D.S.; Brown, S.J. Double-blind fluoxetine trial in comorbid MDD-CUD youth and young adults. *Drug Alcohol Depend.* **2010**, *112*, 39–45. [CrossRef]
57. Gray, K.M.; Sonne, S.C.; McClure, E.A.; Ghitza, U.E.; Matthews, A.G.; McRae-Clark, A.L.; Carroll, K.M.; Potter, J.S.; Wiest, K.; Mooney, L.J.; et al. A randomized placebo-controlled trial of N-acetylcysteine for cannabis use disorder in adults. *Drug Alcohol Depend.* **2017**, *177*, 249–257. [CrossRef]
58. McRae-Clark, A.L.; Sonne, S.C.; McClure, E.A.; Ghitza, U.E.; Matthews, A.G.; McRae-Clark, A.L.; Carroll, K.M.; Potter, J.S.; Wiest, K.; Mooney, L.J.; et al. Vilazodone for cannabis dependence: A randomized, controlled pilot trial. *Am. J. Addict.* **2016**, *25*, 69–75. [CrossRef]
59. McRae-Clark, A.L.; Baker, N.L.; Gray, K.M.; Killeen, T.K.; Wagner, A.M.; Brady, K.T.; DeVane, C.L.; Norton, J. Buspirone treatment of cannabis dependence: A randomized, placebo-controlled trial. *Drug Alcohol Depend.* **2015**, *156*, 29–37. [CrossRef]
60. Smith, P.H.; Bessette, A.J.; Weinberger, A.H.; Sheffer, C.E.; McKee, S.A. Sex/gender differences in smoking cessation: A review. *Prev. Med.* **2016**, *92*, 135–140. [CrossRef]
61. Franconi, F.; Campesi, I.; Occhioni, S.; Antonini, P.; Murphy, M.F. Sex and gender in adverse drug events, addiction, and placebo. *Handb. Exp. Pharmacol.* **2012**, *214*, 107–126.
62. Petkovic, J.; Trawin, J.; Dewidar, O.; Yoganathan, M.; Tugwell, P.; Welch, V. Sex/gender reporting and analysis in Campbell and Cochrane systematic reviews: A cross-sectional methods study. *Syst. Rev.* **2018**, *7*, 113. [CrossRef]
63. Song, M.M.; Imonsen, C.K.; Wilson, J.D.; Jenkins, M.R. Development of a PubMed Based Search Tool for Identifying Sex and Gender Specific Health Literature. *J. Womens Health* **2016**, *25*, 181–187. [CrossRef] [PubMed]
64. Morgan, T.; Williams, L.A.; Gott, M. A Feminist Quality Appraisal Tool: Exposing gender bias and gender inequities in health research. *Crit. Public Health* **2017**, *27*, 263–274. [CrossRef]

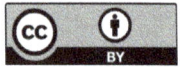

© 2020 by the authors. Licensee MDPI, Basel, Switzerland. This article is an open access article distributed under the terms and conditions of the Creative Commons Attribution (CC BY) license (http://creativecommons.org/licenses/by/4.0/).

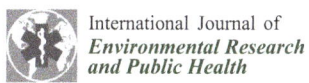

Review

Gender Norms, Roles and Relations and Cannabis-Use Patterns: A Scoping Review

Natalie Hemsing [1,*] and Lorraine Greaves [1,2]

1 Centre of Excellence for Women's Health, Vancouver, BC V6H 3N1, Canada; lgreaves@cw.bc.ca
2 School of Population and Public Health, University of British Columbia, Vancouver, BC V6T 1Z4, Canada
* Correspondence: nhemsing@cw.bc.ca; Tel.: +1-604-875-2633

Received: 31 December 2019; Accepted: 29 January 2020; Published: 4 February 2020

Abstract: Currently, boys and men use cannabis at higher rates than girls and women, but the gender gap is narrowing. With the legalization of recreational cannabis use in Canada and in multiple US states, these trends call for urgent attention to the need to consider how gender norms, roles and relations influence patterns of cannabis use to inform health promotion and prevention responses. Based on a scoping review on sex, gender and cannabis use, this article consolidates existing evidence from the academic literature on how gender norms, roles and relations impact cannabis-use patterns. Evidence is reviewed on: adherence to dominant masculine and feminine norms and cannabis-use patterns among adolescents and young adults, and how prevailing norms can be both reinstated or reimagined through cannabis use; gendered social dynamics in cannabis-use settings; and the impact of gender roles and relations on cannabis use among young adults of diverse sexual orientations and gender identities. Findings from the review are compared and contrasted with evidence on gender norms, roles and relations in the context of alcohol and tobacco use. Recommendations for integrating gender transformative principles in health promotion and prevention responses to cannabis use are provided.

Keywords: cannabis; gender norms; gender roles; gender relations

1. Introduction

Similar to other substances, men and boys have higher rates and frequency of cannabis use [1–6]. Boys and men also report using a greater variety of routes of administration of cannabis use compared to women and girls [7] and are more likely to use high-potency products and cannabis concentrates. These patterns of use have been linked with greater risk of developing cannabis-use dependence [8]. Young men who use cannabis are also more likely to report using alcohol and other substances, which increases the risk of adverse health and social consequences [9]. Researchers have often examined substance use from the purview of men, perceived as primarily an activity of men [10]. While the current cannabis-use patterns and trends might immediately suggest that policy and practice responses should prioritize the needs of boys and men, emerging evidence reveals the gap in cannabis-use prevalence between women and men is narrowing [11], and similar to other substances, trans and gender-diverse individuals report higher prevalence of cannabis use [12,13].

These patterns and trends in cannabis use highlight the need to attend to a range of gender-related factors. Not to be confused or conflated with sex, which refers to a range of biologically based characteristics that are linked to being male or female, gender refers to the socially constructed norms, relations, roles, expressions, behaviours and identities of girls, women, boys, men, and gender diverse people [14]. Gender is often conceptualized as a binary (e.g., woman/man). For example, masculinity and femininity have often been conceptualized in opposition to one another "as a relation of complementary difference" [15]. Yet how people understand, experience, and express gender is far more complex and varied [14]. Furthermore, as argued by Budgeon, the "gender binary which traditionally established gender hierarchy has become more multi-dimensional and complex," (p. 318) as social norms and gender ideologies continue to change and evolve [15]. Gender norms are dynamic and embedded in the social, cultural and political context of social groups. Gender is socially constructed and individually enacted and experienced, but influenced by institutionalized power and the social, political and economic advantages and disadvantages afforded to different genders. It also intersects with other social determinants of health including social class, race, and ethnicity [16]. Therefore, studying gender in the context of cannabis use, or any other substance use, is complex, temporal and culturally specific. For further details on the features of both sex and gender as concepts, and the interaction of sex and gender in the context of cannabis use see the article published in this special issue by Greaves and Hemsing [17].

Gender Norms, Roles and Relations

Of these multiple dimensions of gender that can be examined in the context of substance use, in this paper we focus on gender norms, roles and relations. *Gender norms* refer to societal rules and expectations that dictate the behaviors considered appropriate or desirable for people based on their gender [14]. Men and women often experience different social pressures to engage in behaviours that are reflective of traditional masculine or feminine norms. Traditional masculine norms are also sometimes referred to as hegemonic masculinity, or dominant masculinity. In some cases, extreme or strong versions of hegemonic masculinity are identifiable such as: dominance, aggression, competition, invulnerability, risk taking, stoicism, and physical and emotional control [18]. These expressions of 'hypermasculinity' enacted through substance use may include frequent using, binging and combining substances, all patterns which may increase the risk of negative health and social consequences. In contrast, traditional or hegemonic feminine norms include values and characteristics such as: nurturance, beauty, virtuousness and expressing emotions [19]. Dominant feminine norms tend to "emphasize risk aversion" and are typically negatively associated with substance-use behaviours in various studies [20]. The greater prevalence of substance use among boys and men may reflect differences in access to substances, with social norms affording greater permissibility for boys and men to experiment with, use substances and engage in riskier patterns of use [21].

While these dominant femininities and masculinities are archetypes, and individuals and sub-populations will deviate from them, adherence to these can be measured. The majority of research on gender norms and substance use has examined adherence to hegemonic gender norms, and particularly masculine norms. For example, the dominant masculine norms from the Conformity to Masculine Norms Inventory (CMNI) of "risk taking" and "playboy" have been strongly associated with heavy alcohol use [22,23]. Having said this, Everitt-Penhale and Ratele critique the notion of a single traditional masculinity, arguing that "traditional masculinity" varies by class, race, ethnicity and geographic context. Furthermore, they suggest that "competing traditional masculinities" are likely to exist within a single group or context [24]. In addition, Wilkinson et al. critique narrow conceptualizations of gender as either a trait (e.g., masculine personality traits) or ideology (e.g., beliefs and attitudes regarding the roles of women and men) [25]. They argue that focusing on traits lacks attention to the social construction of gender, while ideological conceptualizations narrowly focus on beliefs—one dimension of gender which does not always align with behaviors.

Gender roles include the expected roles and behaviours attached to the genders. Expectations about gender roles often affects and determines the opportunities available to different genders, based on culture, place and time. For example, there may be different expectations regarding substance use among girls and boys, or mothers and fathers, in different social contexts and among different cultures.

Gender relations refer to the interactions between genders that reflect gendered norms and affect health, behaviours and roles [14]. Femininity and masculinity can be defined both individually and relationally; for example, one's own gender ideology may restrain substance use, while the gender norms of friends or partners, or those embedded in media may promote, or deter, substance-use behaviours [20]. Due to the social, relational and performative nature of gender and its different contexts, qualitative research is instrumental for understanding how gender norms are expressed in gender roles and relations. Therefore, investigating the relational aspects of gender is a critical area of inquiry to understand the relationship between gender and cannabis use.

While there are many cross-sectional studies and surveys analyzing gender 'differences' in cannabis prevalence and consumption patterns, there is limited research exploring the social factors underpinning these patterns of use. Indeed, no reviews are available on the impact of gender related factors on cannabis use. In response to this gap, we conducted a scoping review to explore the available literature on gender and cannabis use, focusing on three dimensions of gender: gender norms (societal norms regarding gender and cannabis use), gender roles (who uses cannabis and in which contexts) and gender relations (how gendered interactions influence cannabis use). In the discussion, we consider this nascent and emerging literature on gender and cannabis in light of evidence from the fields of alcohol and tobacco research and discuss opportunities for responding to various gendered aspects of cannabis use in prevention and harm reduction programming.

2. Methods

This scoping review on gender and cannabis is part of, and based on, a larger scoping review conducted on sex, gender and four substances: cannabis, alcohol, tobacco/nicotine and opioids.

We conducted a scoping review of the academic literature to identify, analyze and synthesize current research in: sex and gender related factors in substance use (initiation/uptake, patterns of use), effects, and prevention, treatment or harm reduction outcomes for four substances (opioids, alcohol, tobacco/nicotine and cannabis); and harm reduction, health promotion/ prevention and treatment interventions and programs that include sex, gender and gender transformative elements to address each of the four substances. A scoping review methodology was used to identify the extent of existing research on sex, gender and the four substances, and existing gaps [26]. Scoping reviews are exploratory, and unlike systematic reviews, have broad inclusion criteria and do not typically assess the quality of individual studies [27]. The scoping review was based on two broad questions:

(1) How do sex and gender related factors impact:

  (a) patterns of use;
  (b) health effects of;
  (c) and prevention/treatment/or harm reduction outcomes for opioid, alcohol, tobacco/nicotine and cannabis use?

(2) *What* harm reduction, health-promotion/prevention and treatment interventions and programs are available *that include sex, gender and gender transformative elements* and how effective are these in addressing opioid, alcohol, tobacco/ nicotine and cannabis use?

We engaged in an iterative academic literature search to identify relevant peer-reviewed studies. The searches were conducted in health-related academic databases with international coverage, including: Medline, Embase, Cochrane Database of Systematic Reviews, and Cochrane Central Register of Controlled Trials via Ovid; The Cumulative Index to Nursing and Allied Health Literature (CINAHL), PsycINFO, Social Work Abstracts, Women's Studies International, and Lesbian, Gay, Bisexual and Transgender (LGBT) Life via EbscoHost; and Social Science Citation Index via Clarivate Analytics.

An information specialist worked with the research team to design, implement and amend the search strategy. The searches were complex, given the multiple substances and levels of intervention of interest, and various components of the concepts sex and gender. The search strategy was amended and refined based on team discussion and analysis of the search returns, articles missed by the searches, and consultation with the information specialist. The initial search covered studies published from January 2007 to August 2017, combining keywords for: sex and gender; substance use and substance-use disorders for each of the four substances (opioids, alcohol, cannabis, tobacco/nicotine); and the three levels of intervention (harm reduction, health promotion and prevention, and treatment).

After reviewing the search returns and consulting with the information specialist, the research team determined that the searches were missing key literature on the health effects of substance use (research question 1b). Therefore, the search was amended in September 2017 to include terms for health effects, and to apply additional sex and gender terms and substance-specific terms. During the process of screening returns from the second search, the research team identified multiple substance-use intervention studies relevant to the review that were not being captured by the first two searches. The information specialist analyzed the keywords used in each of the missed articles, and in April 2018 performed a third literature search with additional sex/gender terms to locate relevant studies and extend the search to cover January 2007 to April 2018. Details on the search terms used in each of these three searches are provided in Appendix A.

The three database searches resulted in $n = 20,121$ unique articles; an additional $n = 11$ records were identified through other sources. The $n = 20,132$ records were first screened by title, then by abstract and finally the full text of remaining papers was retrieved and screened a final time for inclusion. In accordance with the UK National Institute for Health and Care Excellence (NICE) manual *Methods for the Development of NICE Public Health Guidance*, abstract and full paper screening was conducted independently by two reviewers, and inter-rater reliability was compared, recorded and maintained [28]. A screening tool was used by the two reviewers to independently code the inclusion/exclusion of each study screened and the reason for exclusion. The coding decisions of the two reviewers were then compared; they participated in weekly meetings with a third researcher for the duration of abstract and full paper screening to review disagreements over the inclusion or exclusion of articles, and to resolve discrepancies by discussion and consensus.

In alignment with scoping review methods, inclusion criteria were amended post-hoc [26]. Based on increasing familiarity with the literature we used an iterative team approach to select relevant studies. The team had weekly web meetings between March 2018 and April 2019 to discuss the progress and to resolve any coding discrepancies. At the beginning of screening (February 2018) and near the end (April 2019) the team met face to face for full day meetings to discuss the scope of included literature and to further refine the inclusion and exclusion criteria. The final set of inclusion criteria, including the PICO (Population, Intervention, Comparator, Outcomes) details for framing each research question, are provided in Appendix B. Included studies were English language articles from a selection of Organization for Economic Cooperation and Development (OECD) member countries (see Appendix B for this list). The population of interest included: women, girls, men, boys, trans and gender diverse people of all ages and demographics. However, studies conducted primarily with pregnant girls and women were excluded as the research team has conducted multiple evidence reviews on substance use among this population. Studies were included that assessed: patterns of use, beliefs and perceptions regarding substance use, and health effects; and intervention studies that analyzed the impact of sex and gender or described or evaluated sex or gender informed interventions. With regard to the four specific substances of interest: tobacco and nicotine included electronic nicotine delivery systems (ENDS); alcohol use included all use and not just problematic use; opioid use included illicit and prescription opioids; and cannabis included both therapeutic and recreational use.

Before acquiring papers for assessment, the $n = 20,132$ titles were initially scanned by one reviewer who removed the clearly irrelevant studies. Title screening reduced the number of included papers to $n = 11,842$. Initially, a random sample of 10% of these abstracts were independently scrutinized by two reviewers in relation to the inclusion criteria. The two reviewers achieved agreement on 83.19% of the sample of abstracts reviewed; the remaining abstracts were then divided and assessed by a single reviewer. Full papers of the remaining included studies ($n = 9615$) were then retrieved and assessed by two independent reviewers. Inter-rater reliability was monitored quarterly (each quarter of the retrieved papers) throughout the full paper screening stage to ensure the reliability score (Cohen's kappa) remained above $\kappa = 0.6$. The final overall kappa was 0.73. After the full paper review, $n = 5030$

papers were still included (n = 4835 were categorized into Research Question 1 (RQ1), and n = 195 were categorized into Research Question 2 (RQ2)). Figure 1 provides an overview of the literature search returns, the number of papers included and excluded at each level of screening, and the final number of included papers identified.

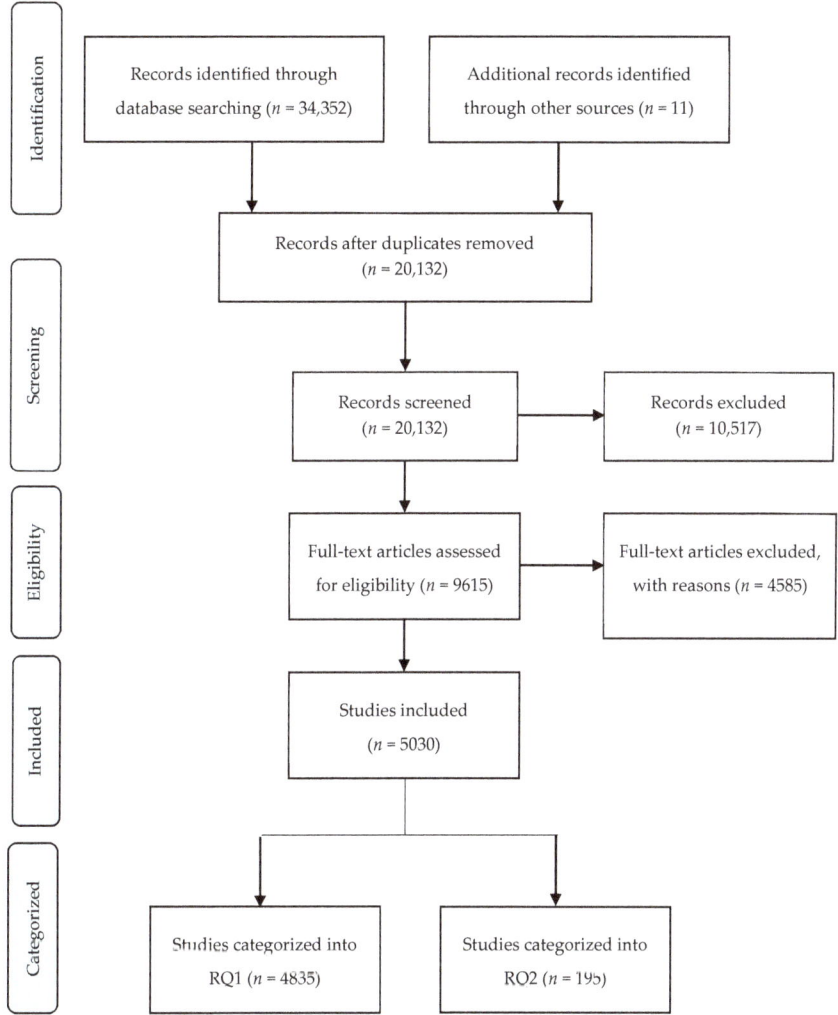

Figure 1. Preferred Reporting Items for Systematic Reviews and Meta-Analyses (Prisma) flow diagram. From Moher D. et al. [29].

Included studies were categorized by one researcher, who coded details on: research question (question one or two); the substance(s) addressed (cannabis, alcohol, opioids, tobacco/nicotine); primary and secondary topic (prevalence/patterns of use; beliefs/perceptions; mechanisms/biological responses; health effects or consequences; prevention intervention; brief intervention; treatment intervention; harm reduction intervention); and whether the study was a quantitative or qualitative design or a systematic review. Because the inclusion criteria were developed iteratively, and amended during screening, a second researcher checked the coding to ensure alignment with the finalized set of inclusion criteria. Once the categories were checked by a second researcher, a final searchable database of included studies was produced, with each included study categorized by substance and topic.

In total, $n = 784$ papers on cannabis were identified in the search. The majority of these papers focused on prevalence and patterns of use ($n = 445$). Additional categories included: $n = 57$ studies on interventions to address cannabis use (including prevention, harm reduction and treatment); $n = 18$ studies on beliefs and perceptions regarding cannabis use; $n = 78$ papers on biological mechanisms; and n = 186 studies on the health effects of cannabis use.

Of these, we identified $n = 15$ studies on cannabis and gender roles, norms and relations. We reviewed the reference lists of these included studies, identifying an additional $n = 6$ relevant studies. In total, we included $n = 21$ studies. Some studies were included that were conducted with one gender group if the authors explored gendered dimensions of cannabis use. While studies were excluded from the original search if they were conducted in Mexico, we chose to include these studies in this scoping review on gender and cannabis use because there were relatively few studies available examining feminine norms and cannabis use.

3. Findings

Details on the $n = 21$ included studies are provided in Table 1, including information on: country, study design, aims, the dimensions of gender included in the study, and key findings regarding cannabis and gender. The 21 studies included were conducted in a range of countries including: Canada, USA, Mexico, Ireland, Norway and the UK. The majority of studies were either qualitative or cross-sectional. The majority of cross sectional studies examined conformity to gender norms (e.g., based on measures of gender typicality), and qualitative studies tended to explore gender roles and relations in the context of cannabis use. A total of $n = 8$ studies included adolescents, $n = 2$ included a longitudinal design and examined cannabis use from adolescence to adulthood; and $n = 11$ included adults. See table for further details.

Findings from the studies on gender norms and cannabis use are summarized narratively in the three sections: *male typicality and cannabis use; conformity to feminine norms*; and *conformity to gender norms, culture and acculturation*. Findings from research on gender roles and relations are summarized in five sections: *reinstating and resisting dominant gender norms; cannabis and gender relations in social networks; cannabis use in intimate relationships; stigma and discrimination; and stigma among mothers and fathers who use cannabis*.

Table 1. Study details.

Author/Year	Country	Study Design	Study Aim	Population	Assessment of Cannabis Use	Dimension of Gender Addressed	Gender and Cannabis Findings
Arnull and Ryder 2019	UK and USA	qualitative comparative study	To prioritize the voices of justice-involved girls in the UK and USA regarding their reasons for substance use	age 13–18 adjudicated girls who had been sentenced for a violent offense; n = 24 girls in USA (primarily identified as "women of color"), n = 35 in UK (primarily White British)	Participants were assessed for eligibility based on self-reported "ever use" of cannabis and alcohol	Gender relations; explored use of alcohol and cannabis, within justice involved girls' social groups.	Girls described pleasure related to their cannabis use with other girls. Within their friend groups they managed physical and sexual risks when using substances.
Belackova and Vaccaro 2013	USA	qualitative	To explore the role of cannabis in friendship groups	n = 44 adult cannabis users and retailers in Florida; n = 32 men and n = 12 women; primarily White	Participants were assessed for eligibility based on self-reported use of cannabis in past 12 months	Gender relations in the context of reasons for/functions of cannabis use.	Some men described opportunities for pursuing intimate interactions with women when using cannabis.
Brady et al. 2016	USA	systematic review	To examine feminine norms and substance use outcomes among women	only n = 2 studies included cannabis use (Kulis 2008; and Kulis 2010, see below)	Not reported	Gender norms; studies were eligible for inclusion if examined feminine norms/ideology or feminine role conflict.	Majority of studies reported that adherence to feminine norms increased substance use, but only two studies included cannabis (included below).
Dahl and Sandberg 2014	Norway	qualitative	To examine how women navigate a gendered cannabis-use culture in Norway	Analyzed data from 2 studies: one with n = 100 cannabis using adults; and one with n = 25 experienced cannabis users (n = 7 women; n = 18 men)	Participants were assessed for eligibility based on self-reported long term cannabis use; included sporadic to heavy use (not quantified)	How adults "do gender" through cannabis use; examined women and men's roles and positions in social networks using cannabis, and their concerns about use.	Dominant femininities and masculinities are both reinstated and reimagined through cannabis use.
Dahl 2015	Norway	qualitative	To examine the change in identity among experienced cannabis users who had quit or reduced their use	n = 7 women, n = 18 men; Age = 23–40 years; former daily cannabis users who had reduced or quit using cannabis without formal drug and alcohol treatment	Participants were assessed for eligibility based on self-reported former daily cannabis use	Gender roles and gender relations in the context of reducing and quitting cannabis se.	New fathers discussed the cannabis user identity as incompatible with their role as father; men discussed changing their use in the context of intimate relationships.

Table 1. *Cont.*

Author/Year	Country	Study Design	Study Aim	Population	Assessment of Cannabis Use	Dimension of Gender Addressed	Gender and Cannabis Findings
Darcy 2019	Ireland	qualitative	To explore how men's illicit substance use patterns and intoxication converge with masculinities	$n = 20$ Irish men who used illicit substances ($n = 17$ heterosexual; 2 homosexual; 1 undeclared)	Participants identified as "recreational illicit drug users"	Gender relations; gender norms; applies a gender lens to examine Irish men's illicit substance using practices in the context of masculinities, and within the context of use with other men.	Men use illicit substances as a way to navigate traditional masculinity in paradoxical ways: both for closeness in friendships, and in competition.
Darcy 2018	Ireland	qualitative	To explore men's substance use as a friendship practice	Same as above	Participants identified as "recreational illicit drug users"	Gender roles and relations; how cannabis is used in friendships and social settings, and in relation to conventional masculine stereotypes.	Cannabis use provided opportunities to "contravene conventional masculine stereotypes" (e.g., by offering a space for bonding with male friends, being more emotionally expressive), as well as reinforced masculine stereotypes (e.g., expressing dominance by obtaining and supplying substances, including cannabis).
Gonzalez, Gallego, and Bockting 2017	USA	cross-sectional	To examine the relationship between gender minority stress and substance use among transgender adults	$n = 1210$ transgender adults ($n = 680$ transgender women; $n = 530$ transgender men)	Participants were asked: "In the last three months, how many days did you use marijuana or hashish (weed, grass, reefers)?"	Gender roles (non-conformity, gender minority stress), gender dysphoria and cannabis use.	Gender dysphoria was associated with cannabis use among both both transgender women and men; among transgender women, gender minority stress was associated with cannabis use.
Haines-Saah et al. 2019	Canada	qualitative	To highlight the perspectives of parents on preventing problematic adolescent cannabis use, and critique notion of 'parents as the best prevention'	$n = 16$ parents of children (over age 13) who used cannabis; mostly women ($n = 12$)	Participants were eligible to participate if they were a parent of a child over age 13 who had experience with cannabis use	Discusses gender roles: expectations of mothers.	Mothers described feeling like failures if they had challenges regarding their child's substance use, and experienced a lack of social support due to judgement and stigma.

Table 1. *Cont.*

Author/Year	Country	Study Design	Study Aim	Population	Assessment of Cannabis Use	Dimension of Gender Addressed	Gender and Cannabis Findings
Haines et al. 2009	Canada	qualitative	To explore how adolescents perceive cannabis-use experiences as influenced by gender	n = 45 adolescents, 13–18 years; n = 26 boys, n = 19 girls	Participants included frequent cannabis users (minimum of past week use)	Gender norms, roles and relations; gender was coded into several sub-themes: styles of use by boys and girls; sex differences in use; gender and access; use in the context of relationships; issues of safety when smoking or "partying". Analysis focused on how students spoke about gender.	Girls and boys described gendered social dynamics in cannabis-use settings and patterns of use.
Hathaway et al. 2011	Canada	qualitative	To examine extra-legal forms of stigma based on interviews with cannabis users	n = 92 (mean age 39) who had used cannabis on 25 or more occasions	Eligibility screening survey identified participants with personal experience with cannabis i (lifetime prevalence)	Gender roles; examines stigma in the context of cannabis use and the disadvantages and benefits of using.	Women described experiencing stigma when using cannabis during pregnancy and as mothers; conflict with the role of "good mother."
Hathaway et al. 2018	Canada	qualitative	To examine patterns of supply of cannabis among students at Canadian universities	n = 130 social sciences students in universities in Ontario and Alberta (55% female; 47% reported ever using cannabis)	Eligibility screening survey identified "regular" or "occasional" cannabis users (not quantified)	Gender relations in the context of cannabis supply.	Buying and maintaining a supply of cannabis was typically a male activity.
Ilan 2012	Ireland	qualitative	To explore the experience of street culture among socio-economically disadvantaged young men in Ireland	n = 7 adolescents and young men engaged in street culture in Dublin	Not reported	Gender relations in the context of male friendships.	Cannabis was used to facilitate male friendships, social bonding.
Kulis et al. 2008	Mexico	cross-sectional	To examine the relationship of femininity and masculinity constructs developed for Mexican-American youth with a range of substance use outcomes	n = 327 adolescents in Mexico	Self-report past 30 day use of cannabis (Likert scale)	Gender norms; assessed four constructs based on Mexican concepts of *marianismo* and *machismo* including; aggressive masculinity, assertive masculinity, affective femininity and submissive femininity.	Aggressive masculinity was associated with greater risk of substance use for most outcome measures, while affective femininity was generally associated with lower risks including less recent use of cannabis.

Table 1. *Cont.*

Author/Year	Country	Study Design	Study Aim	Population	Assessment of Cannabis Use	Dimension of Gender Addressed	Gender and Cannabis Findings
Kulis et al. 2010	USA	cross-sectional	To examine the relationship of femininity and masculinity constructs with substance use among Mexican-American youth	n = 151 Mexican-American adolescents	Self-report past 30 day use of cannabis (Likert scale)	Same as Kulis et al. 2008.	Submissive femininity was significantly associated with alcohol use; no significant association was found for gender role and cannabis use.
Kulis et al. 2012	USA	cross-sectional	To examine the relationship between adaptive and maladaptive constructs of masculinity and femininity, substance misuse and acculturation among Mexican-American youth	n = 1466 Mexican-American adolescents	Self-report past 30 day use of cannabis (Likert scale)	Same as Kulis et al. 2008.	Highly acculturated girls who reported high maladaptive masculinity (aggressive, controlling) reported the highest cannabis use.
Mahalik et al. 2015	USA	cross sectional longitudinal	To examine the relationship between gender, male-typicality, and social norms on longitudinal patterns of alcohol intoxication and cannabis use in US youth	n = 10,588 youth (48% male; 52% female)	Self-report days per month cannabis use (Likert scale)	Gender norms; adherence to male typical behaviours and attitudes among females and males from adolescence to adulthood (based on measure of male typicality from Add Health data).	Greater male typicality among both females and males was associated with substance use including cannabis use; however, the effect was greater for males.
Palamar et al. 2018	USA	qualitative	To examine and compare cannabis users' psychosocial and physical sexual experiences and sexual risk behavior	n = 24 adults (n = 12 women; n = 12 men); all heterosexual	Participants were eligible to participate if they self-reported sexual intercourse while high on cannabis in the past 3 months	Gender relations; cannabis use in the context of heterosexual sexual relations.	Young women reported being more selective regarding sexual partners when they were using cannabis. Participants (female and male) reported feeling more in control on cannabis than alcohol, but also quieter and less social.

Table 1. *Cont.*

Author/Year	Country	Study Design	Study Aim	Population	Assessment of Cannabis Use	Dimension of Gender Addressed	Gender and Cannabis Findings
Robinson 2015	Canada	mixed methods	To examine the impact of anxiety on cannabis use among bisexual women	n = 92 bisexual women ages 18–54	Self-report cannabis use in the past year (Likert scale) using the Drug Use Disorders Identification Test-Extended Version (DUDIT-E)	Non-conformity to gender roles and impact on stress and substance use.	Cannabis may be used as a way to cope with "female gender roles", and discrimination based on gender and sexual orientation.
Robinson, Sanches, and MacLeod 2016	Canada	correlational	To examine the prevalence and mental health correlates of illicit cannabis use among bisexual women	n = 262 bisexual adult women	Self-report cannabis use in the past year (Likert scale) using the Drug Use Disorders Identification Test-Extended Version (DUDIT-E)	Gender relations; non conformity to gender roles and social exclusion.	Cannabis use correlated with social support; bisexual women who often face social exclusion may use cannabis as a tool for social connection.
Wilkinson et al. 2018	USA	cross-sectional longitudinal	To examine the associations between adherence to gender-typical behavior and substance use from adolescence to adulthood	n = 4617 males; n = 5660 females	Self-report number of occurrences (Waves 1 and 3) and days of cannabis use (Wave 4) in the past 30 days	Gender norms; gender typicality based on adherence to gender typical behaviours; behaviours included a range from individual actions (e.g., exercising) to states of being (e.g., getting sad) that correlated with being female or male.	Greater male typicality at wave one was associated with greater odds of high frequency cannabis and cigarette use and increased risk of use of one or more substances at Wave three (during emerging adulthood). Among females, there was a lower change in high frequency use and polysubstance use over time.

4. Gender Norms

4.1. Male Typicality and Cannabis Use

Several studies were identified measuring adherence to "male typicality" in the context of substance use, including cannabis use. Based on the theory that some boys and young men may use substances to support the development of a "male-typical or masculine" identity, Mahalik et al. explored the relationship between gender, male typicality and social norms in regards to alcohol and cannabis use, following a sample of youth from adolescence to adulthood [30]. The gender typicality measure includes 16 items assessing attitudes and behaviours demonstrated to have moderate to strong gender differences among adolescents (e.g., frequency of crying; frequency of being in serious fights) based on data from the National Longitudinal Study of Adolescent Health (Add Health). This measure identified the gender of females and males with 81.7% accuracy. Mahalik et al. applied these measures to predict the probability of each participant being male and analyzed the correlation with substance use. They hypothesized that females and males, but particularly males, who report greater conformity to male-typical behaviours and attitudes would demonstrate greater substance use during adolescence and into adulthood. Confirming their hypothesis, they found males reported greater cannabis use over time. Greater male typicality among both females and males was associated with substance use including cannabis use; however, the effect was greater for males.

Wilkinson and colleagues applied the same Add Health gender diagnostic measures, in relation to substance use from adolescence to young adulthood. However, in contrast to the study by Mahalik et al., they used multiple waves of data collection to assess gender typicality, and they assessed females and males on their adherence to female and male typicality. Similar to Mahalik et al., they also found a stronger relationship between substance use and traditional masculine gender norms for boys. Greater male typicality at wave one was associated with greater odds of high frequency cannabis and cigarette use and increased risk of use of one or more substances at wave three (during emerging adulthood). Among females, there was less change in high frequency use and polysubstance use over time. However, they caution when interpreting these findings that there is individual variability in how masculinity and femininity are understood and enacted.

4.2. Conformity to Feminine Norms

A systematic review examined the role of feminine norms on substance use among women. The authors were interested in individual conformity to traditional feminine norms and the relationship with substance use. The majority of studies used the Bem Sex Role Inventory (BSRI) which measures feminine traits based on societal norms, or the Conformity to Feminine Norms Inventory (CFNI) which assesses conformity to the following eight dominant feminine norms: nice in relationships, thinness, modesty, domestic, care for children, romantic relationship, sexual fidelity, and invest in appearance [19]. Their review found that 74% of studies identified a relationship between feminine norms and substance use. However, while they included search terms for cannabis/marijuana, of the $n = 23$ studies included in their review, only $n = 2$ studies included cannabis use in relation to feminine norms. All authored by Kulis et al., these studies are described in the following section.

4.3. Conformity to Gender Norms, Culture and Acculturation

Kulis and colleagues conducted several studies with Mexican and Mexican-American adolescents examining the impact of gender norms on cannabis use. They developed four gender constructs based on "marianismo" and "machismo"—conceptualizations of femininity and masculinity in Mexico that they argue include both positive and negative dimensions. Accordingly, the authors developed the following four constructs: *assertive masculinity* (self-confidence, personal valor and assertiveness); *affective femininity* (empathy, emotional expression, nurturing); negative masculinity or *aggressive masculinity* (a tendency to control and seek domination in relationships); and negative femininity or *submissive femininity* (dependence and submissiveness). They used 19 items to measure these four dimensions of gender identity, asking students to indicate how often they thought they exhibited gender typical traits and behaviours.

In their 2008 study, Kulis et al. surveyed adolescents in Mexico, and found that affective femininity tended to be associated with lower risks including less recent use of cannabis, while submissive femininity was not related to substance use [31]. Aggressive masculinity was associated with greater substance use including cannabis use, while assertive masculinity was only associated with perceptions of substance use among friends and receiving substance use offers. However, as the study was cross-sectional it is not possible to determine the direction of these relationships. The authors suggest that for youth identifying with aggressive masculinity, substance use may be a tool for demonstrating "toughness." In contrast, they suggest that affective femininity may be associated with lower risk of substance use because using substances may be incompatible with aspects of this construct, such as gentleness and showing attention to others. Furthermore, they suggest that the lack of relationship of assertive masculinity and submissive femininity with substance use may reflect cultural differences between the USA and Mexico. While the USA has a more individualistic culture, in which substance use may relate to measures of assertiveness, Mexico tends to be a more collectivistic society. Similarly, they explain that submissive femininity is more strongly valued and prescribed in Mexico than the USA, and therefore boys and girls who conform to submissive femininity may not experience the same pressures to use some substances (as has been observed in studies conducted in the USA).

Two additional studies led by Kulis et al. used the same measures but with samples of Mexican-American adolescents. In one study, submissive femininity was significantly associated with alcohol use, but no significant association was found for cannabis use [32]. In a second study, they reported the following correlations regarding gender and cannabis use: assertive masculinity (assertive, self-confident, problem-solving) was associated with higher cannabis amount and frequency in girls; while assertive femininity was associated with lower levels of cannabis use in boys. Furthermore, acculturation was largely unrelated to substance use, except for cannabis use in girls [33]; highly acculturated girls who reported high aggressive masculinity (aggressive, controlling) reported the highest cannabis use. They suggest that as adolescent girls became acculturated, they may adopt certain dominant masculine norms that confer greater risk for substance use. According to the authors, *marianismo* (a Mexican conceptualization of traditional femininity) may be protective by limiting social interactions outside controlled family settings, but this protective effect may decrease with acculturation. Another explanation they offer is that as girls become more acculturated, they may be more vulnerable to using cannabis to cope with stress.

5. Gender Roles, Norms and Relations

5.1. Reinstating and Resisting Dominant Gender Norms

Several qualitative studies have explored gender roles, norms and gender relations in the context of cannabis. The performative aspect of gender expresses itself in norms of use, and through the adoption of gendered roles in relation to substance use. There is evidence that adolescents and adults "do gender" through cannabis use, and dominant femininities and masculinities can be both reinstated or resisted through cannabis use [34]. For example, in a Canadian qualitative study, adolescents were hesitant to discuss their cannabis-use behaviours as shaped by gender even though the narratives of adolescents revealed gendered social dynamics in cannabis-use settings and patterns of use [35]. For example, habitual use by girls was described as inappropriate, and girls who did smoke cannabis were often perceived as acting too "silly" and "giggly" when high, while boys who used cannabis regularly were seen as cool and relaxed. Similarly, in the qualitative study by Dahl et al., female cannabis users "did gender" in multiple ways. Predominantly, they "did traditional femininity" by not buying cannabis, remaining in control when using, smoking less and admitting when they felt anxious or too high [34]. However, some participants "did masculinity" by supplying cannabis, rolling joints, being able to consume large amounts, and enjoying being high. In contrast, men were more engaged with dealers and cultivators, often used cannabis with other men, were more likely to maximize their intoxication (e.g., by method or quantity of use) and were more open with their use.

Cannabis may also be used in ways contrary to dominant gender norms as a "way to revise or undermine gender norms" [35] (p. 2035). In the study with Canadian adolescents, boys suggested cannabis use may be associated with more androgynous values, and may represent an alternative and gentler way of "doing masculinity," in comparison to other substance use [35]. For example, some boys described their preference for using cannabis over alcohol because it is a "happy drug" and allowed them to talk honestly and be open with their emotions; in contrast, boys explained that alcohol use among groups of boys often resulted in aggressive behavior and fights. Similarly, in a study conducted in Norway, Dahl and colleagues suggest that the "masculinity embedding cannabis use" combined two ideologies. One is a form of traditional masculinity, which tends to foster substance use, violence and sexism, and the other is a form of masculinity that "combines an ideology of gender equality with relaxation, play, fun and not taking things too seriously" [34] (p. 708). For example, men were accepting and often applauding of women who engaged in cannabis-use patterns perceived as masculine (e.g., using frequently, enjoying the high), yet they also described these behaviours as "manly" or unfeminine.

These studies from Canada [35] and Norway [34] both reveal how female cannabis users can resist dominant feminine ideals, positioning themselves as "one of the boys" by engaging in cannabis-use activities traditionally identified as more masculine. Similarly, a qualitative study by Arnull and Ryder described alcohol and cannabis use among a sample of justice-involved girls in the UK and USA as a way of "doing gender control" by resisting "hegemonic norms [framing] ... [alcohol or drug] use as unusual, unfeminine or non-agentic" [36] (p. 1365). By sharing the girls' narratives, they argue that substance use among girls is both a "pleasurable and boundaried" activity for girls. The authors stress the role of girls as agents in making decisions regarding their alcohol and cannabis use, rather than framing girls' substance use as deviant, "unfeminine" or caused by trauma.

5.2. Cannabis and Gender Relations in Social Networks

Qualitative research reveals gendered social dynamics in accessing cannabis. Hathaway et al. conducted interviews with social sciences students attending universities in Ontario and Alberta regarding their substance use [37]. Young women who used cannabis discussed the benefits of gaining access to cannabis via their male friends. As one young woman said:

"I have never really bought it. I always sort of smoke other people's weed. Like I have this friend of mine. He is a really nice guy, and I usually smoke with him and his friends. They never let me pay, because they say I don't smoke much ... but I really think it's because I am a girl and they are trying to be nice (laughs) (Female, 18)." [37] (p. 1675).

The authors suggest that buying and maintaining a supply of cannabis is typically a male activity, but that some women may access cannabis for free through their relationships with men. Similarly, a qualitative study with Canadian adolescents found that among some participants, girls were perceived (by both girls and boys) as more easily accessing cannabis [35]. While men are usually the dealers or suppliers, girls were described as flirting and using their beauty or "sexuality as a tool" to access cannabis for free. As one male participant explained:

"Because a lot of the dealers are men and women have a lot of power of persuasion over men, especially if they are beautiful women. It's easy for them to get what they want out of men, so there's a bit of manipulation that goes on there" (p. 2034).

There are also gendered social dynamics regarding cannabis use among male friend groups. A qualitative study explored men's greater prevalence of illicit psychoactive substance use in Ireland in relation to masculinities [38]. Darcy argues that men use illicit substances to navigate masculinities in "paradoxical ways." They found that some of the men's substance-using behaviours aligned with hegemonic masculine ideals–including notions of "toughness," competition and endurance of physical and emotional strain. For example, they described "competitive drug taking" scenarios in which experienced cannabis users would consume cannabis using a combination of methods (e.g., bucket bongs, gravity bongs), with the purpose of *"seeing, how high, how far, how fast. Last man standing, whatever it might be"* [38] (p. 11).

Certain ways of consuming cannabis, including the methods used, the intensity, and the combination with other substances may provide opportunities for men to demonstrate their masculinity by showing the control they have over their bodies. The authors argue this is a form of gender performance. However, other ways of performing masculinity, or resisting dominant masculine norms, emerged. For example, men described how using cannabis facilitated closeness and allowed men to express their emotions; in particular, among heterosexual men, cannabis allowed opportunities for men to "contravene conventional gender expectations" regarding expressing emotions and openness between male friends [38].

In a second paper based on qualitative data collected with the same sample of men, the offering and sharing of cannabis with other men was perceived as a sign of friendship [39]. While using cannabis together was described as a "social leveler," possessing and providing cannabis to other men was identified as facilitating an elevated social position and changing the social dynamic. In addition to providing a space where men could perform traditional masculinity via cannabis use (achieving dominance by obtaining and supplying substances including cannabis), cannabis use provided opportunities for bonding with male friends and being more emotionally expressive. Similarly, in an ethnographic study with low income, criminally involved young men living in Ireland, buying, maintaining and consuming cannabis strengthened social bonds with other men, with them consuming cannabis together in "a regularity that approached ritual" [40] (p. 8).

One study explored substance use, including cannabis use, in the context of girls' friendships. Arnull and Ryder argue that public health approaches have focused narrowly on the risks of substance use, avoiding both the pleasurable functions of substance use, and the efforts of people who use substances to manage and minimize risks. By sharing the voices of a group of justice-involved girls, they describe how girls negotiate risks and use substances for social bonding and pleasure. Girls reported having fun with friends while using substances and experiencing pleasure from intoxication. They also described how they relied on their friend group to prevent or reduce physical and sexual risks of alcohol and cannabis use. For example, girls discussed remaining with their girlfriends when they went out partying, ensuring their friends arrived home safe or staying in each other's homes if they were too intoxicated.

5.3. Cannabis Use in Intimate Relationships

There is evidence from qualitative research on cannabis use and gender relations in intimate heterosexual relationships. In a Norwegian study conducted with people who had reduced or quit using cannabis, some participants discussed changing their cannabis-use patterns to please a partner. This theme was central in interviews with young men, but only one woman discussed stopping her daily cannabis use when she began a new relationship with a man who did not use cannabis [41]. Some men described engaging in arguments and conflicts with their partners regarding reducing or quitting cannabis use, while others described their change in use as unproblematic. For example, one man in the study described quitting cannabis when he moved in with his non cannabis-using partner, explaining: *"it would be sort of excluding if I was to be on a different mental level"* (p. 180). Men negotiated the frequency, occasion and context of their cannabis use to please their partners, and several described this shift as a natural progression from youth to adulthood. However, the authors caution that the findings from this study may have limited generalizability as participants were relatively socially advantaged with 19 of the 25 men having a higher education. These findings may not be translatable to cannabis users who are experiencing social disadvantage.

In one qualitative study examining substance use and sexual experiences among young adults, alcohol was commonly used by young men for pursuing potential sexual partners, and young women reported being more accepting of sexual offers from men when using alcohol [42]. In contrast, when using cannabis, young women reported being more selective regarding sexual partners. Both young women and men reported feeling more in control on cannabis than alcohol, but also quieter and less social. Women and men who used cannabis prior to a sexual experience reported greater post-sexual satisfaction compared to those who used alcohol before sex, while participants who drank alcohol reported greater regret following sex. Some participants reported that the illegal nature of cannabis occasionally meant more private use that sometimes facilitated sexual encounters [42].

Similarly, in a qualitative study with cannabis users and retailers in Florida, some men discussed the role of cannabis for facilitating private moments with women they were attracted to [43]:

'Kara is the one that I'm quite fond of, she smokes in my bathroom at all the parties ... So being able to steal Kara was very easy to do with just [saying to her] "Hey why don't you come and have a conversation with me in my bathroom?" (Matthew, age 30) (p. 761).

While these gender relations have been observed in the context of illegal cannabis markets, the hidden nature of use and opportunities for privacy may diminish as cannabis use becomes legal, openly consumed, and socially normalized [42]. Nonetheless, it seems clear that the role of cannabis in intimate heterosexual relationships may be somewhat different than that of alcohol.

5.4. Stigma and Discrimination

There is a lack of research examining the impact of gender roles and relations on cannabis use among people with a range of sexual orientations or diverse gender identities. Yet, several studies suggest cannabis may be used to cope with experiences of stigma and discrimination related to not conforming to predominant gender norms and roles. In a qualitative study on the impact of anxiety on cannabis use among bisexual women in Canada [44], some women described experiencing a lack of belonging, and how this contributed to using cannabis to manage anxiety. The authors suggest that cannabis may be used as a way to cope with not conforming to gender roles, or the stress related to experiencing multiple forms of oppression and discrimination related to being a bisexual woman, including sexism and biphobia. For women who experience these social disadvantages, cannabis may be used as a way to facilitate social belonging. This is also elucidated in their findings from an earlier study in which cannabis use was correlated with higher levels of social support among bisexual women, and described during focus groups as a tool for social connection [45].

Gender identity has also been examined in a study examining the relationship between gender minority stress and substance use among transgender women and men in the USA where the authors found that transgender men reported higher rates of cannabis use compared to transgender women. The authors note that this is similar to findings among general populations of women and men who do not identify as transgender, suggesting that gender socialization may also influence cannabis use among transgender people. Gender dysphoria, defined as the conflict between one's sex assigned at birth and gender identity, was associated with cannabis use among both transgender women and men. Additionally, among transgender women gender minority stress was associated with cannabis use [46]. The authors conclude that transgender individuals may use cannabis to "validate and affirm their gender identities" and identify the need for more research to explore the differences in cannabis use among transgender men and women.

5.5. Stigma among Mothers and Fathers Who Use Cannabis

Substance use tends to be perceived as more socially acceptable for men than women. In particular, gender norms that position women as mothers and caretakers are defined in opposition to substance use. Women who are mothers have identified stigma associated with cannabis use [34]. Women often report stopping cannabis use when they transition to motherhood because of this stigma, and those who do not report experiencing social disapproval [47]. Dahl argues that women experience more social controls at an earlier age compared to men [41]. In a qualitative analysis of cannabis use and stigma among a sample of cannabis users in Canada, Hathaway and colleagues discuss how stopping substance use during pregnancy was expected among women [47]. Women who smoked cannabis during pregnancy reported experiencing social disapproval [47]; as one woman remarked:

> *"When I was pregnant, I had morning sickness all day, every day for nine months, but I smoked only a few times. There was a strong social stigma against me. People told me not to smoke. (Paralegal, 41)"* (p. 462).

Women who were parents of adolescents described being afraid of child welfare involvement and feeling hypocritical if they were using and hiding their cannabis use from their children. In order to manage this, women limited where and when they used cannabis to avoid having their children and others knowing about it. The authors describe the women as internalizing stigma regarding their cannabis use and engaging in practices of "moral regulation" to maintain their mothering role, as well as others' perception of them as a "good mother."

Similarly, in a qualitative study with parents of children who had used cannabis, participants revealed normative gender roles and the expectations that women experience [48]. Mothers described feeling like failures if they had experienced challenges regarding their child's substance use, and often encountered a lack of social support due to the judgement and stigma. While this appeared to be more salient for women, one father also expressed feeling judgement and stigma regarding asking for help with parenting challenges related to substance use. Furthermore, the authors argue that focusing on the parent-child unit as the site for preventing and responding to substance use is problematic because it individualizes substance use and decontextualizes it from the influence of social factors.

One study found that men also perceived cannabis use as incompatible to their role as fathers. In a qualitative study conducted with people who had reduced or quit using cannabis in Norway, participants who were parents or who were expecting a child discussed cannabis use as being incompatible with parenting, particularly due to fear over the consequences of using an illicit substance [41]. One father said it would be "out of the question" to keep cannabis in the home, and multiple men spoke of the dangers of buying and using cannabis in the context of fatherhood. As one man explained:

> *"Smoking hash isn't that dangerous, but being caught and stigmatized as a criminal—a criminal parent of young children; is that what I am? That is quite a poor starting point for being a family man, as you're supposed to be"* (p. 178).

Men who were expectant fathers also discussed reducing or stopping to support the transition in their role to fatherhood. Some men qualified that they do not perceive cannabis use during parenting as necessarily harmful, but with the new responsibility of caring for and protecting their child, they felt uncomfortable with the idea of using cannabis while parenting. However, some men did convey a sense of loss with the shift in identity from cannabis user to a non-using father.

6. Discussion

Based on limited, but emerging evidence, it is clear that gender norms, roles and relations impact patterns of cannabis use in a range of ways. Several correlational studies examined the relationship between adherence to gender norms and cannabis use, reporting an association between measures of masculinity (specifically, male typicality) and cannabis use [20,30]. Most research on adherence to dominant masculine norms or male typicality and health behaviours has reported a negative effect on measures of health, including higher rates of substance use and dependence [22]. However, the relationship between gender norms and behaviours, including those surrounding substance use, is complex. Some masculine norms may actually be associated with health promoting behaviours.

For example, the "winning" and "competition" subscales of the CMNI have been associated with protection from substance use and misuse, and may have application in promoting health among men [49].

Studies examining the relationship of adherence to feminine norms with cannabis use are lacking. However, similar to the research on masculine norms and substance use, there is evidence that some feminine norms may be protective of substance use while others may increase risk. For example, women who conformed to traditional feminine norms identified in the CFNI, including "sexual fidelity" and "modesty," have reported lower likelihood to engage in binge drinking. However, the feminine norm "relational" was associated with increased binge drinking [50]. Adherence to some 'masculine norms' by young women is also associated with substance use [20]. For example, a study with college women in the US found that female adherence to certain masculine norms (as identified in the CMNI), including 'risk-taking' and "emotional control," was associated with binge drinking [50]. Further research is needed to examine the relationship of specific traditional feminine or masculine norms with cannabis use and how they operate across genders.

Studies measuring adherence to gender norms have been critiqued for underestimating the complexity of the relationship of gender norms with various social factors including race, ethnicity, religious identity, and sexual orientation [22]. For example, cross-sectional study designs assessing measures of male typicality or adherence to masculine or feminine norms at specific time-points may erroneously imply that gender norms are fixed [19]. For example, the CMNI and CFNI do not recognize or integrate historical or developmental changes in gender norms or the influence of culture and social and political contexts [20]. Additionally, Wilkinson et al. argue that gender ideologies and the expression of gender norms changes with age, especially during transitional periods from adolescence to adulthood that involve changing relationships, roles, employment, social settings and responsibilities [20]. Recently, there has been much greater understanding of gender as fluid and socially constructed.

Indeed, gender is both socially constructed and individually enacted, and traditional masculinities and femininities can be both reinstated and reimagined through cannabis use. In addition to discussing how adherence to traditional gender norms influences substance use, findings from several qualitative studies show how substances may be used to challenge or disrupt societal gender norms. As described by Robertson and colleagues, masculinities are complex, dynamic, and can be expressed in diverse ways [51].

Research on alcohol use and tobacco use among girls and young women has also explored how substances may be used to transcend and contest certain femininities. For example, a study conducted in Spain describes how female adolescents use alcohol in public spaces as a way of challenging social expectations regarding femininity that have typically restricted their use of public space and substances [52]. Similarly, qualitative research reveals that young women can frame their alcohol [53] and tobacco use [54] as a form of rebellion against traditional gender roles. These complex and sometimes contradictory ascribed meanings of tobacco use can persist into adulthood among women [55,56]. As social norms and gender ideologies continue to evolve [15], further research is needed to examine how gender norms are perceived, expressed and contested, how these meanings persist or change through the life cycle, how they may differ across cultures, and how this influences cannabis-use patterns.

While cannabis use is becoming more socially acceptable, findings from the review suggest that stigma remains high among pregnant women and mothers who use cannabis. This is also true for other forms of substance use. Among women, substance use is considered in conflict with traditional feminine norms and gender roles. Women who use substances during pregnancy and parenting are often perceived as selfish and uncaring, and in opposition to the traditional role of the "good mother" [57]. Applying a feminist embodiment approach to substance use, Ettorre discusses how substance use among women tends to focus narrowly on the health effects for the fetus, with women's bodies reduced to "fetal containers" [58]. Women who use substances are perceived as "unfit to reproduce", and pregnant women who use substances are perceived as "lethal fetal containers" [58]. She stresses the importance of addressing stigma and discrimination and maintaining the basic human right of reproductive choices regardless of substance use. Indeed, it is important to see women's health and substance use as in itself worthy of harm reduction-oriented support, whether during pregnancy or motherhood, or in general. Service approaches that consider three clients as important: the mother, the child, and the mother-child unit are increasingly being advocated [59].

The Norwegian study conducted with women and men who had recently reduced or stopped smoking cannabis found that men described fatherhood as incompatible with cannabis use, although this was discussed largely in the context of fear of legal consequences (in Norway, where cannabis is an illegal substance) rather than social disapproval [41]. Men also described reducing or quitting using cannabis if their partner disapproved of their use, although some men did cite arguments and conflicts. Similarly, researchers in Canada have explored the experiences of fathers who smoke [60] and developed and evaluated gender-sensitive resources for men [61]. In a qualitative study on men's experiences of quitting during the transition to fathering, they found that men often experienced disapproval from their partners and sought to maintain their autonomy while experiencing pressures to stop smoking [49]. Further research is needed to identify opportunities for addressing gender norms in cannabis use in harm reduction and health promotion efforts.

There is a general lack of research on gender norms, roles, relations and cannabis use among non-heterosexual people and people with diverse gender identities. Yet trans and gender-diverse youth report high rates of substance use, mental health issues and violence and trauma, and transgender women and non-binary assigned male at birth youth tend to report greater substance use [62]. Similarly, among young adults, high rates of tobacco use have been reported among both sexual minority females and gender minorities [63]. Further research is needed to understand how substance use among trans and gender diverse people, and cannabis use in particular, is shaped by gender norms, roles and relations. In addition, qualitative research on the experiences related to gender and cannabis use among people of diverse sexual orientations is needed to explore the complex relationships between sexual minority status, heterosexuality and gender roles and norms. Existing evidence highlights the need for integrating social supports in responses to prevent and address cannabis use among both groups: people of non-heterosexual orientations and diverse gender identities.

More research is also required to explore how gender intersects with other social determinants of health to influence cannabis use. In our review, we found several studies exploring the relationship between gender and culture or acculturation and substance use [31]. Some qualitative studies included sub-groups of males or females experiencing social disadvantage, including: low income men [40], and justice involved girls [36]; however, these studies did not analyze the intersection of gender and social disadvantage in relation to cannabis use. Yet evidence from the wider substance use field suggests that other social dimensions of health influence how we act, respond to, or "do gender." For example, in an intersectional analysis of women's smoking, the authors contend that the ability to challenge traditional social constructions of femininity is typically a privilege reserved for women belonging to higher social class [54]. More nuanced research is required to explore how other social determinants of health intersect with gender to shape cannabis-use experiences.

In summary, addressing gender norms, roles and relations in health-promotion messaging regarding cannabis use is critically important. Evidence from the review suggests that these dimensions of gender can have an effect on harms, risk and exposure. As more evidence emerges on gender and cannabis use, it is critical to avoid approaches to either prevention or health promotion that are gender exploitive and reinforce negative gender stereotypes. For example, an analysis of substance use education in Australia describes how school-based substance-use education reproduces harmful feminine and masculine norms by framing young women's substance use as more problematic than men's and blaming women for the physical and sexual victimization they are at risk of while intoxicated [64].

But advancing beyond approaches that merely avoid harmful gender stereotypes, health-promotion responses are needed that actively integrate gender transformative principles. Rather than just reflecting gender-based factors and concerns in messaging, gender transformative health promotion is aimed at improving gender equity *at the same time* as improving health [65]. Evidence from this review suggests there may be substantial opportunities for both gender-responsive and gender-transformative responses to cannabis use. For example, messaging might address shared responsibility for abstinence from cannabis use during pregnancy and parenting, and resources and supports could be developed for men to reduce or quit cannabis use during pregnancy and parenting, emphasizing the role of men as providers and protectors, similar to smoking cessation resources that have been developed for men [61]. In addition, messaging could address gendered risky patterns of use, including: cannabis and alcohol use, competitive use among men, and driving and riding as a passenger after cannabis use. Finally, there is a need for stigma reduction among pregnant women and mothers and fathers who use cannabis. One way stigma can be reduced is by providing accurate information regarding the health effects of cannabis use during pregnancy and parenting, while avoiding language that is judgmental and shaming.

7. Conclusions

While research on gender and cannabis is in its infancy, the available literature indicates that, similar to other substance use, gender norms, roles and relations have the potential to strongly influence patterns of cannabis use. How gender is expressed through cannabis use is complex, culturally specific, multi-faceted, and ever-evolving. As gender norms, roles and relations are constantly in flux, ongoing research is needed to explore the relationship between gender and cannabis use that is situated in the social, cultural and political context. Further research is also needed to understand how people belonging to diverse gender identities perceive and express gender through cannabis use; and that investigates how gender intersects with other social determinants of health including: sexual orientation, class, race and ethnicity. Harm-reduction, health-promotion and prevention messaging approaches are needed that address substance use and gender norms, as well as structural and institutional factors that specifically support harmful gender norms and behaviours. Specifically, gender transformative principles can be integrated in prevention, harm-reduction and health-promotion messaging to advance gender and health equity simultaneously, and erode the impact of negative gender stereotypes and stigmas. All of these gender-related issues need to be visited as cannabis use becomes more regulated, decriminalized or legalized in various jurisdictions around the world.

Author Contributions: Both authors contributed to the analysis of literature review findings and manuscript preparation. All authors have read and agreed to the published version of the manuscript.

Funding: This research was supported by funding from the Canadian Institutes of Health Research Institute of Gender and Health (CIHR-IGH) Knowledge Translation Team Grant, and the CIHR-IGH and Health Canada's Gender Health Unit (GHU) Research-Policy Partnership Grant.

Conflicts of Interest: The authors declare no conflict of interest.

Appendix A. Database Search Strategies

Search (1) August 2017

1	"gender transformative". ti,ab.
2	("gender informed" or "gender integrated" or "gender responsive"). ti,ab.
3	("sex informed" or "sex integrated" or "sex responsive"). ti,ab.
4	("gender equalit *" or "gender equit *" or "gender inequality *" or "gender inequit *"). ti,ab.
5	("sex equalit *" or "sex equit *" or "sex inequality *" or "sex inequit *"). ti,ab.
6	("gender related" or "gender difference *" or "gender disparit *"). ti,ab.
7	("sex related" or "sex difference*" or "sex disparit*").ti,ab.
8	"gender comparison *". ti,ab.
9	"sex comparison *". ti,ab.
10	"compar* gender *". ti,ab.
11	"compar * sex *". ti,ab.
12	"gender based".ti,ab.
13	"sex based".ti,ab.
14	("gender divers *" or "gender minorit *"). ti,ab.
15	"gender analys *". ti,ab.
16	"sex analys *". ti,ab.
17	(transgender * or "trans gender *" or LGBQT or LGBTQ or LGBT or LGB or lesbian * or gay or bisexual * or queer *). ti,ab.
18	("transsexual *" or "trans sexual *").ti,ab.
19	17 or 18
20	(transgender * or "trans gender *" or LGBQT or LGBTQ or LGBT or LGB or lesbian * or gay or bisexual * or queer * or "transsexual *" or "trans sexual *"). ti,ab.
21	("non binary *" or nonbinar *). ti,ab.
22	Homosex *. ti,ab.
23	("woman focused" or "woman focussed" or "girl focused" or "girl focussed" or "woman centred" or "girl centred" or "woman centered" or "girl centered" or "female focused" or "female focussed" or "female centred" or "female centered"). ti,ab.
24	("man focused" or "man focussed" or "boy focused" or "boy focussed" or "man centred" or "boy centred" or "man centered" or "boy centered" or "male focused" or "male focussed" or "male centred" or "male centered"). ti,ab.
25	Transgender Persons/
26	Sexual Minorities/
27	Transsexualism/
28	Bisexuality/
29	exp Homosexuality/
30	Gender Identity/
31	(bigender * or "bi gender *"). ti,ab.
32	("gender identit *" or "gender incongru *"). ti,ab.
33	"differently gendered". ti,ab.
34	or/1–33 [GENDER]
35	exp Opioid-Related Disorders/
36	exp Analgesics, Opioid/
37	(opioid * or opiate *). tl,ab.
38	(fentanyl or phentanyl or Fentanest or Sublimaze or Duragesic or Durogesic or Fentora or "R 4263" or R4263). ti,ab.
39	(oxycontin or oxycodone or oxycodan or percocet or percodan). ti,ab.
40	(heroin or morphine). ti,ab.
41	or/36–40 [OPIOIDS]
42	Prescription Drug Misuse/ or Prescription Drug Overuse/
43	((("prescription drug" or "prescription drugs" or "prescribed drug" or "prescribed drugs") and (dependen * or misuse * or mis-use * or abuse * or overuse * or over-use * or addict *)). ti,ab.
44	exp Substance-Related Disorders/

45	("substance disorder *" or "substance related disorder *" or "substance use disorder *" or "drug use disorder *" or "drug related disorder *"). ti,ab.
46	("over prescription" or "over prescribed"). ti,ab.
47	Drug Overdose/ or (overdose* or over-dose *).ti,ab.
48	or/42–47
49	35 or (41 and 48)
50	exp Alcohol-Related Disorders/
51	exp Alcohol Drinking/
52	(binge drink * or underage drink * or under-age drink * or problem drink * or heavy drink * or harmful drink * or alcoholi* or inebriat * or intoxicat *). ti,ab.
53	("alcohol dependen *" or "alcohol misuse *" or "alcohol mis-use *" or "alcohol abuse *" or "alcohol overuse *" or "alcohol over-use *" or "alcohol addict *"). ti,ab.
54	alcohol. ti,ab. and (44 or 45)
55	Alcohol Abstinence/
56	or/50–55
57	"Tobacco Use Disorder"/
58	Tobacco/
59	Nicotine/
60	exp Tobacco Products/
61	exp "Tobacco Use"/
62	((cigar * or e-cigar * or tobacco or nicotine or smoking or vaping) and (dependenc * or misuse * or mis-use * or abuse * or overuse * or over-use * or addiction *)). ti,ab.
63	(58 or 59 or 60 or 61) and (44 or 45)
64	exp "Tobacco Use Cessation"/
65	exp "Tobacco Use Cessation Products"/
66	((tobacco or smoking) and cessation). ti,ab.
67	or/57,62–66
68	Marijuana Abuse/
69	Cannabis/
70	Marijuana Smoking/
71	exp Cannabinoids/
72	(marijuana or marihuana or hashish or ganja or bhang or hemp or cannabis or cannabinoid * or cannabidiol or tetrahydrocannabinol). ti,ab.
73	(69 or 70 or 71 or 72) and (43 or 44 or 45)
74	or/68,73
75	or/49,56,67,74
76	Harm Reduction/
77	("harm reduction" or "reducing harm" or "reducing harmful" or "harm minimization" or "minimizing harm" or "minimizing harmful" or "harm minimisation" or "minimising harm" or "minimising harmful"). ti,ab.
78	exp Risk Reduction Behavior/
79	("risk reduction" or "reducing risk" or "reducing risks" or "risk minimization" or "minimizing risk" or "minimizing risks" or "risk minimisation" or "minimising risk" or "minimising risks"). ti,ab.
80	or/76–79
81	exp Health Promotion/
82	("health promotion" or "promoting health" or "promoting healthy" or "promoting wellness" or "patient education" or "consumer education" or "client education" or outreach or "wellness program" or "wellness programs" or "wellness programme" or "wellness programmes"). ti,ab.
83	81 or 82
84	Preventive Health Services/
85	Consumer Health Information/ or Health Literacy/
86	Secondary Prevention/
87	(prevention or "preventive health" or "preventive healthcare"). ti,ab.
88	or/84-87
89	(prevention or preventive). ti,ab.
90	88 or 89

91	Rehabilitation/
92	(abstain * or abstinence or detox * or rehab * or sobriety or sober or temperance or intervention * or cessation or recovery). ti,ab.
93	Methadone/tu [Therapeutic Use]
94	"methadone maintenance". ti,ab.
95	Opiate Substitution Treatment/
96	("opiate substitution" or "opioid substitution" or "withdrawal management" or "managing withdrawal"). ti,ab.
97	(treatment* or treating or therapy or therapies). ti,ab.
98	Intervention *. ti,ab.
99	or/91–98
100	or/80,83,88,99
101	or/80,83,90,99
102	34 and 75 and 101
103	limit 102 to (english language and yr = "2007–2017") [Limit not valid in Cochrane Database of Systematic Reviews (CDSR); records were retained]
104	(Animals/ or Animal Experimentation/ or "Models, Animal"/ or (animal * or nonhuman * or non human * or rat or rats or mouse or mice or rabbit or rabbits or pig or pigs or porcine or dog or dogs or hamster or hamsters or fish or chicken or chickens or sheep or cat or cats or raccoon or raccoons or rodent * or horse or horses or racehorse or racehorses or beagle *). ti,ab.) not (Humans/ or (human * or participant * or patient or patients or child * or seniors or adult or adults). ti,ab.)
105	103 not 104
106	(editorial or comment or letter or newspaper article). pt.
107	105 not 106
108	(conference or conference abstract or conference paper or "conference review" or congresses). pt.
109	107 not 108EBM Reviews- Cochrane Database of Systematic Reviews < 2005 to 2 August 2017 >Embase < 1980 to 3 August 2017 >Ovid MEDLINE(R) Epub Ahead of Print, In-Process and Other Non-Indexed Citations, Ovid MEDLINE(R) Daily and Ovid MEDLINE(R) < 1946 to Present >EBM Reviews- Cochrane Central Register of Controlled Trials < July 2017 >
110	remove duplicates from 109EBM Reviews- Cochrane Database of Systematic Reviews < 2005 to 2 August 2017 >Embase < 1980 to 3 August 2017 >Ovid MEDLINE(R) Epub Ahead of Print, In-Process and Other Non-Indexed Citations, Ovid MEDLINE(R) Daily and Ovid MEDLINE(R) < 1946 to Present>EBM Reviews- Cochrane Central Register of Controlled Trials < July 2017 >
111	110 use ppez [MEDLINE]
112	110 use emezd [EMBASE]
113	110 not (111 or 112) [selected 2 only as 13 were conference abstracts]

Search 2: September 2017

After reviewing the returns from the original search in August 2017, we amended the search in September 2017 to identify studies on the health effects of substance use (for cannabis, alcohol, opioids, tobacco/nicotine). In addition, we added sex/gender terms and substance-specific terms. The search was amended as follows:

1. Health effects terms were added to the search terms.

("health effect" or "heath effects" or "effect on health" or "effects on health" or "affect * health" or "affect * the health" or "heath impact *" or "impact * on health" or "impact * health"). ti,ab. [HEALTH EFFECTS]

These terms were searched in combination with the gender terms and substance terms as follows:
Concept 1—Gender/sex
AND
Concept 2—Substances (opioids, alcohol, tobacco, cannabis)
AND
Concept 3—health effects

1. "gender determinant*" or "gender specific" were added to the gender/sex terms (see lines 1–33 in original search strategy)
2. "alcohol use" or "use of alcohol" and "risky drink" were added to the alcohol terms

Search 3: April 2018

After identifying multiple papers relevant to our review that were not being captured by the original searches, we conducted a third search in April 2018. Based on analysis of the keywords in the articles that were missed, we amended the search as follows:

1. The following terms were added to the gender/sex terms:

    (woman or man or women or men or girl or boy or girls or boys or trans or transgender or transgendered or female or male or sex or gender). ti. [GENDER IN TI]

    A search was then conducted of the article titles only, combining the following concepts:

    Search strategy:

    Concept 1—Gender/sex terms

    AND

    Concept 2—Substances (opioids, alcohol, tobacco, cannabis) terms

    AND

    Concept 3—Harm reduction, health promotion, prevention, treatment, health effects terms
2. "heat not burn" was added to the tobacco terms.
3. The search included studies published up until April 2018

Appendix B. Final Inclusion Criteria

Study Design:

- randomised-controlled trials (RCTs) (not already covered in an included systematic review)
- case-control studies
- interrupted time series
- cohort studies
- cross sectional studies
- observational studies
- systematic reviews
- qualitative studies
- grey literature sources
- case series

    Note:

- Narrative reviews will not be included but saved as context.
- Case studies will be excluded.

    The following types of literature will be included in the grey literature review:

- book chapters
- reports
- practice guidelines
- health policy documents
- unpublished research, theses

Note: magazines and books will be excluded from the grey literature.

Countries of studies:

- Australia, Austria, Belgium, Canada, Denmark, Finland, France, Germany, Greece, Iceland, Ireland, Italy, Luxembourg, Netherlands, New Zealand, Norway, Portugal, Spain, Sweden, Switzerland, United Kingdom, United States
- Studies published in all other countries will be excluded, including animal studies.
- Studies including data from multiple countries, that include an out of scope country, will be excluded if the data is not disaggregated.
- Systematic reviews which include studies from multiple countries will be included if reporting on one or more studies published in an eligible country.

Date of publication:

- The literature search will cover studies published between 2007 to 2017

Language:

- Only studies published in the English language will be included.

Research Q1: PICO (Population, Intervention, Comparator, Outcome)
Q(1) *How* do sex- and gender-related factors impact:

(a) patterns of use;
(b) health effects of;
(c) and prevention/treatment/or harm reduction outcomes for opioid, alcohol, tobacco and cannabis use?

Population:

- Women, girls, men, boys, trans people/ gender diverse people
  - All ages, demographics within the defined populations
- Studies that are conducted primarily with pregnant girls and women will be excluded.
- Studies addressing the fetal health effects of maternal/ paternal substance use will be excluded.
- Studies addressing the health effects of substance use on the infant among women who are breastfeeding will be excluded.
- Studies comparing heterosexual populations to LGBT populations, without sex or gender disaggregation will be excluded.

Intervention:

Q1 (a) and (b) includes non-intervention studies (e.g., patterns of use, health effects):

- Inclusive of tobacco in general (include e-cigarettes)
- Inclusive of all alcohol use (not just binge drinking)
- Inclusive of all opioid use issues (include illicit use/heroin, prescription opioids, etc.)
  - ■ Opioid use for cancer pain management will be excluded
- Inclusive of all purposes (therapeutic and recreational), forms and modes of ingestion of cannabis (e.g., smoking, vaping, edibles, extracts, etc.).
- Studies that report on "substance use" but do not disaggregate results by one or more of the four substances in our review will be excluded.

Q1 (c) Harm reduction, health promotion, prevention, treatment (including brief intervention) responses to opioids, alcohol, cannabis, tobacco/e-cigarettes

- Studies that report on "substance use" but do not disaggregate results by one or more of the four substances in our review will be excluded.
- Opioid substitution therapy for substances other than opioids (e.g., cocaine, methamphetamine) will be excluded

Comparator:

- Many Q1 (a) and (b) studies will be descriptive/ prevalence studies (not intervention studies) and may not include a comparator.
- Many qualitative and grey literature sources will likely not include comparators
- Q1 (c) studies *must* include a comparison between gender groups e.g., women vs. men; sub-groups of women/ men OR if sex- or gender- based factors are described or discussed in the study (e.g., masculinity norms, hormones etc.). Q1c studies that do not compare gender groups or describe sex- or gender-based factors will be excluded.

Outcome:

- <u>For non-intervention studies:</u> prevalence/patterns of use (frequency of use, form and method of ingestion, etc.);
- <u>For intervention studies (Q1c):</u> outcomes reported in the reviews will be the outcomes that are reported in the individual papers that are reviewed. Relevant outcomes from the included studies might include:

    - Changes in substance use (uptake/initiation, harms associated with use cessation, reduction)
    - Changes in client perceptions/attitudinal change
    - Changes in service provider perceptions
    - Changes in retention/treatment completion
    - Increased use of services
    - improved health and quality of life outcomes

Note: Studies that report on one or more of the four substances in relation to sex/gender *only* in the baseline characteristics of the sample will be excluded, even if statistical significance is reported.

Research Q2: PICO (Population, Intervention, Comparator, Outcome)

(Q2) *What* harm reduction, health promotion/prevention and treatment interventions and programs are available *that include sex, gender and gender transformative elements* and how effective are these in addressing opioid, alcohol, tobacco and cannabis use?

Population:

- Women, girls, men, boys, trans people/gender-diverse people

    - All ages, demographics within the defined populations

- Studies that are conducted primarily with pregnant girls and women will be excluded.
- Studies addressing the fetal health effects of maternal/paternal substance use will be excluded.
- Studies addressing the health effects of substance use on the infant among women who are breastfeeding will be excluded.

Intervention:

- Harm reduction, health promotion, prevention, treatment (including brief intervention) responses to opioids, alcohol, cannabis, tobacco/e-cigarettes including some *sex, gender and/or gender transformative elements*

- Studies that report on 'substance use' will be included if they potentially contain one of the four substances. However, if substance use is defined, and does not contain alcohol, tobacco, opioids or cannabis it will be excluded.
- Opioid substitution therapy for substances other than opioids (e.g., cocaine, methamphetamine) will be excluded.

- Examples of sex specific elements (address biological differences in substance use and dependence):
  - administering different types or quantities of pharmacotherapies based on evidence of biological differences in drug metabolism/effectiveness
  - timing tobacco-cessation intervention for young women based on the menstrual cycle (hormonal fluctuations impact withdrawal)

- Examples of possible gender/gender-transformative elements:
  - address gender-based violence
  - provide social support
  - address caregiving
  - address poverty
  - address negative gender stereotypes
  - include education or messaging on gender norms/relations
  - address employment issues/work-related stress
  - address discrimination and violence related to gender identity

Interventions to address these four substances are:

- Inclusive of tobacco in general (include e-cigarettes)
- Inclusive of all alcohol use (not just binge drinking)
- Inclusive of all opioid use issues (include illicit use/heroin, prescription opioids, etc.)

  - Opioid use for cancer pain management will be excluded

- Inclusive of all purposes (therapeutic and recreational), forms and modes of ingestion of cannabis (e.g., smoking, vaping, edibles, extracts, etc).

Note: Methadone maintenance therapy will only be included if it is provided to opioid users (i.e., exclude if provided to treat substances outside of scope such as cocaine).

Comparator:

- No intervention or usual practice (i.e., interventions that are not gender-informed/ gender-transformative, sex-specific), or the comparison of two intervention types.
  - Many qualitative and grey literature sources will likely not include comparators.

Outcome:

- Outcomes reported in the reviews will be the outcomes that are reported in the individual papers that are reviewed. Relevant outcomes from the included studies might include:
  - Changes in substance use (uptake/initiation, harms associated with use, cessation, reduction)
  - Changes in client perceptions/attitudinal change
  - Changes in service provider perceptions
  - Changes in retention/treatment completion

- Increased use of services
- improved health and quality of life outcomes
- changes in health and gender equity

Note: Studies that report on one or more of the four substances in relation to sex/gender *only* in the baseline characteristics of the sample will be excluded, even if statistical significance is reported.

References

1. Cranford, J.A.; Eisenberg, D.; Serras, A.M. Substance use behaviors, mental health problems, and use of mental health services in a probability sample of college students. *Addict. Behav.* **2009**, *34*, 134–145. [CrossRef]
2. Carliner, H.; Mauro, P.M.; Brown, Q.L.; Shmulewitz, D.; Rahim Juwel, R.; Sarvet, A.L.; Wall, M.M.; Martins, S.S.; Carliner, G.; Hasin, D.S. The widening gender gap in marijuana use prevalence in the U.S. During a period of economic change, 2002–2014. *Drug Alcohol Depend.* **2017**, *170*, 51–58. [CrossRef] [PubMed]
3. Felton, J.W.; Collado, A.; Shadur, J.M.; Lejuez, C.W.; MacPherson, L. Sex differences in self-report and behavioral measures of disinhibition predicting marijuana use across adolescence. *Exp. Clin. Psychopharmacol.* **2015**, *23*, 265–274. [CrossRef] [PubMed]
4. Farmer, R.F.; Kosty, D.B.; Seeley, J.R.; Duncan, S.C.; Lynskey, M.T.; Rohde, P.; Klein, D.N.; Lewinsohn, P.M. Natural course of cannabis use disorders. *Psychol. Med.* **2015**, *45*, 63–72. [CrossRef] [PubMed]
5. Johnson, R.M.; Fairman, B.; Gilreath, T.; Xuan, Z.M.; Rothman, E.F.; Parnham, T.; Furr-Holden, C.D.M. Past 15-year trends in adolescent marijuana use: Differences by race/ethnicity and sex. *Drug Alcohol Depend.* **2015**, *155*, 8–15. [CrossRef] [PubMed]
6. Cuttler, C.; Mischley, L.K.; Sexton, M. Sex differences in cannabis use and effects: A cross-sectional survey of cannabis users. *Cannabis Cannabinoid Res.* **2016**, *1*, 166–175. [CrossRef]
7. Baggio, S.; Deline, S.; Studer, J.; Mohler-Kuo, M.; Daeppen, J.B.; Gmel, G. Routes of administration of cannabis used for nonmedical purposes and associations with patterns of drug use. *J. Adol. Health* **2014**, *54*, 235–240. [CrossRef]
8. Daniulaityte, R.; Zatreh, M.Y.; Lamy, F.R.; Nahhas, R.W.; Martins, S.S.; Sheth, A.; Carlson, R.G. A twitter-based survey on marijuana concentrate use. *Drug Alcohol Depend.* **2018**, *187*, 155–159. [CrossRef]
9. Weiss, K.G.; Dilks, L.M. Marijuana, gender, and health-related harms: Disentangling marijuana's contribution to risk in a college "party" context. *Sociol. Spectr.* **2015**, *35*, 254–270. [CrossRef]
10. Hunt, G.; Asmussen Frank, V.; Moloney, M. Rethinking gender within alcohol and drug research. *Subst. Misuse* **2015**, *50*, 685–692. [CrossRef]
11. Legleye, S.; Piontek, D.; Pampel, F.; Goffette, C.; Khlat, M.; Kraus, L. Is there a cannabis epidemic model? Evidence from France, Germany and USA. *Int. J. Drug Policy* **2014**, *25*, 1103–1112. [CrossRef] [PubMed]
12. Day, J.K.; Fish, J.N.; Perez-Brumer, A.; Hatzenbuehler, M.L.; Russell, S.T. Transgender youth substance use disparities: Results from a population-based sample. *J. Adol. Health* **2017**, *20*, 729–735. [CrossRef] [PubMed]
13. Keuroghlian, A.S.; Reisner, S.L.; White, J.M.; Weiss, R.D. Substance use and treatment of substance use disorders in a community sample of transgender adults. *Drug Alcohol Depend.* **2015**, *152*, 139–146. [CrossRef]
14. Schmidt, R.; Poole, N.; Greaves, L.; Hemsing, N. *New terrain: Tools to Integrate Trauma and Gender Informed Responses into Substance Use Practice and Policy 2018*; Centre of Excellence for Women's Health: Vancouver, BC, Canada, 2018.
15. Budgeon, S. The dynamics of gender hegemony: Femininities, masculinities and social change. *Sociology* **2014**, *48*, 317–334. [CrossRef]
16. Berkowitz, D.; Manohar, N.N.; Tinkler, J.E. Walk like a man, talk like a woman: Teaching the social construction of gender. *Teach. Sociol.* **2010**, *38*, 132–143. [CrossRef]
17. Greaves, L.; Hemsing, N. Sex and gender interactions on the use and impact of recreational cannabis. *Int. J. Environ. Res. Public Health* **2020**, *17*, 509. [CrossRef] [PubMed]
18. Creighton, G.; Oliffe, J.L. Theorising masculinities and men's health: A brief history with a view to practice. *Health Sociol. Rev.* **2010**, *19*, 409–418. [CrossRef]
19. Brady, J.; Iwamoto, D.K.; Grivel, M.; Kaya, A.; Clinton, L. A systematic review of the salient role of feminine norms on substance use among women. *Addict. Behav.* **2016**, *62*, 83–90. [CrossRef]

20. Wilkinson, A.L.; Fleming, P.J.; Halpern, C.T.; Herring, A.H.; Harris, K.M. Adherence to gender-typical behavior and high frequency substance use from adolescence into young adulthood. *Psychol. Men Masc.* **2018**, *19*, 145–155. [CrossRef]
21. McHugh, R.K.; Votaw, V.R.; Sugarman, D.E.; Greenfield, S.F. Sex and gender differences in substance use disorders. *Clin. Psychol. Rev.* **2018**, *66*, 12–23. [CrossRef]
22. Gerdes, Z.T.; Levant, R.F. Complex relationships among masculine norms and health/well-being outcomes: Correlation patterns of the conformity to masculine norms inventory subscales. *Am. J. Men Health* **2018**, *12*, 229–240. [CrossRef] [PubMed]
23. Iwamoto, D.K.; Corbin, W.; Lejuez, C.; MacPherson, L. College men and alcohol use: Positive alcohol expectancies as a mediator between distinct masculine norms and alcohol use. *Psychol. Men Masc.* **2014**, *15*, 29–39. [CrossRef] [PubMed]
24. Everitt-Penhale, B.; Ratele, K. Rethinking 'traditional masculinity' as constructed, multiple, and hegemonic masculinity. *S. Afr. J. Psychol.* **2015**, *46*, 4–22.
25. Wilkinson, A.L.; Halpern, C.T.; Herring, A.H.; Shanahan, M.; Ennett, S.T.; Hussey, J.M.; Harris, K.M. Testing longitudinal relationships between binge drinking, marijuana use, and depressive symptoms and moderation by sex. *J. Adol. Health* **2016**, *59*, 681–687. [CrossRef]
26. Arksey, H.; O'Malley, L. Scoping studies: Towards a methodological framework. *Int. J. Soc. Res. Methodol.* **2005**, *8*, 19–32. [CrossRef]
27. Levac, D.; Colquhoun, H.; O'Brien, K.K. Scoping studies: Advancing the methodology. *Implement. Sci.* **2010**, *5*, 69. [CrossRef]
28. National Institute for Health and Care Excellence. *Methods for the Development of NICE Public Health Guidance*; NICE: London, UK, 2012.
29. Moher, D.; Liberati, A.; Tetzlaff, J.; Altman, D.G.; Group, P. Reprint—Preferred reporting items for systematic reviews and meta-analyses: The PRISMA statement. *Phys. Ther.* **2009**, *89*, 873–880. [CrossRef]
30. Mahalik, J.R.; Lombardi, C.M.; Sims, J.; Coley, R.L.; Lynch, A.D. Gender, male-typicality, and social norms predicting adolescent alcohol intoxication and marijuana use. *Soc. Sci. Med.* **2015**, *143*, 71–80. [CrossRef]
31. Kulis, S.; Marsiglia, F.F.; Lingard, E.C.; Nieri, T.; Nagoshi, J. Gender identity and substance use among students in two high schools in Monterrey, Mexico. *Drug Alcohol Depend.* **2008**, *95*, 258–268. [CrossRef]
32. Kulis, S.; Marsiglia, F.F.; Nagoshi, J.L. Gender roles, externalizing behaviors, and substance use among Mexican-American adolescents. *J. Soc. Work Pract. Addict.* **2010**, *10*, 283–307. [CrossRef]
33. Kulis, S.; Marsiglia, F.F.; Ayers, S.L.; Booth, J.; Nuno-Gutierrez, B.L. Drug resistance and substance use among male and female adolescents in alternative secondary schools in Guanajuato, Mexico. *J. Stud. Alcohol Drug.* **2012**, *73*, 111–119. [CrossRef] [PubMed]
34. Dahl, S.L.; Sandberg, S. Female cannabis users and new masculinities: The gendering of cannabis use. *Sociology* **2015**, *49*, 696–711. [CrossRef]
35. Haines, R.J.; Johnson, J.L.; Carter, C.I.; Arora, K. "I couldn't say, I'm not a girl"–adolescents talk about gender and marijuana use. *Soc. Sci. Med.* **2009**, *68*, 2029–2036. [CrossRef] [PubMed]
36. Arnull, E.; Ryder, J. 'Because it's fun': English and American girls' counter-hegemonic stories of alcohol and marijuana use. *J. Youth Stud.* **2019**, *22*, 1361–1377. [CrossRef]
37. Hathaway, A.D.; Mostaghim, A.; Erickson, P.G.; Kolar, K.; Osborne, G. "It's really no big deal": The role of social supply networks in normalizing use of cannabis by students at Canadian universities. *Deviant Behav.* **2018**, *39*, 1672–1680. [CrossRef]
38. Darcy, C. A psychoactive paradox of masculinities: Cohesive and competitive relations between drug taking Irish men. *Gend. Place Cult.* **2019**, 1–21. [CrossRef]
39. Darcy, C. 'You're with your ten closest mates ... and everyone's kind of in the same boat': Friendship, masculinities and men's recreational use of illicit drugs. *J. Friendsh. Stud.* **2018**, *5*, 43–57.
40. Ilan, J. Street social capital in the liquid city. *Ethnography* **2012**, *14*, 3–24. [CrossRef]
41. Dahl, S.L. Remaining a user while cutting down: The relationship between cannabis use and identity. *Drugs Educ. Prev. Policy* **2015**, *22*, 175–184. [CrossRef]
42. Palamar, J.J.; Acosta, P.; Ompad, D.C.; Friedman, S.R. A qualitative investigation comparing psychosocial and physical sexual experiences related to alcohol and marijuana use among adults. *Arch. Sex. Behav.* **2018**, *47*, 757–770. [CrossRef]

43. Belackova, V.; Vaccaro, C.A. "A friend with weed is a friend indeed": Understanding the relationship between friendship identity and market relations among marijuana users. *J. Drug Issues* **2013**, *43*, 289–313. [CrossRef]
44. Robinson, M. The role of anxiety in bisexual women's use of cannabis in Canada. *Psychol. Sex. Orientat. Gend. Divers.* **2015**, *2*, 138–151. [CrossRef]
45. Robinson, M.; Sanches, M.; MacLeod, M.A. Prevalence and mental health correlates of illegal cannabis use among bisexual women. *J. Bisex.* **2016**, *16*, 181–202. [CrossRef]
46. Gonzalez, C.A.; Gallego, J.D.; Bockting, W.O. Demographic characteristics, components of sexuality and gender, and minority stress and their associations to excessive alcohol, cannabis, and illicit (noncannabis) drug use among a large sample of transgender people in the United States. *J. Prim. Prev.* **2017**, *38*, 419–445. [CrossRef] [PubMed]
47. Hathaway, A.D.; Comeau, N.C., Erickson, P.G. Cannabis normalization and stigma: Contemporary practices of moral regulation. *Criminol. Crim. Justice* **2011**, *11*, 451–469. [CrossRef]
48. Haines-Saah, R.J.; Mitchell, S.; Slemon, A.; Jenkins, E.K. 'Parents are the best prevention'? Troubling assumptions in cannabis policy and prevention discourses in the context of legalization in Canada. *Int. J. Drug Policy* **2019**, *68*, 132–138. [CrossRef]
49. Kwon, J.-Y.; Oliffe, J.L.; Bottorff, J.L.; Kelly, M.T. Masculinity and fatherhood: New fathers' perceptions of their female partners' efforts to assist them to reduce or quit smoking. *Am. J. Men Health* **2014**, *9*, 332–339. [CrossRef]
50. Kaya, A.; Iwamoto, D.K.; Grivel, M.; Clinton, L.; Brady, J. The role of feminine and masculine norms in college women's alcohol use. *Psychol. Men Masc.* **2016**, *17*, 206–214. [CrossRef]
51. Robertson, S.; Williams, B.; Oliffe, J. The case for retaining a focus on "masculinities". *Int. J. Men Health* **2016**, *15*, 52–67.
52. Romo-Avilés, N.; Marcos-Marcos, J.; Tarragona-Camacho, A.; Gil-García, E.; Marquina-Márquez, A. "I like to be different from how i normally am": Heavy alcohol consumption among female Spanish adolescents and the unsettling of traditional gender norms. *Drugs Educ. Prev. Policy* **2018**, *25*, 262–272. [CrossRef]
53. Yang, Y.; Tang, L. Understanding women's stories about drinking: Implications for health interventions. *Health Educ. Res.* **2018**, *33*, 271–279. [CrossRef] [PubMed]
54. Triandafilidis, Z.; Ussher, J.M.; Perz, J.; Huppatz, K. Doing and undoing femininities: An intersectional analysis of young women's smoking. *Fem. Psychol.* **2017**, *27*, 465–488. [CrossRef]
55. Greaves, L. Can tobacco control be transformative? Reducing gender inequity and tobacco use among vulnerable populations. *Int. J. Environ. Res. Public Health* **2014**, *11*, 792–803. [CrossRef] [PubMed]
56. Greaves, L. *Smoke Screen: Women's Smoking and Social Control*; Scarlet Press: London, UK, 1996.
57. Reid, C.; Greaves, L.; Poole, N. Good, bad, thwarted or addicted? Discourses of substance-using mothers. *Crit. Soc. Policy* **2008**, *28*, 211–234. [CrossRef]
58. Ettorre, E. Embodied deviance, gender, and epistemologies of ignorance: Re-visioning drugs use in a neurochemical, unjust world. *Subst. Use Misuse* **2015**, *50*, 794–805. [CrossRef]
59. Andrews, N.C.Z.; Motz, M.; Pepler, D.J.; Jeong, J.J.; Khoury, J. Engaging mothers with substance use issues and their children in early intervention: Understanding use of service and outcomes. *Child Abuse Neg.* **2018**, *83*, 10–20. [CrossRef]
60. Greaves, L.; Oliffe, J.L.; Ponic, P.; Kelly, M.T.; Bottorff, J.L. Unclean fathers, responsible men: Smoking, stigma and fatherhood. *Health Sociol. Rev.* **2010**, *19*, 522–533. [CrossRef]
61. Bottorff, J.L.; Oliffe, J.L.; Sarbit, G.; Kelly, M.T.; Cloherty, A. Men's responses to online smoking cessation resources for new fathers: The influence of masculinities. *Res. Protocol.* **2015**, *4*, e54. [CrossRef]
62. Newcomb, M.E.; Hill, R.; Buehler, K.; Ryan, D.T.; Whitton, S.W.; Mustanski, B. High burden of mental health problems, substance use, violence, and related psychosocial factors in transgender, non-binary, and gender diverse youth and young adults. *Arch. Sex. Behav.* **2019**, *4*. [CrossRef]
63. Delahanty, J.; Ganz, O.; Hoffman, L.; Guillory, J.; Crankshaw, E.; Farrelly, M. Tobacco use among lesbian, gay, bisexual and transgender young adults varies by sexual and gender identity. *Drug Alcohol Depend.* **2019**, *201*, 161–170. [CrossRef]

64. Farrugia, A. Gender, reputation and regret: The ontological politics of Australian drug education. *Gend. Educ.* **2017**, *29*, 281–298. [CrossRef]
65. Greaves, L.; Pederson, A.; Poole, N. *Making It Better: Gender Transformative Health Promotion*; Canadian Scholars' Press: Toronto, ON, Canada, 2014.

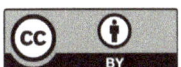

© 2020 by the authors. Licensee MDPI, Basel, Switzerland. This article is an open access article distributed under the terms and conditions of the Creative Commons Attribution (CC BY) license (http://creativecommons.org/licenses/by/4.0/).

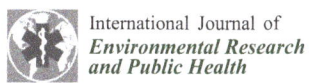

Review

Gender Informed or Gender Ignored? Opportunities for Gender Transformative Approaches in Brief Alcohol Interventions on College Campuses

Lindsay Wolfson [1,2,*], Julie Stinson [1] and Nancy Poole [1]

[1] Centre of Excellence for Women's Health, Vancouver, BC V6H 3N1, Canada; juliestinson7@gmail.com (J.S.); npoole@cw.bc.ca (N.P.)
[2] Canada Fetal Alcohol Spectrum Disorder Research Network, Vancouver, BC V5R 0A4, Canada
* Correspondence: lindsay.wolfson@gmail.com; Tel.: +1-647-270-4048

Received: 22 December 2019; Accepted: 6 January 2020; Published: 7 January 2020

Abstract: Brief alcohol interventions are an effective strategy for reducing harmful and risky alcohol use and misuse. Many effective brief alcohol interventions include information and advice about an individual's alcohol use, changing their use, and assistance in developing strategies and goals to help reduce their use. Emerging research suggests that brief interventions can also be expanded to address multiple health outcomes; recognizing that the flexible nature of these approaches can be helpful in tailoring information to specific population groups. This scoping review synthesizes evidence on the inclusion of sex and gender in brief alcohol interventions on college campuses, highlighting available evidence on gender responsiveness in these interventions. Furthermore, this scoping review offers strategies on how brief alcohol interventions can be gender transformative, thereby enhancing the effectiveness of brief alcohol interventions as harm reduction and prevention strategies, and in promoting gender equity.

Keywords: alcohol; brief intervention; college campus; gender; gender transformative; gender equity

---

1. Introduction

Alcohol use, misuse, and related consequences experienced by students on college campuses have been widely documented in the alcohol literature. Individual and environmental factors associated with increased use include alcohol expectancies, drinking motives, and perceived norms; involvement in fraternities or sororities; type of residence; college size; location; and alcohol availability [1]. The growing body of literature and public health concern over heavy drinking and alcohol related consequences as individuals transition into college has resulted in increasing research on effective alcohol reduction interventions [2–4].

While the prevalence of alcohol use remains higher among boys and men, the gender gap is narrowing particularly among young Canadians [5,6]. In 2016, rates of heavy drinking among all age groups were 24% for men and 14% for women; however, among young women ages 18–24, rates of heavy drinking were much higher (23% of young women compared with 34% of young men) [5]. On college campuses, important sex factors and gender influences must be considered. These include sex differences in metabolizing alcohol [7], prompting the different recommendations for low risk alcohol use [4]; a greater likelihood of women reporting substance use as a coping mechanism [8] or in connection to experiences of sexual violence [4,9]; and male students being less likely to use harm reduction or protective behavioural strategies [10] due to the perceptions of masculinity on alcohol use [11].

Sex and gender considerations can be integrated into alcohol interventions when designing the intervention (i.e., taking into account sex- and gender-related factors on drinking), when implementing the intervention (i.e., taking into account gendered barriers into intervention engagement and retention), and in addressing equity issues (i.e., identifying and addressing stigma related to women who drink heavily and have unprotected sex, or engaging boys and men in supporting girls' and women's health, as well as their own) [11]. Strategies that are gender responsive illustrate the ways in which health interventions can accommodate and/or address gendered influences in the design, delivery, and evaluation of the intervention. Gender transformative interventions are those that consider gender norms, roles, and relations; challenge rigid gender norms; and promote gender equity [11,12].

There has been extensive work to implement and evaluate alcohol prevention and reduction strategies on college campuses. Reviews from Larimer and colleagues have demonstrated that brief interventions (also known as brief motivational interventions) have been an effective strategy in individual or group formats, or using in-person, mail-in, or technological mediums [1,13].

Brief interventions are short interactions between individuals and their health care providers that often involve personalized feedback on a health concern and discussion of strategies to improve health [14,15]. They can be done in a variety of health settings by health or social care providers to increase students' motivation to change their alcohol use and increase their awareness and understanding of their patterns of use, alcohol expectancies and related consequences, peer normative beliefs, and protective behavioural strategies to reduce harm [16].

On college campuses in North America, the Brief Alcohol Screening and Intervention for College Students (BASICS) program [17] has been used as the prototypical intervention to address college drinking. Based on motivational interviewing [18] and cognitive behavioural relapse prevention, BASICS consists of two in-person 45- to 60-min individual sessions for high risk drinkers [16]. In the first session, students complete an assessment to identify topics relevant to their substance use or change behaviour; and in session two, participants review personalized feedback generated from their responses from session one. Brief interventions on college campuses have since been adapted in a number of ways, including integrating personalized behavioural strategies, reducing the number of in-person sessions, targeting specific subpopulations and low-risk drinkers, using standalone personalized normative feedback (PNF) web or mail-in interventions to highlight peer drinking norms as a comparator to individual use, and delivering interventions in a group format that is facilitated by either care providers or peers [16,19].

While there has been extensive work to review the efficacy of brief alcohol interventions on college campuses [1], there has been less effort to consider how these interventions are gender responsive beyond considering the moderating effects of gender on existing interventions [16,19]. The purpose of this scoping review was to examine gender considerations in brief alcohol interventions on college campuses and offer opportunities to expand the scope of brief alcohol interventions to become gender transformative.

2. Materials and Methods

This scoping review is based on a subset of data collected as part of a larger scoping review conducted to identify and synthesize current research on sex- and gender-related factors connected to opioid, alcohol, tobacco, and cannabis use. A scoping review methodology was used to identify the breadth of existing literature that responded to two questions:

1. How do sex- and gender-related factors impact (a) patterns of use; (b) health effects of; and (c) prevention, treatment, and harm reduction outcomes for the four substances?
2. What harm reduction, health promotion, prevention, and treatment interventions and programs are available that include sex, gender, and gender-transformative elements, and how effective are these interventions in addressing opioid, alcohol, tobacco, and cannabis use?

A scoping review methodology was used to identify the breadth of existing literature relating to sex, gender, and the four substances as well as to summarize and analyze the research [20]. This methodology was selected due to the exploratory nature that, unlike systematic reviews, have broad inclusion criteria [21].

An iterative search of peer-reviewed literature was conducted in health-related academic databases, including Medline, Embase, Cochrane Database of Systematic Reviews, and Cochrane Central Register of Controlled Trials via Ovid, CINAHL, PyscINFO, Social Work Abstracts, Women's Studies International, and LGBT Life via EbscoHost, and Social Science Citation Index via Clarivate Analytics.

The scoping review included English language articles published from 2007 to 2017 from a selection of Organizational for Economic Cooperation and Development member countries, including Australia, Austria, Belgium, Canada, Denmark, Finland, France, Germany, Greece, Iceland, Ireland, Italy, Luxembourg, Netherlands, New Zealand, Norway, Portugal, Spain, Sweden, Switzerland, United Kingdom, and United States. The population of interest included women, girls, men, boys, trans, and gender-diverse individuals of all ages and demographics. Articles related to substance use in pregnancy were excluded in the original scoping review.

For the full methods and search strategy of the original scoping review see Hemsing et al. (forthcoming) [22].

A total of 5030 articles were included in the original scoping review. These articles were organized in an Endnote library by substance (alcohol, tobacco, opioid, cannabis, general substance use, or containing multiple substances) as well as by research focus (i.e., prevalence, health consequences, and intervention type). Drawing on the original findings, this scoping review examined a subset of the original data collected to further examine how gender was integrated into brief alcohol interventions on college campuses. A scoping review methodology was chosen for this to explore the breadth of the literature on gender responsive brief interventions on college campuses.

As with the original review, this scoping review included English language articles published from 2007 to 2017 from the aforementioned Organizational for Economic Cooperation and Development member countries. The population of interest included women, girls, men, boys, trans, and gender-diverse individuals of all ages and demographics. Using a scoping review methodology allowed for inclusion criteria to be amended post-hoc based on familiarity with the literature [20]. From the original findings, the authors excluded literature on cannabis, opioids, tobacco, and polysubstance use, as well as literature about other intervention approaches, including broader prevention or treatment efforts, which left the authors with 54 articles on brief alcohol intervention to review. Titles and abstracts were read and screened by one researcher (LW) and checked by a second researcher (JS) to ensure that relevant studies were included. Alcohol brief interventions that did not take place on college campuses were excluded. The final sample included 21 articles on brief alcohol interventions on college campuses. A flow diagram detailing the number of studies included and excluded at each stage is provided in Figure 1.

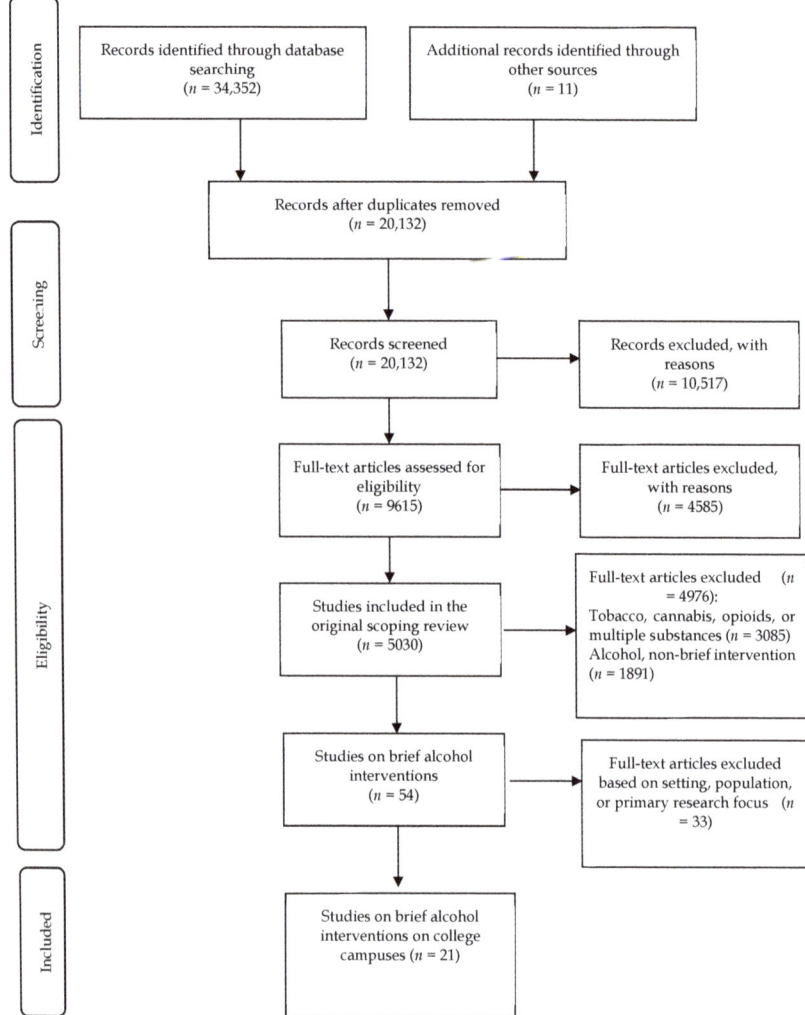

Figure 1. The Preferred Reporting Items for Systematic Reviews and Meta-analysis (PRISMA) flow diagram adapted from Moher et al. (2009) [23] for the scoping review process [24].

The authors extracted data from the 21 included studies in Microsoft Excel, including information on location and setting, methodology and measures, number of participants and eligibility criteria, research aims, and key findings (see Table 1). As is typical in scoping reviews, the authors did not conduct a quality assessment [25], but rather focused on identifying and analyzing sex and gender inclusion and considerations in brief alcohol interventions on college campuses, and offered opportunities to expand the scope of brief alcohol interventions to be gender transformative.

Table 1. Description of included studies.

Author	Location	Research Aim	Participants	Measures (Excluding Baseline Demographic)	Intervention Overview	Key Findings
Bountress et al. 2017 [38]	United States	To examine the effects of sexual assault history on alcohol and sexual risk behaviours (SRBs) and the effect of a web-based alcohol BI to reduce alcohol use and SRBs	n = 160 female college students, 18–20 years old (yo), who engaged in past-month HED	Questions on number of male sexual partners, and HED occasions; Sexual Assertiveness Survey (Pregnancy STD Prevention Subscale); revised Childhood Sexual Abuse (CSA) questionnaire; and Sexual Experiences Survey (SES)	Web-based intervention using personalized and gender-specific feedback, including protective strategies	Increased levels of condom use assertiveness; no effect on number of sexual partners; higher alcohol use among individuals with adolescent sexual assault histories
Brahms et al., 2011 [43]	United States	To analyze the effects of sexual violence on Brief Alcohol Screen in College Students (BASiCS) outcomes	n = 351 female college students reporting significant alcohol and/or drug use	Sexual Risk Behaviour Questionnaire; Brief Symptom Inventory; Daily Drinking Questionnaire (DDQ); and Quantity Frequency Scale	Two 45–60-min BASICS sessions	Reduced alcohol consumption; reduced coping skills in women who experienced sexual violence, but not with women who had not experienced sexual violence
Clinton-Sherrod et al., 2011 [41]	United States	To examine the effect of sexual victimization on an alcohol brief intervention	n = 229 first year, female college students	Prior victimization measures; questions on past-month drinks and drinking-occasions; Young Adult Alcohol Problems Screening Test; Stages of Change Readiness; and Treatment Eagerness Scale and Ambivalence and Recognition subscales	Four intervention conditions: (a) MI only included exploring alcohol-related consequences and change readiness; (b) feedback only included personalized feedback norms, estimated level of risk, a list of relevant resources; (c) MI with feedback (MIFB) which included strategies from both conditions; and d) control	Ambivalence to change was associated with sexual coercion; decreased alcohol use for women in MI and MIFB conditions; women with history of sexual violence in MIFB condition had steeper declines in three-month violence outcomes compared to women without a history of sexual violence
Gajecki et al., 2014 [39]	Sweden	To explore the effect of two smartphone alcohol BI on university students with established levels of risky alcohol consumption	n = 1929 university student union members with Alcohol Use Disorders Identification Test (AUDIT) scores ≥ 6 for women and ≥ 8 for men and a smartphone	DDQ and AUDIT	Two smartphone apps: (a) Promillekoll (Check Your BAC) included real time e-Blood Alcohol Content (BAC) and protective and behavioural strategies; (b) PartyPlanner included event simulation, skillfulness and behavioural strategies, and pre-party simulated and real-time BAC.	Increased drinking frequency among male Promillekoll users
Gilmore et al., 2015 [36]	United States	To assess the efficacy of a web-based alcohol BI, sexual assault risk reduction (SARR) intervention, or combined intervention reducing alcohol use and SRBs	n = 264 female college students, 18–20 yo, who engaged in past-month HED	Questions on alcohol use during sexual experiences, HED, and estimation of sexual violence; revised Dating Self-Protection against Rape Scale; DDQ; SES; Drinking Norms Rating Form; and Protective Behavioural Strategies Surveys (PBSS)	Four intervention conditions: (a) SARR only included sexual assault education and resistance strategies; (b) alcohol only included alcohol psychoeducation, personalized feedback, and PNF; (c) combined intervention which included strategies from both conditions; and (d) control	Reduced alcohol-related sexual violence among the combined condition; reduced HED among women with more severe sexual violence histories in the combined condition; increased perceived likelihood of alcohol-related sexual violence in the SARR condition
Gilmore et al., 2016 [27]	United States	To assess the efficacy of a web-based alcohol and SARR intervention on female college students who are drinking as a coping mechanism	n = 264 female college students, 18–20 yo, who engaged in past-month HED	Questions on HED and Greek affiliation; SES; Readiness to Change questionnaire for brief interventions; and Drinking Motives Questionnaire—Revised Short-Form	See Gilmore et al., 2015	Increased readiness to change among individuals with severe sexual assault histories; reduced drinking to cope for individuals with HED in the combined intervention; no effects on alcohol or SARR interventions on drinking to cope

77

Table 1. *Cont.*

Author	Location	Research Aim	Participants	Measures (Excluding Baseline Demographic)	Intervention Overview	Key Findings
Kaysen et al., 2009 [31]	United States	To explore the effect MI on participants' readiness to change (RTC) and drinking behaviours	n = 182 first year female college students who consumed alcohol at least once in the previous month	Questions on intention to drink; 3-month Timeline Followback (TLFB); and Readiness to Change Ruler	Two-hour group sessions with 8–12 participants including individual TLFB assessment, discussion on alcohol expectancies and positive and negative consequences, normative feedback, sex-specific considerations, and personal goal setting	Correlation between missing to report and increased drinking; correlation between RTC and decreased future drinking; increased RTC among intervention group
Kenney et al., 2014 [32]	United States	To increase protective behavioural strategies (PBS) through a cognitive behaviour skills intervention focusing on decreasing risky drinking and related consequences	n = 226 first year female college students who engaged in past-month HED	Online survey on health behaviours and beliefs related to alcohol and mental health; PBSS and Strategy Questionnaire; DDQ; Rutgers Alcohol Problem Index (RAPI); Beck Anxiety Inventory; and Centre for Epidemiologic Studies Depression Scale	Two-hour group sessions with 8–12 participants using cognitive behavioural skills to discuss alcohol-related consequences, skills to use PBS, and PBS-related goals. Personalized PBS feedback sheets provided to participants with past-month PBS.	Increased PBS at 1- and 6-month follow up; higher PBS among high anxiety participants in intervention group
LaBrie et al., 2007 [7]	United States	To explore female-specific reasons for drinking and the impact of a group brief motivational intervention (BMI) on alcohol consumption and alcohol-related negative consequences	n = 115 female college students who were first time offenders of campus alcohol policies	Questions on alcohol use over the past month; Drinking Motives Questionnaire (DMQ) and Conformity, Coping, Enhancement, and Social Motives subscales; and RAPI	Two-hour group sessions with 8–12 participants using cognitive behavioural skills to discuss alcohol-related consequences and skills to use PBS. Twelve follow-up diaries were used to calculate behavioural outcomes and to assess alcohol-related consequences.	Decreased drinks per month, number of drinking days per month, average drinks, and maximum drinks; significant reductions in all alcohol use behaviours except for number of drinking days per month
LaBrie et al., 2008 [33]	United States	To examine the effect of a single BMI with a focus on female-specific reasons for drinking	n = 220 first year female college students	DMQ and Conformity, Coping, Enhancement, and Social Motives subscales; TLFB; and RAPI	See Kaysen et al., 2009	Reduced binge drinking episodes and alcohol related consequences; most significant decreases with women with stronger social and enhancement drinking motives
LaBrie et al., 2008 [42]	United States	To assess the role of relational health in alcohol consumption and alcohol-related consequences	n = 214 first year female college students	RAPI; TLFB; Relational Health Indices; and DMQ and Conformity, Coping, Enhancement, and Social Motives subscales	Group session to learn about and discuss alcohol-related consequences	Women with stronger peer relationships and community connection drank more but experienced fewer alcohol-related consequences
LaBrie et al., 2009 [44]	United States	To explore the efficacy of a group BMI on female alcohol consumption	n = 285 first year female college students	TLFB; DMQ and Conformity, Coping, Enhancement, and Social Motives subscales; and RAPI	See Kaysen et al., 2009	Reduced drinks per week, maximum drinks, and heavy episodic events; women with strong social drinking motives were more likely to reduce their drinks per week compared to those with weak social motives; results no longer significant at 6-month follow-up

Table 1. *Cont.*

Author	Location	Research Aim	Participants	Measures (Excluding Baseline Demographic)	Intervention Overview	Key Findings
LaBrie et al., 2010 [14]	United States	To validate the effectiveness of a group BMI intervention on adjudicated male students, and develop a gender-specific intervention for men	n = 230 male college students who violated campus alcohol policies	Questions on drinking behaviours and motivations; TLFB; and DMQ and Conformity, Coping, Enhancement, and Social Motives subscales	One 60–75-min group session with 8 to 15 participants to discuss their school sanctions, perceived drinking norms, alcohol-related consequences, and skills to respond to adverse consequences. Twelve follow-up diaries were used to calculate behavioural outcomes and to assess alcohol-related consequences.	Decreased drinks per month, RAPI scores, and recidivism rates
Lewis et al., 2007 [26]	United States	To evaluate if gender specificity in computer-generated personalized normative feedback (PNF) intervention would shift alcohol norms and reduce alcohol consumption	n = 165 college students who engaged in past-month HED	Drinking Norms Rating Form (and the gender-specific version); Alcohol Consumption Inventory; DDQ; Quantity Frequency Scale; and revised Collective Self-Esteem Scale	Three intervention groups: (a) gender-specific PNF and (b) gender-neutral PNF, which included with 1–2 min computer feedback and printout on personal drinking, perceptions of student drinking, and drinking norms; and (c) control	Reduced drinking among both PNF conditions; gender-specific PNF was more effective on reducing drinking among women who strongly identified with their gender; higher gender-specific normative misperceptions among men with medium effect sizes for women
Lewis et al., 2007 [34]	United States	To determine if a gender-specific computer-generated PNF intervention would be more effective than gender-neutral PNF intervention in shifting alcohol norms and reducing alcohol consumption	n = 209 first year college students who engaged in past-week HED	Questions on past-month alcohol consumption, DDQ and Drinking Norms Rating Form (and the gender-specific version)	Three intervention groups: (a) gender-specific PNF and (b) gender-neutral PNF, which included with 1–2-min computer feedback and printout on personal drinking, perceptions of student drinking, and drinking norms; and (c) control	Freshmen and opposite-sex norms were not related to drinks per week; same-sex freshmen norms were associated with increased risks per week; reduced drinks in both intervention groups but with more consistent changes among the gender-specific PNF
Lojewski et al., 2010 [35]	United States	To determine if gender-specific normative feedback will be more effective than a gender-neutral intervention in decreasing alcohol use misperceptions on campus and reducing alcohol consumption	n = 246 college students	Drinking Norms Rating Form; AUDIT; College Alcohol Problem Scale-revised	Three intervention groups: (a) gender-specific PNF and (b) gender-neutral PNF, where participants were provided normative feedback and detailed representation of norms and drinking behaviours; and (c) control	No gender interaction on perceptions of drinking; age was negatively correlated with peer drinking perceptions and reduced alcohol per episode
Merrill et al., 2014 [15]	United States	To determine the effect of gender and depression on the efficacy of an alcohol BI	n = 330 college freshmen, sophomores or juniors, 18–25 yo that engaged in ≥1 episode of past-week HED or ≥4 episodes of past-month HED	Questions on Greek affiliation; Epidemiologic Studies Depression Scale; DDQ; and RAPI	Five intervention groups stratified by gender: (a) TLFB interview; (b) TLFB control; (c) control; (d) basic BMI; and (e) BMI with decisional other	BMI conditions significantly reduced weekly drinking and heavy frequency among men with high depression scores and women with low depression scores; association with higher levels of depression and alcohol-related consequences
Murgraff et al., 2007 [36]	United Kingdom	To evaluate the efficacy of a leaflet intervention in reducing Friday and Saturday risky single-occasion drinking	n = 347 college students who engaged in moderate alcohol consumption	Questions on standard drink consumption and to measure cognitions on intention, self-efficacy and action-specific self-efficacy	Leaflet with recommended daily limits, strategies for reduced alcohol consumption, and implementation intention prompts	Increased self-efficacy on actions to reduce alcohol consumption for men; reduced risky single-occasion drinking for women

Table 1. *Cont.*

Author	Location	Research Aim	Participants	Measures (Excluding Baseline Demographic)	Intervention Overview	Key Findings
Neighbors et al., 2012 [37]	United States	To evaluate the efficacy of a pamphlet and personalized letter on reducing peak alcohol consumption	$n = 818$ college students who engaged in past-month HED	Alcohol Frequency-Quantity Questionnaire	Two intervention groups: (a) personalized letter with their reported BAC, peak drinking occasions, and information about alcohol and other substance use and available resources; and (b) non-personalized letter including information about alcohol and other substance use, available resources, and a BAC calculator	Personalized letter reduced peak BAC in women and students with higher alcohol use
Suffoletto et al., 2016 [40]	United States	To describe the impact of a six-week text-message intervention on weekend drinking and binge drinking episodes	$n = 224$ college students who violated campus alcohol policies	Questions on alcohol consumption and willingness to commit to a drinking limit	Six-week text message intervention that collected data on Thursday and Sunday to understand their weekend drinking patterns, commit to weekend drinking limits, and change attitudes and perceived norms	Decreased binge drinking and number of drinks consumed
Thompson et al., 2018 [29]	Canada	To evaluate the impact of the e-CHECKUP TO GO (e-CHUG) on drinking outcomes and perceived norms in first year university resident students	$n = 245$ first year college students in residence who engaged in alcohol consumption	Questions on alcohol use, alcohol-related harm, and social norm misperceptions; and AUDIT	Web-based BMI with PNF	Decreased norm misperceptions; reduced norm misperceptions associated with reduced drinking outcomes

3. Results

Twenty-one studies were included in the scoping review that integrated sex, gender, or gender-transformative considerations in brief alcohol interventions on college campuses. The included studies are summarized within the following categories: interventions using social norms and PNF; technology-based interventions; dual interventions; and mail-in interventions. Several of the interventions fit into multiple categories, such as those that used PNF and technology-based or mail-in mediums, but are discussed based on the study's primary focus. Details on the study location, research aim, measures used, participants, and key findings are presented in Table 1.

3.1. Interventions Using Social Norms and Personalized Normative Feedback

Twelve studies integrated social norms or PNF as the brief intervention approach. These interventions relied on correcting misperceptions and overestimations of peer drinking in order to reduce drinking or alcohol-related consequences [26]. The medium in which the interventions were delivered varied greatly, with five-interventions using a web-based medium [26–30], six interventions conducted in-person or in group settings [7,31–35], and one using a mail-in medium [36]. Of the twelve interventions, five included only female students, one included only male students, and five included both male and female students.

The identified studies had differing ways in which they reported on the efficacy of using social norms and PNF. While many studies included normative feedback as part of the intervention, few reported on changes in norm perceptions or the effect of norm-based components on alcohol use. Of those that included such findings, the results suggest that norm-based alcohol reduction interventions often had significant effects regardless of the medium in which they were delivered [26,30,35,37].

Four web-based interventions, three from the United States [26,28,30] and one from Canada [29], found that PNF significantly lowered perceptions of normative drinking. In one study, the authors found that while the PNF resulted in corrections to normative misperceptions, particularly amongst male participants, the PNF had a small-to-medium effect on norms at one-month follow-up [26]. However, in two studies from Canada and the United States, the authors found that the reductions in norm misperceptions at the three-month follow-up were a significant predictor of reduced drinking outcomes at the five-month follow-up [29,30].

In studies that explored the impact of gender-specific PNF (whereby PNF components are based on same-gender norms rather than opposite-gender norms), researchers suggested that gender-specific normative misperceptions were evident for both men and women [26,30]. However, there were varied results in the efficacy of gender-specific PNF. In one study from the United States, the authors found that gender-specific PNF resulted in significantly reduced alcohol use in comparison to the control condition, and that gender-specific PNF resulted in stronger, and more consistent, drinking reductions compared to the gender-neutral or control conditions. However, reductions in alcohol use from the gender-specific PNF were not statistically significant compared to the gender-neutral PNF [30]. In another study from the United States, gender-specific PNF was most effective amongst women who strongly identified with their gender, whereas gender identity was not associated with changes in alcohol use in the gender-neutral or control conditions [26]. In a third study from the United States, the authors found that that while normative feedback was effective in reducing misperceptions around alcohol use, there was no significant effect of gender-specific PNF [35].

3.2. Technology-Based Interventions

Eight interventions were technology-based. Six of the studies were web-based or computerized [26–30,38] and two were mobile health interventions using smartphone applications (apps) [39] and short message service (SMS) [40]. All of the web-based and computerized interventions were validated and modeled on previously described and evaluated interventions [27–29,38]. Computerized brief interventions can be disseminated widely for a low cost, without high human resource requirements or participant demands [27–29,38]. These interventions also allow participants to anonymously report information that they may not feel comfortable sharing in a face-to-face setting [28]. This was specifically of note for the three interventions that were only inclusive of women, where the interventions required women to disclose prior experience(s) of sexual violence.

Only one computerized intervention evaluated the impact of the medium on alcohol use reduction. The study, from Canada, found that while the focus on norm misperceptions had salient effects, there were no significant effects of e-CHECKUP TO GO (e-CHUG) on drinking outcomes at follow-up, indicating that additional sessions may be required to sustain the efficacious elements of the intervention [29].

Two studies examined mobile phone interventions, both of which were directed to students regardless of their gender. In one study from Sweden, the authors examined the uptake and efficacy of two smartphone apps amongst university students. The *Promillekoll* (Check Your Blood Alcohol Content (BAC)) app allowed users to find their real time BAC by registering their alcohol use and providing suggested strategies to maintain a safe level of consumption. The PartyPlanner app was developed to modify drinking behaviour through event simulation, allowing users to visualize their drinking intentions and adapt their risk perceptions to real-life situations. The app also provided an electronic display of BAC at distinct points through the simulation and real-time occasion. Both of the apps had high attrition rates. Women were more likely to continue using the program and complete the follow-up. Unexpectedly, the *Promillekoll* app showed increased drinking frequency among male users, possibly as a result of men using the app as a competitive drinking game rather than as a risk reduction tool; the same effect was not found for the PartyPlanner app [39].

The other mobile phone intervention, from the United States, combined an SMS intervention called PantherTRAC with two in-person sessions to increase students' understanding of their own weekend drinking, change their attitudes and self-efficacy, and commit students to reduced drinking. The software would commence a text-based dialogue starting on Thursday to prompt users to reflect on their drinking plans and goals, and end on Sunday with a prompt for students to report the number of drinks consumed, which would allow for the intervention to provide tailored feedback based on participants' consumption. The intervention resulted in change behaviour, with participants reporting a decrease of binge drinking behaviour and reporting decreased binge drinking on weekends where they had committed to a weekend drinking goal. There were no gender differences in alcohol reduction [40].

3.3. Dual Interventions

Four studies explored the efficacy of interventions for alcohol and other health concerns. All of the studies were from the United States, were inclusive of only female college students, and all explored the efficacy of interventions targeting alcohol and sexual risk reduction [27,28,38,41].

Two studies explored the effect of a brief alcohol intervention on sexual risk behaviours. In one web-based brief intervention, the authors found a positive intervention effect on condom use assertiveness among those with a history of childhood sexual assault [38]. In another study exploring changes in alcohol use and victimization, the authors found that the motivational interviewing and motivational interviewing with feedback conditions decreased alcohol use, with the latter condition resulting in steeper decreases in unwanted sexual activity. Alcohol use and ambivalence to change were associated with unwanted sexual activity [41].

Two studies explored the efficacy of a dual web-based alcohol and sexual assault risk reduction brief intervention compared to a singularly focused alcohol or sexual assault risk reduction intervention. Female students in the combined condition reported decreased sexual assault risk or rape at the three-month follow-up, and women in the combined condition with a history of adult sexual assault reported decreases in heavy episodic drinking (HED) [28]. The combined intervention also resulted in reduced "drinking to cope" amongst those with higher baseline levels of drinking to cope, as a result of having information, protective strategies, and resources to both reduce HED and sexual assault risk [27].

3.4. Mail-In Interventions

Two studies used pamphlets or a letter to reduce single occasion and peak alcohol use. The studies, from the United Kingdom [36] and United States [37], were inclusive of male and female students who reported alcohol use and heavy episodic drinking, respectively.

Both pamphlets included standard drink sizes and recommended daily limits [36,37]. In the British study, the pamphlet also included peer drinking norms, strategies to reduce alcohol consumption, and prompting information on implementation intentions. The pamphlet intervention resulted in reduced risky weekend drinking among women and increased self-efficacy in relation to actions that could be used to promote alcohol reduction among men [36].

In the American study, in addition to the aforementioned information, the pamphlet also included general information about substance use, resources and referrals, and a BAC handout. In a second intervention condition, the authors examined the efficacy of the pamphlet sent along with a personalized letter expressing concern over students' drinking patterns, their BAC, assurance of confidentiality, and contact information if individuals wanted additional information. The latter condition resulted in reducing peak BAC among women and those with higher reported alcohol use, but not with men. However, there were no significant differences between those that were sent the combined letter and pamphlet compared to those that just received the pamphlet [37].

3.5. Gender Inclusion and Considerations

As part of the scoping review inclusion criteria, all of the studies had to consider sex, gender, or have gender responsive [12] elements in their alcohol brief intervention. Few of the articles included sex considerations, and where it was included, it was as part of the brief intervention to describe the physiology of how men and women metabolize alcohol [7,34,42]. However, all of the articles included gender responsive aspects and were directed to specific gender groups.

Of the 21 studies included, 11 interventions included women only [7,27,28,31–33,38,41–44], one inclusive of males only [34], and nine were inclusive of both men and women [26,29,30,35–37,39,40,45]. No studies identified other forms of inclusion beyond the gender binary or addressed other intersections of equity, such as race/ethnicity or sexual orientation.

Five studies from LaBrie and colleagues employed group brief motivational interventions that examined gender-specific reasons for drinking. Four of the interventions were geared to female college students, where the interventions examined the positive and negative aspects of drinking, normative feedback, and the moderating effects on women's drinking. The authors found that social and enhancement motivations were positively associated with drinking [33]. As such, women with strong social motivations were more likely to experience reductions in drinking outcomes [44] and that participation in the gender-specific intervention resulted in significant reductions in drinking outcomes, including drinks per month, drinking days, average drinks, and alcohol-related negative consequences [7,42]. Using the same model, LaBrie and colleagues developed a gender-specific program for adjudicated male students that found significant reductions in drinks per month and alcohol-related consequences [34].

These findings demonstrate support for the efficacy of brief alcohol interventions, as well as the growing evidence supporting the efficacy of group-based and gender-specific interventions, which address gendered motivations and influences, not only normative behaviours for drinkers in a gender group.

4. Discussion

While gender and sex have been integrated into existing interventions and research on brief alcohol interventions on college campuses, further work is needed to bring attention and address sex and gender influences on alcohol use for college students. Moreover, there is an immense need to consider sex and gender in the design and implementation of the brief alcohol intervention—and the intervention's capacity to address gender equity issues.

Six of the included studies reported only differences in intervention efficacy among male and female students, as opposed to exploring any sex and gender factors and influences [29,36,37,39,40,45]. Two studies even conflate sex and gender, with one study discussing sex-related norms (for a gender-specific PNF) [30] and the other study reporting on the moderating effects of sex rather than gender [29]. This misuse of language emphasizes the critical need for researchers to develop an understanding of sex and gender to further the efficacy of health promotion interventions [12].

Only three interventions designed for male and female students incorporated gender-based analysis beyond an examination of the moderating effects on outcome overall [26,30,35]. In research from Lewis et al., evaluating the efficacy of a gender-specific and gender-neutral PNF, the findings demonstrated that while both PNF conditions resulted in reduced drinking, the gender-specific PNF resulted in more consistent reductions [30] and was more effective in reducing alcohol consumption among women who strongly identified with their gender [26]. These findings may suggest the potential benefits for the gender-specific elements extend beyond reinforcing stereotypical gender norms [12] to address other aspects of gender, such as the role of gender relations in affecting alcohol use when developing and evaluating brief alcohol interventions [30].

LaBrie and colleagues examined the efficacy of interventions on female- [7,33,44] and male-specific [34] reasons for drinking. Participants discussed the normative and "good" and "not-so-good" things about alcohol use, such as the social benefits for drinking, alcohol expectancies and related consequences, and identified strategies, skills, or coping mechanisms to reduce alcohol use and related consequences [7,33,34,44]. The authors further developed a female-specific intervention to examine the role of relational health in alcohol consumption and related consequences [42]. These studies, which underpinned motivations for alcohol consumption, were particularly effective in responding to the relational components of men's and women's alcohol use. Similar to the work of Smith and Berger [46], the findings suggest that female college students, particularly in their freshmen year, primarily drank to fulfill the need for social connection [42].

Five interventions for women were dual interventions for alcohol and sexual assault risk reduction [27,28,38,41] or to examine the moderating effects of sexual violence on the brief alcohol intervention [43]. Often, these studies integrated protective behavioural strategies, such as finding personal transportation or meeting in a public place [28,32,38], that can help reduce alcohol-related consequences and risk of sexual violence [9]. While research suggests that women are more likely to experience sexual violence on days of heavy drinking [9,27,28,41], and that women may be more likely to use protective behavioural strategies compared to men [19], such interventions put the onus on women to reduce their risk of assault or their number of sexual partners, rather than addressing the sexual violence as a gender equity issue. As such, brief alcohol interventions must also be developed for men that are inclusive of their own change behaviour, norms about both alcohol use and sexual violence, and that promote respect, safety, and consent in all sexual relations. Such learnings could be built upon the male-only interventions from LaBrie et al. [34] or future interventions that are geared towards men.

4.1. Future Considerations

Of the studies included, those that explored gendered motivations for substance use (i.e., female students drinking to enhance social connection) and responded by creating brief alcohol interventions that addressed the relational elements of substance use were in the best position to address gender inequities [7,33,44]. These interventions considered gender from the onset; they were developed bearing gender considerations in mind and were implemented in group settings, which allowed for harm reduction and prevention strategies that facilitated connection outside of a drinking context. Future interventions should follow a similar trajectory in developing and responding to gender norms and relations.

There are other examples of gender transformative interventions on college campuses. In Canada, the Caring Campus project was developed to promote male students' health by empowering first year male students to take on leadership roles to advance men's mental health and transform campus drinking norms. The intervention used an empowerment-based health promotion framework to encourage individuals' self-esteem and self-efficacy, with the goals of prompting community action and confidence to affect change. By targeting first year males, the intervention was able to respond to how the transition into college can be a time of increasingly risky drinking, how masculine norms affect drinking and access to health and wellness services. Moreover, through developing a peer-led model, Caring Campus allowed for the normalization and destigmatization of mental health and substance-use concerns, which allowed both men and women to more readily access services which otherwise would have seemed inaccessible [47].

Another Canadian initiative, What's Your Cap at the University of Saskatchewan, is a student run harm reduction initiative to raise awareness about alcohol-related consequences. What's Your Cap shares campus-specific PNF and raises awareness of the harms related to risky alcohol consumption on their website, social media, and through peer facilitation [48]. Some of their materials, such as the "Blindsided by the Alcohol Industry" infographic, have been designed to empower women to question the alcohol industry's gendered marketing approaches that promote alcohol consumption by women, by linking alcohol consumption to attractiveness, sexuality, and relational success [49]. Through such initiatives, the potential can be seen for mail-in or web-based interventions to promote examination of, and change in, gender norms and inequities as a means of achieving goals of reducing alcohol use and promoting health.

These two examples from Canada are illustrative of the essence of gender-transformative approaches—to change negative gender norms that adversely affect health, engage men and boys in new ways, and empower girls and women at multiple levels. And to do this while working on alcohol issues, as a proactive way of improving health related to alcohol use by integrating gender equity critique and collective action.

There is an increasing interest and commitment by governments and research bodies to adopt sex, gender, and equity analysis (SGBA+), a process that analyzes research from perspectives of individuals and groups who differ by sex, gender, sexual orientation, etc., and to apply this understanding in a systematic way to achieve equity [50]. See, for example, Status of Women Canada [51], Canadian Institutes of Health Research [52], European Gender Medicine [53], and National Institutes of Health [54]. Universities and colleges must lead with the same commitment and momentum. Such analysis and gender-transformative approaches are integral to most effectively facilitate cultural change and respond to the needs of the students that these interventions are targeting. Moreover, future interventions should also consider intersecting areas of equity, which interact with gender and sex in significant ways but were sparsely included in the literature.

4.2. Limitations

This scoping review only included studies where brief alcohol interventions on college campuses were the primary focus. As such, it is possible that there are gender-transformative brief alcohol interventions that were excluded, such as those that were occurring off-campus [55,56], where the brief alcohol intervention was included as a control condition [57,58], or for women in the pregnancy or post-partum periods. However, the scoping review demonstrated that there is a tremendous need to expand to address gender inequities, as well as to expand the scope of the work to include men, trans, and gender-diverse individuals.

5. Conclusions

Gender transformative interventions can shift gender norms and correct power imbalances so that individuals are able to better reach their health potential. Despite extensive work on brief alcohol interventions on college campuses, there has been no such work to review these studies and analyze their attention to a full range of gendered influences on use, engagement, outcomes, and improvement in equity. This scoping review demonstrates the need to further gender responsiveness in brief alcohol interventions on college campuses and the ways in which interventions can be gender transformative through advancing gender equity while also addressing alcohol use. Future work must move beyond reinforcing prescriptive and stereotypical notions of gender to demonstrate an understanding of the differences between sex and gender. By integrating sex, gender, and other equity considerations, brief alcohol interventions can better respond to the systemic influences that perpetuate negative gender roles, expectations, relations, and regulations that underlie alcohol use among college students. In doing so, interventions will be able better facilitate both individual health, safety, and equity, as well as systems-level change as students transition into, and out of, college.

Author Contributions: Conceptualization, L.W. and N.P.; methodology, L.W.; formal analysis, L.W.; data curation, L.W. and J.S.; writing—original draft preparation, L.W.; writing—review and editing, L.W., J.S., and N.P.; visualization, L.W.; supervision, N.P.; funding acquisition, N.P. All authors have read and agreed to the published version of the manuscript.

Funding: This research was supported by the Canadian Institutes of Health Research (CIHR)—Institute of Gender and Health Team Grant #384548.

Acknowledgments: The authors wish to acknowledge the project team of the "Integrating and measuring the effect of sex, gender, and gender transformative approaches to substance use treatment, prevention, and harm reduction in Canada" project.

Conflicts of Interest: The authors declare no conflict of interest.

References

1. Larimer, M.; Cronce, J.M.; Lee, C.M.; Kilmer, J.R. Brief intervention in college settings. *Alcohol Res. Health* **2004**, *28*, 94–104. [PubMed]
2. O'Malley, P.M.; Johnston, L.D. Epidemiology of alcohol and other drug use among American college students. *J. Stud. Alcohol* **2002**, *63*, 23–39. [CrossRef] [PubMed]
3. Sher, K.J.; Rutledge, P.C. Heavy drinking across the transition to college: Predicting first-semester heavy drinking from precollege variables. *Addict. Behav.* **2007**, *32*, 819–835. [CrossRef] [PubMed]
4. Canadian Centre on Substance Use and Addiction. *Reducing the Harms Related to Alcohol on College Campuses*; Canadian Centre on Substance Use and Addiction: Ottawa, ON, Canada, 2016.
5. Statistics Canada. *Heavy Drinking, 2016*; Statistics Canada: Ottawa, ON, Canada, 2017.
6. Thompson, M.P.; Spitler, H.; McCoy, T.P.; Marra, L.; Sutfin, E.L.; Rhodes, S.D.; Brown, C. The moderating role of gender in the prospective associations between expectancies and alcohol-related negative consequences among college students. *Subst. Use Misuse* **2009**, *44*, 934–942. [CrossRef] [PubMed]
7. LaBrie, J.W.; Thompson, A.D.; Huchting, K.; Lac, A.; Buckley, K. A group Motivational Interviewing intervention reduces drinking and alcohol-related negative consequences in adjudicated college women. *Addict. Behav.* **2007**, *32*, 2549–2562. [CrossRef] [PubMed]
8. Kuntsche, E.; Muller, S. Why do young people start drinking? Motives for first-time alcohol consumption and links to risky drinking in early adolescence. *Eur. Addict. Res.* **2012**, *18*, 34–39. [CrossRef]
9. Neilson, E.C.; Gilmore, A.K.; Pinsky, H.T.; Shepard, M.E.; Lewis, M.A.; George, W.H. The Use of Drinking and Sexual Assault Protective Behavioral Strategies: Associations With Sexual Victimization and Revictimization Among College Women. *J. Interpers. Violence* **2018**, *33*, 137–158. [CrossRef]
10. Demartini, K.S.; Carey, K.B.; Lao, K.; Luciano, M. Injunctive norms for alcohol-related consequences and protective behavioral strategies: Effects of gender and year in school. *Addict. Behav.* **2011**, *36*, 347–353. [CrossRef]
11. Schmidt, R.; Poole, N.; Greaves, L.; Hemsing, N. *New Terrain: Tools to Integrate Trauma and Gender Informed Responses into Substance Use Practice and Policy*; Centre of Excellence for Women's Health: Vancouver, BC, Canada, 2018.
12. Pederson, A.; Greaves, L.; Poole, N. Gender-transformative health promotion for women: A framework for action. *Health Promot. Int.* **2015**, *30*, 140–150. [CrossRef]

13. Larimer, M.E.; Cronce, J.M. Identification, prevention and treatment: A review of individual-focused strategies to reduce problematic alcohol consumption by college students. *J. Stud. Alcohol Suppl.* **2002**, *14*, 148–163. [CrossRef]
14. Nathoo, T.; Poole, N.; Wolfson, L.; Schmidt, R.; Hemsing, N.; Gelb, K. *Doorways to Conversation: Brief Intervention on Substance Use with Girls and Women*; Centre of Excellence for Women's Health: Vancouver, BC, Canada, 2018.
15. Nathoo, T.; Wolfson, L.; Gelb, K.; Poole, N. New approaches to brief intervention on substance use during pregnancy. *Can. J. Midwifery Res. Pract.* **2019**, *18*, 10–21.
16. Huh, D.; Mun, E.Y.; Larimer, M.E.; White, H.R.; Ray, A.E.; Rhew, I.C.; Kim, S.Y.; Jiao, Y.; Atkins, D.C. Brief motivational interventions for college student drinking may not be as powerful as we think: An individual participant-level data meta-analysis. *Alcohol. Clin. Exp. Res.* **2015**, *39*, 919–931. [CrossRef] [PubMed]
17. Dimeff, L.A.; Baer, J.S.; Kivlahan, D.R.; Marlatt, G.A. *Brief Alcohol Screening and Intervention for College Students (BASICS): A Harm Reduction Approach*; Guilford Press: New York, NY, USA, 1999.
18. Miller, W.R.; Rollnick, S. *Motivational Interviewing: Preparing People to Change Addictive Behaviour*; Guilford Press: New York, NY, USA, 2002.
19. LaBrie, J.W.; Lac, A.; Kenney, S.R.; Mirza, T. Protective behavioral strategies mediate the effect of drinking motives on alcohol use among heavy drinking college students: Gender and race differences. *Addict. Behav.* **2011**, *36*, 354–361. [CrossRef] [PubMed]
20. Arksey, H.; O'Malley, L. Scoping studies: Towards a methodological framework. *Int. J. Soc. Res. Methodol.* **2005**, *8*, 19–32. [CrossRef]
21. Levac, D.; Colquhoun, H.; O'Brien, K.K. Scoping studies: Advancing the methodology. *Implement. Sci.* **2010**, *5*, 69. [CrossRef]
22. Hemsing, N.; Greaves, L. Gender norms, roles, and relations and cannabis use patterns: A scoping review. *Int. J. Environ. Res. Public Health* **2020**. Forthcoming.
23. Moher, D.; Liberati, A.; Tetzlaff, J.; Altman, D.J.; The PRISMA Group. Preferred reporting items for systematic reviews and meta-analyses: The PRISMA Statement. *PLoS Med.* **2009**, *6*. [CrossRef]
24. Peters, M.D.J.; Godfrey, C.M.; Khalil, H.; McInerney, P.; Parker, D.; Baldini Soares, C. Guidance for conducting systematic scoping reviews. *Int. J. Evid. Based Healthc.* **2015**, *13*, 141–146. [CrossRef]
25. Daudt, H.M.; Van Mossel, C.; Scott, S.J. Enhancing the scoping study methodology: A large, inter-professional team's experience with Arskey and O'Malley's framework. *BMC Med. Res. Methodol.* **2013**, *13*, 48. [CrossRef]
26. Lewis, M.A.; Neighbors, C. Optimizing personalized normative feedback: The use of gender-specific referents. *J. Stud. Alcohol Drugs* **2007**, *68*, 228–237. [CrossRef]
27. Gilmore, A.K.; Bountress, K.E. Reducing drinking to cope among heavy episodic drinking college women: Secondary outcomes of a web-based combined alcohol use and sexual assault risk reduction intervention. *Addict. Behav.* **2016**, *61*, 104–111. [CrossRef] [PubMed]
28. Gilmore, A.K.; Lewis, M.A.; George, W.H. A randomized controlled trial targeting alcohol use and sexual assault risk among college women at high risk for victimization. *Behav. Res. Ther.* **2015**, *74*, 38–49. [CrossRef] [PubMed]
29. Thompson, K.; Burgess, J.; MacNevin, P.D. An Evaluation of e-CHECKUP TO GO in Canada: The Mediating Role of Changes in Social Norm Misperceptions. *Subst. Use Misuse* **2018**, *53*, 1849–1858. [CrossRef] [PubMed]
30. Lewis, M.A.; Neighbors, C.; Oster-Aaland, L.; Kirkeby, B.S.; Larimer, M.E. Indicated prevention for incoming freshmen: Personalized normative feedback and high-risk drinking. *Addict. Behav.* **2007**, *32*, 2495–2508. [CrossRef] [PubMed]
31. Kaysen, D.L.; Lee, C.M.; Labrie, J.W.; Tollison, S.J. Readiness to change drinking behavior in female college students. *J. Stud. Alcohol Drugs* **2009**, 106–114. [CrossRef]
32. Kenney, S.R.; Napper, L.E.; LaBrie, J.W.; Martens, M.P. Examining the Efficacy of a Brief Group Protective Behavioral Strategies Skills Training Alcohol Intervention with College Women. *Psychol. Addict. Behav.* **2014**, *28*, 1041–1051. [CrossRef]
33. LaBrie, J.W.; Huchting, K.; Tawalbeh, S.; Pedersen, E.R.; Thompson, A.D.; Shelesky, K.; Larimer, M.; Neighbors, C. A randomized motivational enhancement prevention group reduces drinking and alcohol consequences in first-year college women. *Psychol. Addict. Behav.* **2008**, *22*, 149–155. [CrossRef]
34. LaBrie, J.W.; Cail, J.; Pedersen, E.R.; Migliuri, S. Reducing alcohol risk in adjudicated male college students: Further validation of a group motivational enhancement intervention. *J. Child Adolesc. Subst. Abus.* **2011**, *20*, 82–98. [CrossRef]

35. Lojewski, R.; Rotunda, R.J.; Arruda, J.E. Personalized normative feedback to reduce drinking among college students: A social norms intervention examining gender-based versus standard feedback. *J. Alcohol Drug Educ.* **2010**, *54*, 19–40.
36. Murgraff, V.; Abraham, C.; McDermott, M. Reducing friday alcohol consumption among moderate, women drinkers: Evaluation of a brief evidence-based intervention. *Alcohol Alcohol.* **2007**, *42*, 37–41. [CrossRef]
37. Neighbors, C.; Pedersen, E.R.; Kaysen, D.; Kulesza, M.; Walter, T. What Should We Do When Participants Report Dangerous Drinking? The Impact of Personalized Letters Versus General Pamphlets as a Function of Sex and Controlled Orientation. *Ethics Behav.* **2012**, *22*, 1–15. [CrossRef] [PubMed]
38. Bountress, K.E.; Metzger, I.W.; Maples-Keller, J.L.; Gilmore, A.K. Reducing sexual risk behaviors: Secondary analyses from a randomized controlled trial of a brief web-based alcohol intervention for underage, heavy episodic drinking college women. *Addict. Res. Theory* **2017**, *25*, 302–309. [CrossRef] [PubMed]
39. Gajecki, M.; Berman, A.H.; Sinadinovic, K.; Rosendahl, I.; Andersson, C. Mobile phone brief intervention applications for risky alcohol use among university students: A randomized controlled study. *Addict. Sci. Clin. Pract.* **2014**, *9*, 11. [CrossRef] [PubMed]
40. Suffoletto, B.; Merrill, J.E.; Chung, T.; Kristan, J.; Vanek, M.; Clark, D.B. A text message program as a booster to in-person brief interventions for mandated college students to prevent weekend binge drinking. *J. Am. Coll. Health* **2016**, *64*, 481–489. [CrossRef]
41. Clinton-Sherrod, M.; Morgan-Lopez, A.A.; Brown, J.M.; McMillen, B.A.; Cowell, A. Incapacitated sexual violence involving alcohol among college women: The impact of a brief drinking intervention. *Violence Women* **2011**, *17*, 135–154. [CrossRef]
42. LaBrie, J.W.; Thompson, A.D.; Ferraiolo, P.; Garcia, J.A.; Huchting, K.; Shelesky, K. The differential impact of relational health on alcohol consumption and consequences in first year college women. *Addict. Behav.* **2008**, *33*, 266–278. [CrossRef]
43. Brahms, E.; Ahl, M.; Reed, E.; Amaro, H. Effects of an alcohol intervention on drinking among female college students with and without a recent history of sexual violence. *Addict. Behav.* **2011**, *36*, 1325–1328. [CrossRef]
44. LaBrie, J.W.; Huchting, K.K.; Lac, A.; Tawalbeh, S.; Thompson, A.D.; Larimer, M.E. Preventing risky drinking in first-year college women: Further validation of a female-specific motivational-enhancement group intervention. *J. Stud. Alcohol Drugs* **2009**, 77–85. [CrossRef]
45. Merrill, J.E.; Reid, A.E.; Carey, M.P.; Carey, K.B. Gender and depression moderate response to brief motivational intervention for alcohol misuse among college students. *J. Consult. Clin. Psychol.* **2014**, *82*, 984–992. [CrossRef]
46. Smith, M.A.; Berger, J.B. Women's ways of drinking: College women, high-risk alcohol use, and negative consequences. *J. Coll. Stud. Dev.* **2010**, *51*, 35–49. [CrossRef]
47. Stuart, H.; Chen, S.-P.; Krupa, T.; Narain, T.; Horgan, S.; Dobson, K.; Stewart, S. The caring campus project overview. *Can. J. Community Ment. Health* **2019**, *37*, 69–82. [CrossRef]
48. Student Wellness Centre. Alcohol 101. Available online: https://students.usask.ca/articles/alcohol.php (accessed on 10 December 2019).
49. Saskatchewan Prevention Institute. *Blindsided by the Alcohol Industry?* Saskatchewan Prevention Institute: Saskatoon, SK, Canada, 2016.
50. Canadian Centre on Substance Use and Addiction. *Sex, Gender, and Equity Analyses*; Canadian Centre on Substance Use and Addiction: Ottawa, ON, Canada, 2019.
51. Status of Women Canada. Government of Canada's Gender-Based Analysis Plus Approach. Available online: https://cfc-swc.gc.ca/gba-acs/approach-approche-en.html (accessed on 10 December 2019).
52. Canadian Institutes of Health Research. Sex, Gender, and Health Research. Available online: https://cihr-irsc.gc.ca/e/50833.html (accessed on 10 December 2019).
53. European Gender Medicine. *Final Report Summary—EUGENMED (European Gender Medicine Network)*; Charité—Universitätsmedizin Berlin: Berlin, Germany, 2016.
54. National Institutes of Health Office of Research on Women's Health. Sex & Gender. Available online: https://orwh.od.nih.gov/sex-gender (accessed on 10 December 2019).
55. Kelley-Baker, T.; Johnson, M.B.; Romano, E.; Mumford, E.A.; Miller, B.A. Preventing victimization among young women: The SafeNights intervention. *Am. J. Health Stud.* **2011**, *26*, 185–195. [PubMed]
56. Grossbard, J.R.; Mastroleo, N.R.; Geisner, I.M.; Atkins, D.; Ray, A.E.; Kilmer, J.R.; Mallett, K.; Larimer, M.E.; Turrisi, R. Drinking norms, readiness to change, and gender as moderators of a combined alcohol intervention for first-year college students. *Addict. Behav.* **2016**, *52*, 75–82. [CrossRef] [PubMed]

57. Labrie, J.; Lamb, T.; Pedersen, E. Changes in drinking patterns across the transition to college among first-year college males. *J. Child Adolesc. Subst. Abus.* **2008**, *18*, 1–15. [CrossRef]
58. Starosta, A.J.; Cranston, E.; Earleywine, M. Safer sex in a digital world: A Web-based motivational enhancement intervention to increase condom use among college women. *J. Am. Coll. Health* **2016**, *64*, 184–193. [CrossRef]

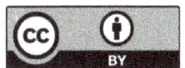

© 2020 by the authors. Licensee MDPI, Basel, Switzerland. This article is an open access article distributed under the terms and conditions of the Creative Commons Attribution (CC BY) license (http://creativecommons.org/licenses/by/4.0/).

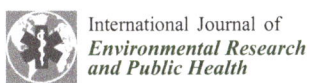

Article

Multi-Dimensional Factors Associated with Illegal Substance Use Among Gay and Bisexual Men in Taiwan

Dian-Jeng Li [1,2], Shiou-Lan Chen [1] and Cheng-Fang Yen [1,3,*]

[1] Graduate Institute of Medicine, College of Medicine, Kaohsiung Medical University, Kaohsiung 80708, Taiwan; u108800004@kmu.edu.tw (D.-J.L.); shioulan@kmu.edu.tw (S.-L.C.)
[2] Department of Addiction Science, Kaohsiung Municipal Kai-Syuan Psychiatric Hospital 80276, Kaohsiung 80708, Taiwan
[3] Department of Psychiatry, Kaohsiung Medical University Hospital, Kaohsiung 80708, Taiwan
* Correspondence: chfaye@cc.kmu.edu.tw; Tel.: +(886)-7-3121101 (ext. 6822)

Received: 8 October 2019; Accepted: 11 November 2019; Published: 14 November 2019

Abstract: Illegal substance use in sexual minorities is an important health issue worldwide. The present cross-sectional study aimed to investigate the multi-dimensional factors associated with illegal substance use among gay and bisexual men in Taiwan. This questionnaire-survey study recruited 500 gay or bisexual men aged between 20 and 25 years. Their experiences of using eight kinds of illegal substances in the preceding month were collected. Their previous experiences of homophobic bullying, satisfaction with academic performance, truancy, perceived family and peer support in childhood and adolescence, and social-demographic characteristics, were also collected. Potential factors associated with illegal substance use were identified using univariate logistic regression, and further selected into a forward stepwise logistic regression model to identify the factors most significantly related to illegal substance use. A total of 22 (4.4%) participants reported illegal substance use in the preceding month, and mean age was 22.9 ± 1.6. Forward stepwise logistic regression revealed that being victims of homophobic cyberbullying in childhood and adolescence (odds ratio (OR) = 1.26; $p = 0.011$), disclosure of sexual orientation at junior high school (OR = 4.67; $p = 0.001$), and missing classes or truancy in senior high school (OR = 2.52; $p = 0.041$) were significantly associated with illegal substance use in early adulthood. Multi-dimensional factors in childhood and adolescence that were significantly associated with illegal substance use in early adulthood among gay and bisexual men were identified. Besides traditional bullying, the effect of cyberbullying and school performance on illegal substance use should not be ignored. This study is limited to the cross-sectional design and possible recall bias. Mental health professionals must routinely assess these significant factors to prevent and intervene in illegal substance use among gay and bisexual men.

Keywords: sexual minorities; illegal substance use; homophobic bullying

1. Introduction

1.1. Substance Use in Sexual Minorities

Substance use has become a major public health concern. According to the 2018 World Drug Report, 2.75 hundred million people have used illegal drugs at least once, which comprises 5.6% of the general population aged between 15 and 64 years [1]. Among them, 31 million people have been diagnosed with substance use disorder. Substance use often results in socio-economical and health burdens, including domestic violence [2,3], increased crime rates [4], suicide [5], comorbidity with mental illnesses [6], and comorbidity with physical illnesses, such as blood-borne disease [7]. Substance abuse is also a key public health issue worldwide for sexual minorities. An epidemiologic study derived from the National Epidemiologic Survey on Alcohol and Related Conditions-III, reported a higher prevalence of drug abuse at some point during their lifetime, for gay/lesbian (19.6%) and bisexual (26.5%) individuals, compared with heterosexual individuals (12.1%) [8]. In Taiwan, a cross-sectional study indicated 16% of recreational drug use in the previous 6 months within men who have sex with men (MSM; 98.6% of them are gay/bisexual men) [9], and it is also higher than an epidemiological study, which reported 0.17% of past-1-year prevalence for club drug use in general population [10]. To be specific, methamphetamine along with ketamine and marijuana are popular according to a national survey [10]; however, such investigation for sexual minorities is insufficient. A previous study indicated that poly drug use among gay and bisexual men, is significantly associated with HIV infection, high-risk sexual practices, and partner violence [11]. Meyer proposed the minority stress theory (MST) to illustrate the association between multiple stressors and mental health status in sexual minorities [12]. This model was tested for substance use and it showed a good level of application in sexual minorities [13]. Investigation of the factors affecting substance use in sexual minorities can serve as the basis for developing prevention and intervention programs.

1.2. Factors Related to Substance Use in Sexual Minorities

According to the ecological systems theory developed by Bronfenbrenner [14], substance use in sexual minority individuals is an ecological phenomenon, which has been established and perpetuated over time because of the complex interactions between individual and social factors. With regards to individual factors associated with substance use, previous studies have indicated that bisexual individuals have a higher rate of substance use compared with gay/lesbian and heterosexual individuals [15,16]. Moreover, some studies have found that disclosure of sexual orientation was associated with significantly greater substance use [17–19], while other studies do not support this finding [20,21]. To the best of our knowledge, whether disclosure of sexual orientation at a specific life stage is associated with substance use in sexual minority individuals has not been previously examined. Given that different individuals may have various abilities and strategies to cope with stress at various life stages [22,23], and that substance use is one common but improper coping strategy [24,25], it is possible that disclosure of sexual orientation at a specific life stage may increase the risk of substance use in sexual minority individuals.

With regard to social factors associated with substance use, social support from peers and family contributes to the mental health of sexual minority individuals [26,27]. Illegal substance use in sexual minority individuals has been previously reported to be associated with family rejection [28]. Individuals who perceived high levels of peer support were more likely to use legal substances, such as cigarettes, compared with those who perceived low levels of peer support [29–31]. In addition to family and peers, schools are also an important social environment that can affect the growth of most individuals. Research has revealed that low academic performance in school is associated with substance use and emotional distress in sexual minority individuals [32]. Moreover, missing classes, truancy, and substance use are presentations of a poor adjustment to school life [33]. However, no study has taken the association between illegal substance use and multiple social factors, including social family support, peer support, satisfaction with academic performance, missing classes, and truancy, into consideration in sexual minority individual.

1.3. Association between Homophobic Bullying and Substance Abuse in Sexual Minority Individuals

Homophobic bullying is also a noteworthy issue for sexual minorities. Homophobia is defined as negative beliefs, attitudes, and behaviors toward Lesbian, gay, bisexual and transgender (LGBT) individuals [34]. A meta-analytic study revealed higher rates of depression and suicide in LGBT individuals [35]. Mental health problems are reported to be mainly a result of negative life experiences, including homophobic bullying [36]. Sexual minority individuals may encounter stress associated with unfriendly social environments full of prejudice and discrimination, which may lead to mental health problems [37,38]. Furthermore, homophobic bullying in childhood and adolescence has been reported to be harmful to future psychosocial and health outcomes in adulthood [39]. Therefore, investigation into the effects of homophobic bullying can help clinicians with early intervention.

The results of previous studies on the association between homophobic bullying and substance abuse in sexual minority individuals are mixed. Although a recent study found that homophobic bullying and victimization were not significantly associated with current substance use among sexual minorities [40], another study demonstrated that lesbian, gay, and bisexual youths reporting a high level of at-school victimization reported more severe substance use than those experiencing a low level or no victimization [41]. Moreover, previous studies mainly examined the role of traditional bullying victimization for substance abuse, whereas the role of cyberbullying victimization, a new type of harassment that has emerged in the digital age [42], in substance abuse warrants further study. It has been previously reported that sexual minority youths experience higher online peer victimization compared with heterosexual youths [43]. The potential association between both traditional homophobic bullying and cyberbullying with illegal substance use in sexual minority individuals, warrants further investigation.

1.4. Aims of the Study

The aim of the present cross-sectional study was to investigate multi-dimensional factors of illegal substance use in gay and bisexual men in Taiwan. The authors suppose that there are multi-dimensional factors, including homophobic bullying victimization, sexual orientation characteristics, and family, peer, and school factors that are associated with illegal substance use in early adulthood among gay and bisexual men.

2. Materials and Methods

2.1. Participants

In the current study, we recruited participants using an online advertisement that was posted on a bulletin board system, Facebook, and the home pages of five health promotion and counseling centers for sexual minorities in Taiwan. Print versions of the advertisement were mailed to the LGBT student clubs at 25 colleges in Taiwan. Those who exhibited any cognitive impairment (e.g., substance intoxication or intellectual disability) that prevented them from understanding the goal of the study or from completing the questionnaires were not included in this study. In total, 500 gay or bisexual men aged between 20 and 25 years were recruited into this study. Before assessment, informed consent was obtained from all participants. Before the recruitment, the study was also approved by the Institutional Review Board of Kaohsiung Medical University Hospital (KMUHIRB-F(I)-20150026).

2.2. Measures

2.2.1. Illegal Substance Use

The D-score of Drug Use Disorders Identification Test-Extended (DUDIT-E) was used to identify the history of illegal substance use for all individuals. It had been developed for the sequential clinical assessment of drug use. The concurrent validity of the D-score is reported to be acceptable, and test-retest reliability is 0.79, indicating an excellent intraclass correlation [44]. The participants were asked about any previous experiences where they used marijuana, methamphetamine, cocaine, heroin, ketamine, ecstasy, hallucinogens, volatile organic compounds, and other drugs in the preceding month. Participants who had used any kind of illegal substance were classified as having illegal substance use.

2.2.2. Experiences of Homophobic Bullying and Victimization

Six items from the Chinese version of the self-report School Bullying Experience Questionnaire (C-SBEQ) [45] were used to assess the experiences of the participants with regard to traditional bullying in primary (grades 1–6), junior high (grades 7–9), and senior high (grades 10–12) schools, based on their gender role nonconformity and sexual orientation at school, tutoring schools, after-school classes, and part-time workplaces. Multiple forms of traditional homophobic bullying victimization were evaluated, including name calling, social exclusion, ill speaking, forced work, physical abuse, and confiscation of money, school supplies, and snacks. The responses for these six items were graded on a 4-point Likert scale as following: 0 = never, 1 = just a little, 2 = often, and 3 = all the time. A previous investigation on C-SBEQ psychometrics revealed that the C-SBEQ has acceptable validity and reliability [45]. The Cronbach α value of the scale for evaluating the homophobic bullying victimization was 0.82. In this study, participants who rated 2 to 3 for any item were identified as self-reported victims of homophobic traditional bullying. In order to group the subtype of traditional bullying, we categorized social exclusion into "social bullying", name calling along with ill speaking into "verbal bullying", physical along with forced work into "physical abuse", and confiscation of money/supplies into "snatching of belongings".

Three items from the Cyberbullying Experiences Questionnaire [46] were also used to evaluate the participants' cyber bullying experiences in elementary, junior high, and senior high schools based on their gender role nonconformity and sexual orientation. These three items described the experiences of others posting mean or hurtful comments, others posting upsetting photos, pictures, or videos, and online rumor-spreading through blogs, emails, social media platforms (Facebook, Twitter, Plurk), and pictures or videos. An example of the questions is as follows: "How often have other students posted mean or hurtful comments about you through emails, blogs, or social media because they thought of you as a sissy (they found you homosexual or bisexual)?" The responses to these items were graded on a 4-point Likert scale, with scores ranging from 0 (never) to 3 (all the time). The Cronbach α value of the scales for evaluating homophobic cyberbullying victimization was 0.81. In this study, participants who rated 1 for any item were marked as self-reported victims of homophobic cyberbullying.

2.2.3. Demographic and Family Characteristics

Data were recorded on the participants' age, educational level, parental marriage status, and paternal and maternal education levels. We divided included participants were into those with high education levels (college or above) and those with low education levels (high school or below). We also grouped participants into those with high parental education levels (parents completed 9 years of compulsory fundamental education) and those with low parental education levels (parents did not complete 9 years of compulsory fundamental education).

2.2.4. Sexual Orientation Characteristics

The sexual orientation of participants (homosexual or bisexual) and disclosure of sexual orientation to others at primary school, junior high school, senior high school, and college, was recorded.

2.2.5. Social Support

The Chinese version of the 5-item self-administered Family Adaptation, Partnership, Growth, Affection, Resolve (APGAR) Index was used to estimate participants' satisfaction with different domains of family support during their childhood and adolescence [47,48]. Each item was rated on a 4-point Likert scale, with scores ranging from 0 (never) to 3 (always). The Family APGAR Index was also transformed into the Peer APGAR Index to identify the participants' satisfaction with different domains of their peer support during childhood and adolescence. Higher total scores on the Family and Peer APGAR indices stood for higher levels of family and peer support, respectively. The Cronbach α values for the Family and Peer APGAR indices in the present study were 0.86 and 0.87, respectively.

2.2.6. School Characteristics

We invited participants to retrospectively remind their subjective satisfaction with their academic performance in primary, junior high, and senior high schools using the 4-point Likert scale, ranging from 0 (very satisfied) to 3 (not satisfied at all). In this study, participants who answered 2 or 3 were identified as dissatisfied with their academic performance. The tendency to miss classes or truancy in elementary, junior high, and senior high schools was evaluated using a 4-point Likert scale, ranging from 0 (never) to 3 (very frequent). In this study, all participants who did not answer 0 on any item were classified as having a tendency to miss classes or truancy.

2.3. Procedure

This study was performed as a paper-and-pencil questionnaire. Assistants in our research team individually explained the procedures and methods for completing the research questionnaires to the participants. The participants could ask any question when they faced difficulties in completing the questionnaires, and the research assistants would answer them.

2.4. Statistical Analysis

Initially, we summarized the demographic, sexual orientation, family, school, and social support characteristics in Table 1. In order to estimate the odds ratio (OR) for multiple variables, univariate logistic regression was used to identify potential predictors associated with illegal substance use. Second, all potential predictive variables ($p < 0.05$) identified from the first step were selected in a forward stepwise logistic regression model to determine the best predictors for illegal substance use. All tests were 2-tailed, and statistical significance was set at $p < 0.05$. All data were processed using SPSS version 23.0 for Windows (SPSS Inc., Chicago, IL, USA).

Table 1. Demographic factors and sexual orientation-related experiences associated with illegal substance use examined by univariate logistic regression ($N = 500$).

Variables	Mean	SD	B	OR	95% CI	p
Age (years)	22.94	1.57	0.13	1.14	0.86–1.51	0.370
	n	%	B	OR	95.0% of CI	p
Education level						
High (college or above)	450	90				
Low (high school or below)	50	10	1.31	3.70	1.38–9.94	**0.009**
Sexual orientation identity						
Gay	371	74.2				
Bisexual	129	25.8	−0.47	0.63	0.21–1.89	0.407
Time to disclose sexual orientation						
At elementary school						
No	476	95.2				
Yes	24	4.8	0.73	2.07	0.46–9.43	0.346
At junior high school						
No	365	73				
Yes	135	27	1.64	5.16	2.11–12.6	**<0.001**
At senior high school						
No	215	43				
Yes	285	57	0.98	2.66	0.97–7.34	0.058
At college or above						
No	53	10.6				
Yes	447	89.4	0.94	2.56	0.34–19.45	0.363
Victims of homophobic bullying						
Traditional bullying						
No	310	62				
Yes	190	38	1.10	3.00	1.24–7.32	**0.015**
Cyberbullying						
No	299	59.8				
Yes	201	40.2	1.44	4.22	1.62–10.98	**0.003**

CI = Confidence interval; OR = Odds ratio, ratio of odds of illegal substance use versus non-use among participants; SD = Standard deviation; bold values indicate statistical significance.

3. Results

3.1. Patient Variables

A total of 500 males, 371 gay men and 129 bisexual men participated in the current study. The mean age of the participants was 22.94 ± 1.57, and 22 (4.4%) men reported using illegal substances in the preceding month. Illegal substance use by the participants included cannabis ($n = 4$; 0.8%), methamphetamines ($n = 7$; 1.4%), ketamine ($n = 1$; 0.2%), inhalants ($n = 1$; 0.2%), and poly-substance use ($n = 9$; 1.8%). The frequency of illegal substance use was as follows: marijuana (never used: 99%; ever used but less than once per month: 1%), methamphetamine (never used: 97%; ever used but less than once per month: 1.8%; once per month but less than twice per month: 0.2%; twice to four times per month: 1%), ketamine (never used: 98.6%; ever used but less than once per month: 1.2%; once per month but less than twice per month: 0.2%), ecstasy (never used: 98.8%; ever used but less than once per month: 1%; once per month but less than twice per month: 0.2%), volatile organic compounds (never used: 99.6%; ever used but less than once per month: 0.2%; twice to thrice per week: 0.2%). The frequency of bullying was as follows: traditional bullying (never: 13%; just a little: 49%; often/all the time: 38%) and cyberbullying (never: 59.8%; just a little: 32.6%; often/all the time: 7.6%). The demographic and sexual orientation characteristics of all individuals are listed in Table 1. The family and school characteristics and social support findings are listed in Table 2.

Table 2. Family, peer, and school factors associated with illegal substance use examined by univariate logistic regression ($N = 500$).

Variables	Mean	SD	B	OR	95% CI	p
Perceived family support on the APGAR	8.49	3.83	−0.08	0.93	0.83–1.03	0.179
Perceived peer support on the APGAR	11.42	2.89	−0.02	0.98	0.85–1.13	0.807
	n	%	B	OR	95.0% CI	p
Parental marital status						
Married and living together [a]	328	65.6	-	-	-	-
Separated or divorced	136	27.2	−0.11	0.90	0.34–2.35	0.830
Widowed	36	7.2	−18.23	<0.001	<0.01–<0.01	0.998
Paternal education level						
High (senior high school or above)	385	77				
Low (junior high school or below)	115	23	−0.02	0.98	0.36–2.72	0.975
Maternal education level						
High (senior high school or above)	388	77.6				
Low (junior high school or below)	112	22.4	0.28	1.32	0.51–3.45	0.576
Satisfaction with academic performance						
In elementary school						
High	401	80.2				
Low	99	19.8	0.18	1.20	0.43–3.34	0.725
In junior high school						
High	336	67.2				
Low	164	32.8	0.75	2.21	0.9–5.01	0.085
In senior high school						
High	310	62.0				
Low	190	38.0	0.32	1.38	0.58–3.26	0.463
Miss classes or truancy						
In elementary school						
No	456	91.2				
Yes	44	8.8	0.52	1.68	0.48–5.93	0.418
In junior high school						
No	414	82.8				
Yes	86	17.2	0.07	1.07	0.35–3.25	0.901
In senior high school						
No	359	71.8				
Yes	141	28.2	0.99	2.68	1.13–6.32	**0.025**

CI = Confidence interval; OR = Odds ratio; SD = Standard deviation; [a]: reference; bold values indicate statistical significance; bold values indicate statistical significance.

3.2. Predictors of Illegal Substance Use

The results of the univariate logistic regression analysis showed that victims of homophobic traditional bullying in school (OR = 3.00; p = 0.015), victims of homophobic cyberbullying in school (OR = 4.22; p = 0.003), disclosure of sexual orientation at junior high school (OR = 5.16; p < 0.001), lower education level (OR = 3.70; p = 0.009), and missing classes or truancy in senior high school (OR = 2.68; p = 0.025) were significantly associated with the use of illegal substances (Tables 1 and 2). Moreover, the association between subtypes of traditional bullying and specific illegal substance were also identified by univariate logistic regression. We found that social bullying was significantly associated with use of methamphetamine (OR = 5.52; p = 0.028). On the other hand, there was an insignificant trend of association between use of marijuana versus snatching of belongings (OR = 10.00; p = 0.051), and use of methamphetamine versus verbal bullying (OR = 4.79; p = 0.063).

The results of the forward stepwise logistic regression revealed that victims of homophobic cyberbullying in school (OR = 1.26; p = 0.011), disclosure of sexual orientation at junior high school (OR = 4.67; p = 0.001), and missing classes or truancy in senior high school (OR = 2.52; p = 0.041) were significantly associated with the use of illegal substances (Table 3).

Table 3. Predictors of illegal substance use examined using forward stepwise logistical regression.

Variables	B	OR	95% CI	p
Disclosure of sexual orientation at junior high school	1.54	4.67	1.88–11.58	0.001
Miss classes or truancy in senior high school	0.93	2.52	1.04–6.13	0.041
Victims of homophobic cyberbullying	1.26	3.51	1.33–9.30	0.011

OR = Odds ratio; bold values indicate statistical significance.

4. Discussion

The present study reports that 4.4% of gay and bisexual men used illegal substances in the preceding month, and that multi-dimensional factors were associated with illegal substance use among gay and bisexual men, including homophobic cyberbullying victimization in childhood and adolescence, disclosure of sexual orientation at junior high school, and missing classes or truancy in senior high school.

4.1. Rate of Illegal Substance Use in Sexual Minorities

The reported prevalence of illegal substance use in gay and bisexual men varies depending on the participants' age and periods of substance use surveyed. For example, a national survey in the United States showed a lifetime prevalence of substance-dependence of 5.7% for gay and bisexual men [49]. Whereas O'Cleirigh and colleagues reported a drug use rate of 53.1% among HIV-infected gay and bisexual men over the past three months [50]. The present study focused on a group of gay and bisexual men aged between 20 and 25 years. The rate of illegal substance use among gay and bisexual men of different ages in Taiwan warrants further study.

4.2. Homophobic Traditional and Cyber Victimization and Illegal Substance Use in Sexual Minorities

The results of the univariate logistic regression in the present study revealed that homophobic traditional victimization in childhood and adolescence was significantly associated with illegal substance use in early adulthood among gay and bisexual men. Sexual minority adolescents were more likely to experience homophobic bullying and illegal substance use compared with heterosexual individuals [40]. Another study proved the association between homophobic bullying victimization in school and substance abuse among LGBT adolescents [51]. Although in the present study, the association between homophobic traditional bullying and illegal substance use became insignificant after the multivariate logistic regression, the negative effects of homophobic traditional bullying on mental health and illegal substance use in sexual minority individuals still warrants monitoring and intervention. Research has found that anti-homophobic bullying policies, which are properly carried out, can significantly decrease the risk of alcohol and drug use among sexual minorities [52].

The present study found that homophobic cyberbullying victimization in childhood and adolescence is a powerful predictor of illegal substance use in early adulthood. Cyberbullying has different characteristics compared with traditional bullying, such as anonymity and individualistic activity [53]. Cyberbullies have lower neuroticism and higher agreeableness in comparison with traditional bullies [54]. For victims, a study of general adolescents demonstrated that compared with those who were only traditionally bullied, those who were cyberbullied were more likely to have depression, anxiety, and aggression [55]. The present study further supported the unique role of homophobic cyberbullying victimization in childhood and adolescence, in the use of illegal substances in early childhood. These results demonstrate the necessity of prevention, early detection, and intervention for homophobic cyberbullying among sexual minority individuals. Anti-bullying policies that are inclusive of sexual orientation [56] and Gay-Straight Alliances [57] are beneficial for LGBT individuals who suffer from traditional or cyber bullying. On the other hand, the significant association between homophobic bullying and illegal substance use can also be explained by MST [12]. Chronic stressors will accumulate and make subjects unable to tolerate and adopt, resulting in mental and substance use disorder [58]. In specific to sexual minorities, MST suggests that both distal (social) and proximal (psychological) stress are predominantly associated with poor health outcomes [38]. The result of the current study echoes the association between social stressors (homophobic bullying) and mental health concerns.

4.3. Disclosure of Sexual Orientation and Illegal Substance Use in Sexual Minorities

The present study found that disclosure of sexual orientation at junior high school was significantly associated with illegal substance use in early adulthood. Gay and bisexual adolescents at junior high school may lack effective coping strategies because of immature neurocognitive functions [59] and social skills [60]. Those individuals who come out in early adolescence may be less able to cope effectively with stressors related to the stigma of sexual minority identification, and they may struggle to deal with bullying incidents compared with those who reach sexual orientation milestones in their late adolescence or young adulthood. This can lead to negative mental health outcomes such as depression and anxiety [61,62]. Illegal substance use may be an ineffective strategy used by them to cope with stress. It is interesting to note that disclosure of sexual orientation at elementary school was not significantly associated with illegal substance use in early adulthood. The rate of participants in the present study who disclosed their sexual orientation at elementary school was less than 5%, which may limit the ability to draw conclusions on the relationship between disclosure of sexual orientation at elementary school and later illegal substance use. In addition, sexual orientation may not be the focus of attention among students at elementary school; therefore, sexual minorities may encounter severe difficulties in sexual orientation related adjustment that may increase their risk of later illegal substance use.

4.4. School Factors Associated with Illegal Substance Use in Sexual Minorities

Researchers have previously investigated the role of school performance and issues of mental health among sexual minorities [63]. The present study found that missing classes or truancy in senior high school was significantly associated with illegal substance use in early adulthood. For school children and adolescents, truancy was found to be significantly associated with substance use [64], and another study showed similar results [65]. However, no further studies have explored this association among sexual minorities, and the present study fills this gap in the literature. The univariate logistic regression analysis in the present study found that a low education level was significantly associated with illegal substance use in early adulthood, although the association became insignificant following multiple adjusted logistic regression analysis. A previous study reported that men with a lower educational level were at a higher risk of being hazardous drinkers and heavy cannabis users [66]. The cross-sectional research design of the present study limited the ability to determine the temporal causal relationship between a low education level and illegal substance use in gay and bisexual men. Further prospective studies are needed to examine whether both low education level and illegal substance use are the results of minority stress encountered by gay and bisexual men.

4.5. Family and Peer Support and Illegal Substance Use in Sexual Minorities

Family acceptance to sexual minorities predicts greater self-esteem and general health status among LGBT individuals [67]. More LGBT-supportive environments in school and communities may also predict less substance use for LGBT adolescents [68]. However, the present study did not find a significant association between family and peer support during childhood and adolescence, and illegal substance use in early adulthood. Although support from peers and family during childhood and adolescent was measured, the individuals current support was not measured, which may strongly contribute to current substance use.

4.6. Limitations

Several limitations of the current study should be addressed. First, as a cross-sectional study, it was not possible to determine causal relationships between homophobic bullying victimization and school factors in childhood and adolescence and illegal substance use in early adulthood. Second, the study data were exclusively self-reported. Therefore, the use of only a single data source could have influenced the findings and may have resulted in shared-method variances. Third, the study obtained data on participants' homophobic bullying victimization, school factors, and family and peer support retrospectively, and therefore, recall bias might have been introduced. Finally, only gay and bisexual men were recruited into this study. Potential implications for lesbian or other sexual minorities is lacking. Therefore, the generalizability of this study is limited.

5. Conclusions

The present study revealed that homophobic cyberbullying victimization in childhood and adolescence, disclosure of sexual orientation at junior high school, and missing classes or truancy in senior high school were significantly associated with illegal substance use in early adulthood. Based on the results of the current study, the authors suggest that mental health professionals should routinely assess the experiences and impact of homophobic cyberbullying victimization in childhood and adolescence when approaching gay and bisexual men with illegal substance use. Timely referral to gay-affirmative cognitive behavioral therapy [69] for victims of homophobic bullying during their youth, could help prevent those using illegal substances to cope with these traumatic experiences. Moreover, the underlying reasons behind the significant association between disclosure of sexual orientation at junior high school and missing classes or truancy in senior high school with illegal substance use in early adulthood, warrants further investigation. These findings could then provide knowledge for the development of a prevention and early intervention strategy for illegal substance use in gay and bisexual men.

Author Contributions: D.-J.L., the first author, takes the responsibility of writing this manuscript. S.-L.C., contributes to data analysis and revises the manuscript. C.-F.Y., the corresponding author, takes all the responsibility of collecting all the information from the other authors, revising the manuscript, and submitting the manuscript.

Funding: The present study was supported by the Ministry of Science and Technology, Taiwan, R.O.C. (grant no. MOST 104-2314-B-037-024-MY3) and the Kaohsiung Medical University Hospital (grant nos. KMUH104-4R60, KMUH105-5R59 and KMUH106-6R67).

Conflicts of Interest: The authors declare no conflict of interest.

References

1. United Nations Office on Drugs and Crime. *World Drug Report*; UN iLiarary: New York, NY, USA, 2018.
2. Choenni, V.; Hammink, A.; van de Mheen, D. Association Between Substance Use and the Perpetration of Family Violence in Industrialized Countries: A Systematic Review. *Trauma Violence Abus.* **2017**, *18*, 37–50. [CrossRef] [PubMed]
3. Nordfjaern, T. Violence involvement among nightlife patrons: The relative role of demographics and substance use. *Aggress. Behav.* **2017**, *43*, 398–407. [CrossRef] [PubMed]
4. Skjaervo, I.; Skurtveit, S.; Clausen, T.; Bukten, A. Substance use pattern, self-control and social network are associated with crime in a substance-using population. *Drug Alcohol Rev.* **2017**, *36*, 245–252. [CrossRef] [PubMed]
5. Hawton, K.; van Heeringen, K. Suicide. *Lancet* **2009**, *373*, 1372–1381. [CrossRef]
6. Tolliver, B.K.; Anton, R.F. Assessment and treatment of mood disorders in the context of substance abuse. *Dialogues Clin. Neurosci* **2015**, *17*, 181–190.
7. Hagan, H.; Des Jarlais, D.C. HIV and HCV infection among injecting drug users. *Mt. Sinai J. Med.* **2000**, *67*, 423–428.
8. Kerridge, B.T.; Pickering, R.P.; Saha, T.D.; Ruan, W.J.; Chou, S.P.; Zhang, H.; Jung, J.; Hasin, D.S. Prevalence, sociodemographic correlates and DSM-5 substance use disorders and other psychiatric disorders among sexual minorities in the United States. *Drug Alcohol Depend.* **2017**, *170*, 82–92. [CrossRef]
9. Ko, N.Y.; Koe, S.; Lee, H.C.; Yen, C.F.; Ko, W.C.; Hsu, S.T. Online sex-seeking, substance use, and risky behaviors in Taiwan: Results from the 2010 Asia Internet MSM Sex Survey. *Arch. Sex. Behav.* **2012**, *41*, 1273–1282. [CrossRef]
10. Chen, W.J.; Wu, S.C.; Tsay, W.I.; Chen, Y.T.; Hsiao, P.C.; Yu, Y.H.; Ting, T.T.; Chen, C.Y.; Tu, Y.K.; Huang, J.H.; et al. Differences in prevalence, socio-behavioral correlates, and psychosocial distress between club drug and hard drug use in Taiwan: Results from the 2014 National Survey of Substance Use. *Int. J. Drug Policy* **2017**, *48*, 99–107. [CrossRef]
11. Stall, R.; Mills, T.C.; Williamson, J.; Hart, T.; Greenwood, G.; Paul, J.; Pollack, L.; Binson, D.; Osmond, D.; Catania, J.A. Association of co-occurring psychosocial health problems and increased vulnerability to HIV/AIDS among urban men who have sex with men. *Am. J. Public Health* **2003**, *93*, 939–942. [CrossRef]
12. Meyer, I.H. Minority stress and mental health in gay men. *J. Health Soc. Behav.* **1995**, *36*, 38–56. [CrossRef] [PubMed]
13. Goldbach, J.T.; Schrager, S.M.; Dunlap, S.L.; Holloway, I.W. The application of minority stress theory to marijuana use among sexual minority adolescents. *Subst. Use Misuse* **2015**, *50*, 366–375. [CrossRef]
14. Bronfenbrenner, U. Six theories of child development: Revised formulations and current issues. In *Ecological Systems Theory*; Vasta, R., Ed.; Jessica Kingsley: Philadelphia, UK, 2002; pp. 221–288.
15. Demant, D.; Hides, L.; Kavanagh, D.J.; White, K.M.; Winstock, A.R.; Ferris, J. Differences in substance use between sexual orientations in a multi-country sample: Findings from the Global Drug Survey 2015. *J. Public Health (Oxf.)* **2017**, *39*, 532–541. [CrossRef] [PubMed]
16. Dermody, S.S. Risk of polysubstance use among sexual minority and heterosexual youth. *Drug Alcohol Depend.* **2018**, *192*, 38–44. [CrossRef] [PubMed]
17. Kipke, M.D.; Weiss, G.; Ramirez, M.; Dorey, F.; Ritt-Olson, A.; Iverson, E.; Ford, W. Club drug use in los angeles among young men who have sex with men. *Subst. Use Misuse* **2007**, *42*, 1723–1743. [CrossRef] [PubMed]
18. Klitzman, R.L.; Greenberg, J.D.; Pollack, L.M.; Dolezal, C. MDMA ('ecstasy') use, and its association with high risk behaviors, mental health, and other factors among gay/bisexual men in New York City. *Drug Alcohol Depend.* **2002**, *66*, 115–125. [CrossRef]
19. Wong, C.F.; Kipke, M.D.; Weiss, G. Risk factors for alcohol use, frequent use, and binge drinking among young men who have sex with men. *Addict. Behav.* **2008**, *33*, 1012–1020. [CrossRef]
20. Rosario, M.; Schrimshaw, E.W.; Hunter, J. Predictors of substance use over time among gay, lesbian, and bisexual youths: An examination of three hypotheses. *Addict. Behav.* **2004**, *29*, 1623–1631. [CrossRef]
21. Wright, E.R.; Perry, B.L. Sexual identity distress, social support, and the health of gay, lesbian, and bisexual youth. *J. Homosex.* **2006**, *51*, 81–110. [CrossRef]

22. Hamarat, E.; Thompson, D.; Zabrucky, K.M.; Steele, D.; Matheny, K.B.; Aysan, F. Perceived stress and coping resource availability as predictors of life satisfaction in young, middle-aged, and older adults. *Exp. Aging Res.* **2001**, *27*, 181–196. [CrossRef]
23. Zimmer-Gembeck, M.J.; Skinner, E.A. Review: The development of coping across childhood and adolescence: An integrative review and critique of research. *Int. J. Behav. Dev.* **2011**, *35*, 1–17. [CrossRef]
24. Holahan, C.J.; Moos, R.H.; Holahan, C.K.; Cronkite, R.C.; Randall, P.K. Drinking to cope, emotional distress and alcohol use and abuse: A ten-year model. *J. Stud. Alcohol* **2001**, *62*, 190–198. [CrossRef]
25. Mauro, P.M.; Canham, S.L.; Martins, S.S.; Spira, A.P. Substance-use coping and self-rated health among US middle-aged and older adults. *Addict. Behav.* **2015**, *42*, 96–100. [CrossRef]
26. McConnell, E.A.; Birkett, M.; Mustanski, B. Families Matter: Social Support and Mental Health Trajectories Among Lesbian, Gay, Bisexual, and Transgender Youth. *J. Adolesc Health* **2016**, *59*, 674–680. [CrossRef]
27. Prestage, G.; Brown, G.; Allan, B.; Ellard, J.; Down, I. Impact of Peer Support on Behavior Change Among Newly Diagnosed Australian Gay Men. *J. Acquir. Immune Defic. Syndr.* **2016**, *72*, 565–571. [CrossRef]
28. Ryan, C.; Huebner, D.; Diaz, R.M.; Sanchez, J. Family rejection as a predictor of negative health outcomes in white and Latino lesbian, gay, and bisexual young adults. *Pediatrics* **2009**, *123*, 346–352. [CrossRef]
29. Kirke, D.M. Chain reactions in adolescents' cigarette, alcohol and drug use: Similarity through peer influence or the patterning of ties in peer networks? *Soc. Netw.* **2004**, *26*, 3–28. [CrossRef]
30. Wang, C.; Hipp, J.R.; Butts, C.T.; Jose, R.; Lakon, C.M. Coevolution of adolescent friendship networks and smoking and drinking behaviors with consideration of parental influence. *Psychol. Addict. Behav.* **2016**, *30*, 312–324. [CrossRef]
31. Wills, T.A.; Vaughan, R. Social support and substance use in early adolescence. *J. Behav. Med.* **1989**, *12*, 321–339. [CrossRef]
32. Pearson, J.; Muller, C.; Wilkinson, L. Adolescent Same-Sex Attraction and Academic Outcomes: The Role of School Attachment and Engagement. *Soc. Probl.* **2007**, *54*, 523–542. [CrossRef]
33. Henry, K.L.; Thornberry, T.P. Truancy and escalation of substance use during adolescence. *J. Stud. Alcohol Drugs* **2010**, *71*, 115–124. [CrossRef]
34. Wright, L.W.; Adams, H.E.; Bernat, J. Development and Validation of the Homophobia Scale. *J. Psychopathol. Behav. Assess.* **1999**, *21*, 337–347. [CrossRef]
35. Marshal, M.P.; Dietz, L.J.; Friedman, M.S.; Stall, R.; Smith, H.A.; McGinley, J.; Thoma, B.C.; Murray, P.J.; D'Augelli, A.R.; Brent, D.A. Suicidality and depression disparities between sexual minority and heterosexual youth: A meta-analytic review. *J. Adolesc Health* **2011**, *49*, 115–123. [CrossRef]
36. Sandfort, T.G.; Melendez, R.M.; Diaz, R.M. Gender nonconformity, homophobia, and mental distress in latino gay and bisexual men. *J. Sex. Res.* **2007**, *44*, 181–189. [CrossRef]
37. Burton, C.M.; Marshal, M.P.; Chisolm, D.J.; Sucato, G.S.; Friedman, M.S. Sexual minority-related victimization as a mediator of mental health disparities in sexual minority youth: A longitudinal analysis. *J. Youth Adolesc* **2013**, *42*, 394–402. [CrossRef]
38. Meyer, I.H. Prejudice, social stress, and mental health in lesbian, gay, and bisexual populations: Conceptual issues and research evidence. *Psychol. Bull.* **2003**, *129*, 674–697. [CrossRef]
39. Birkett, M.; Newcomb, M.E.; Mustanski, B. Does it get better? A longitudinal analysis of psychological distress and victimization in lesbian, gay, bisexual, transgender, and questioning youth. *J. Adolesc Health* **2015**, *56*, 280–285. [CrossRef]
40. Mereish, E.H.; Goldbach, J.T.; Burgess, C.; DiBello, A.M. Sexual orientation, minority stress, social norms, and substance use among racially diverse adolescents. *Drug Alcohol Depend.* **2017**, *178*, 49–56. [CrossRef]
41. Bontempo, D.E.; D'Augelli, A.R. Effects of at-school victimization and sexual orientation on lesbian, gay, or bisexual youths' health risk behavior. *J. Adolesc Health* **2002**, *30*, 364–374. [CrossRef]
42. Kowalski, R.M.; Limber, S.; Agatston, P.W. *Cyberbullying: Bullying in the Digital Age*, 2nd ed.; Wiley-Blackwell: Malden, MA, USA, 2012.
43. Ybarra, M.L.; Mitchell, K.J.; Palmer, N.A.; Reisner, S.L. Online social support as a buffer against online and offline peer and sexual victimization among U.S. LGBT and non-LGBT youth. *Child Abuse Negl.* **2015**, *39*, 123–136. [CrossRef]
44. Berman, A.H.; Palmstierna, T.; Kallmen, H.; Bergman, H. The self-report Drug Use Disorders Identification Test: Extended (DUDIT-E): Reliability, validity, and motivational index. *J. Subst. Abuse Treat.* **2007**, *32*, 357–369. [CrossRef]

45. Yen, C.F.; Kim, Y.S.; Tang, T.C.; Wu, Y.Y.; Cheng, C.P. Factor structure, reliability, and validity of the Chinese version of the School Bullying Experience Questionnaire. *Kaohsiung J. Med. Sci.* **2012**, *28*, 500–505. [CrossRef]
46. Yen, C.F.; Chou, W.J.; Liu, T.L.; Ko, C.H.; Yang, P.; Hu, H.F. Cyberbullying among male adolescents with attention-deficit/hyperactivity disorder: Prevalence, correlates, and association with poor mental health status. *Res. Dev. Disabil.* **2014**, *35*, 3543–3553. [CrossRef]
47. Chen, Y.C.; Hsu, C.C.; Hsu, S.H.; Lin, C.C. A Preliminary Study of Family Apgar Index. *Acta Paediatr. Sin.* **1980**, *21*, 210–217.
48. Smilkstein, G. The family APGAR: A proposal for a family function test and its use by physicians. *J. Fam. Pract.* **1978**, *6*, 1231–1239.
49. Cochran, S.D.; Ackerman, D.; Mays, V.M.; Ross, M.W. Prevalence of non-medical drug use and dependence among homosexually active men and women in the US population. *Addiction* **2004**, *99*, 989–998. [CrossRef]
50. O'Cleirigh, C.; Magidson, J.F.; Skeer, M.R.; Mayer, K.H.; Safren, S.A. Prevalence of Psychiatric and Substance Abuse Symptomatology Among HIV-Infected Gay and Bisexual Men in HIV Primary Care. *Psychosomatics* **2015**, *56*, 470–478. [CrossRef]
51. Flores, J.M.; Santos, G.M.; Makofane, K.; Arreola, S.; Ayala, G. Availability and Use of Substance Abuse Treatment Programs Among Substance-Using Men Who Have Sex With Men Worldwide. *Subst. Use Misuse* **2017**, *52*, 666–673. [CrossRef]
52. Konishi, C.; Saewyc, E.; Homma, Y.; Poon, C. Population-level evaluation of school-based interventions to prevent problem substance use among gay, lesbian and bisexual adolescents in Canada. *Prev. Med.* **2013**, *57*, 929–933. [CrossRef]
53. Dehue, F.; Bolman, C.; Vollink, T. Cyberbullying: youngsters' experiences and parental perception. *Cyberpsychol. Behav.* **2008**, *11*, 217–223. [CrossRef]
54. Resett, S.; Gamez-Guadix, M. Traditional bullying and cyberbullying: Differences in emotional problems, and personality. Are cyberbullies more Machiavellians? *J. Adolesc.* **2017**, *61*, 113–116. [CrossRef]
55. Waasdorp, T.E.; Bradshaw, C.P. The overlap between cyberbullying and traditional bullying. *J. Adolesc. Health* **2015**, *56*, 483–488. [CrossRef]
56. Hatzenbuehler, M.L.; Keyes, K.M. Inclusive anti-bullying policies and reduced risk of suicide attempts in lesbian and gay youth. *J. Adolesc. Health* **2013**, *53*, S21–S26. [CrossRef]
57. Toomey, R.B.; Ryan, C.; Diaz, R.M.; Russell, S.T. High School Gay-Straight Alliances (GSAs) and Young Adult Well-Being: An Examination of GSA Presence, Participation, and Perceived Effectiveness. *Appl. Dev. Sci.* **2011**, *15*, 175–185. [CrossRef]
58. Brady, K.T.; Sinha, R. Co-occurring mental and substance use disorders: The neurobiological effects of chronic stress. *Am. J. Psychiatry* **2005**, *162*, 1483–1493. [CrossRef]
59. Casey, B.J.; Jones, R.M.; Hare, T.A. The adolescent brain. *Ann. N. Y. Acad. Sci.* **2008**, *1124*, 111–126. [CrossRef]
60. Alikasifoglu, M.; Erginoz, E.; Ercan, O.; Uysal, O.; Albayrak-Kaymak, D. Bullying behaviours and psychosocial health: Results from a cross-sectional survey among high school students in Istanbul, Turkey. *Eur. J. Pediatr.* **2007**, *166*, 1253–1260. [CrossRef]
61. Friedman, M.S.; Marshal, M.P.; Stall, R.; Cheong, J.; Wright, E.R. Gay-related development, early abuse and adult health outcomes among gay males. *AIDS Behav.* **2008**, *12*, 891–902. [CrossRef]
62. Katz-Wise, S.L.; Rosario, M.; Calzo, J.P.; Scherer, E.A.; Sarda, V.; Austin, S.B. Associations of Timing of Sexual Orientation Developmental Milestones and Other Sexual Minority Stressors with Internalizing Mental Health Symptoms Among Sexual Minority Young Adults. *Arch. Sex. Behav.* **2017**, *46*, 1441–1452. [CrossRef]
63. Poteat, V.P.; Scheer, J.R.; Mereish, E.H. Factors affecting academic achievement among sexual minority and gender-variant youth. *Adv. Child Dev. Behav.* **2014**, *47*, 261–300.
64. Peltzer, K. Prevalence and correlates of substance use among school children in six African countries. *Int. J. Psychol.* **2009**, *44*, 378–386. [CrossRef]
65. Egger, H.L.; Costello, E.J.; Angold, A. School refusal and psychiatric disorders: A community study. *J. Am. Acad. Child Adolesc Psychiatry* **2003**, *42*, 797–807. [CrossRef]
66. Teixido-Compano, E.; Espelt, A.; Sordo, L.; Bravo, M.J.; Sarasa-Renedo, A.; Indave, B.I.; Bosque-Prous, M.; Brugal, M.T. Differences between men and women in substance use: The role of educational level and employment status. *Gac. Sanit.* **2018**, *32*, 41–47. [CrossRef]

67. Ryan, C.; Russell, S.T.; Huebner, D.; Diaz, R.; Sanchez, J. Family acceptance in adolescence and the health of LGBT young adults. *J. Child Adolesc Psychiatr. Nurs.* **2010**, *23*, 205–213. [CrossRef]
68. Eisenberg, M.E.; Erickson, D.J.; Gower, A.L.; Kne, L.; Watson, R.J.; Corliss, H.L.; Saewyc, E.M. Supportive Community Resources Are Associated with Lower Risk of Substance Use among Lesbian, Gay, Bisexual, and Questioning Adolescents in Minnesota. *J. Youth Adolesc.* **2019**, 1–13. [CrossRef]
69. Craig, S.L.; Austin, A.; Alessi, E. Gay affirmative cognitive behavioral therapy for sexual minority youth: A clinical adaptation. *Clin. Soc. Work J.* **2013**, *41*, 258–266. [CrossRef]

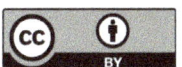

© 2019 by the authors. Licensee MDPI, Basel, Switzerland. This article is an open access article distributed under the terms and conditions of the Creative Commons Attribution (CC BY) license (http://creativecommons.org/licenses/by/4.0/).

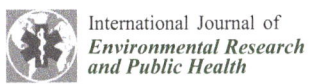

Article

Sex and Polytobacco Use among Spanish and Turkish University Students

Sílvia Font-Mayolas [1,*], Mark J. M. Sullman [2] and Maria-Eugenia Gras [1]

1. Quality of Life Research Institute, Universitat de Girona, 17071 Girona, Spain; eugenia.gras@udg.edu
2. Department of Social Sciences, University of Nicosia, Nicosia 2417, Cyprus; sullman.m@unic.ac.cy
* Correspondence: silvia.font@udg.edu

Received: 29 September 2019; Accepted: 7 December 2019; Published: 11 December 2019

Abstract: Polytobacco use has become increasingly popular among young adults, particularly males, and can be defined as the concurrent use of regular cigarettes and other tobacco products (e.g., e-cigarettes). The present study investigated the use of legal smoking products (cigarettes, waterpipe and electronic cigarettes) among young adults (n = 355) in Spain and Turkey. The survey measured demographics, lifetime and past month tobacco use, waterpipe and e-cigarette use, whether waterpipes and e-cigarettes contained nicotine and reasons for using these substances. The majority of the Turkish (men = 80% and women = 63.9%) and Spanish sample (men = 61.4% and women = 69.3%) were polytobacco users. The most common reason for using e-cigarettes was "to experiment, to see what is like" (Turkish sample: men 66.7% and women 57.1; Spanish sample: men 72.7% and women 93.8%). The most common reason to use regular cigarettes was "to relax and relieve tension" (Turkish sample: men 88.9% and women 77.6%; Spanish sample: men 78.1% and women 76%), while for waterpipe users, the most common reason was "to experiment, to see what it is like" (Turkish sample: men 93.3% and women 80%; Spanish sample: men 78.9% and women 93.8%). The implications for prevention and future research are discussed.

Keywords: electronic cigarettes; cigarettes; waterpipe; hookah; polytobacco use; young adults; sex; cognitions; attitudes

1. Introduction

Polydrug use is defined as the consumption of more than one type of drug by an individual [1]. The use of at least two different psychoactive substances among young adults is common and significantly contributes to the addiction problem [2–4].

The polydrug use phenomenon has also been described specifically among nicotine users, in what some authors have called "Polytobacco use" or the concurrent use of cigarettes and other tobacco products [5]. Alternative nicotine and tobacco products (ANTP) include electronic-cigarettes and waterpipes (also known as hookah, shisha or narghile), which have recently increased in popularity [6–9]. Hookah use has been identified as a predictor of the subsequent use of tobacco products, such as e-cigarettes [10]. Hookah use has also been found to be associated with lung cancer and other types of respiratory illness [11–13]. Furthermore, although in lower concentrations than in regular cigarettes, a number of toxic substances, including carcinogens, have been found in the vapor from electronic cigarettes [14].

The WHO Study Group on Tobacco Products Regulation identified regional patterns of waterpipe smoking with traditional use in the Eastern Mediterranean region (e.g., Turkey) and emerging use in the European region (e.g., Spain). Turkey and Spain have developed public policies to reduce cigarette use and more recently e-cigarette use. Turkey has also developed policies to reduce waterpipe use, such as the addition of warning labelling on waterpipe bowls [10], but there has been little research about waterpipe use in Spain. Investigating the current pattern of polytobacco use in those two countries could contribute to our understanding of the polytobacco use phenomenon in these two regions.

Previous research in North America has found substantial gender differences in polytobacco use, in that more males (than females) were polytobacco users and male lifetime polytobacco users were more likely to use alcohol and drugs than women [6,15]. The findings regarding waterpipe and e-cigarette use have been inconsistent, with some research finding men were more frequent users [16] and others finding no association [17,18]. Examining the different typologies of polytobacco use by sex may be a useful strategy to understand this behavior and to develop tailored interventions [19].

The main aim of the present study was to describe lifetime and current use of electronic cigarettes, regular cigarettes, waterpipes and current polytobacco use among young adults by sex and by country. The second aim was to investigate whether e-cigarettes and waterpipes were used to smoke nicotine and whether there were any sex differences. The third purpose was to examine reasons for differences in the use of e-cigarettes, regular cigarettes and waterpipes by sex and by country.

2. Materials and Methods

2.1. Participants and Procedure

A convenience sample of university students ($n = 355$) completed an online survey. Data were collected during the 2018/19 academic year. Participants were recruited using the university online platform "Moodle" in Spain and by emailing students attending a Turkish university in Northern Cyprus (Turkish).

This cross-sectional survey involved emailing a link to the students taking two compulsory courses. After clicking on the link, the students were presented with an information sheet that was followed by a page asking for their informed consent. Then students were asked to complete an online questionnaire about the prevalence of the three types of smoking behaviors. Students could complete the questionnaire in the privacy of their own rooms or homes. After completing the questionnaire, they were presented with a debriefing page and provided with details regarding how to contact the researcher, if they wanted to withdraw their data, had additional questions or wanted to know about the results. This study was approved by the Human Research Ethics Committee at Middle East Technical University—Northern Cyprus Campus.

2.2. Measures

2.2.1. Demographics

Respondents reported their sex, age and ethnicity.

2.2.2. Lifetime Use of Electronic Cigarettes, Regular Cigarettes and Waterpipe/Hookah

Participants answered the following items: "Have you ever smoked electronic cigarettes (e-cigarettes) or vaped?", "Have you ever smoked tobacco from a waterpipe (also known as hookah, shisha, narguile)?" and "Have you ever smoked regular cigarettes?". Response options were "yes/no".

2.2.3. Use of E-Cigarettes, Regular Cigarettes and Waterpipe/Hookah in the Past 30 Days

Students responded to the question "How frequently have you smoked e-cigarettes during the past 30 days?". The same question was adapted to hookah and regular cigarettes. Response options were "never", "occasionally", "once a week", "more than once a week, but not every day", and "every day".

2.2.4. E-Cigarettes and Waterpipe Nicotine Contents

Participants were asked whether they had smoked e-cigarettes during the past 30 days and whether the e-cigarettes were: "with nicotine", "without nicotine" and "with and without nicotine" [20] (Ministry of Health, Social Services and Equality, 2017). Participants that had used waterpipe/hookah during the past 30 days were also asked whether the waterpipe(s) were: "with tobacco", "with non-tobacco or herbal shisha" and "with marijuana or hashish" [21].

2.2.5. Reasons for Vaping/Smoking

Participants who reported having vaped or smoked at some time were asked "What were your main reasons for using an e-cigarette/regular cigarette/waterpipe?" [22]. Thirteen possible reasons were given: "to experiment, to see what it is like", "because it tastes good", "because of boredom, nothing else to do", "to have a good time with my friends", "to relax or relieve tension", "because it looks cool", "to help me quit regular cigarettes", "to get high", "because I am "hooked"—I have to have it", "because friends or family member used them", "because e-cigarettes/waterpipe without nicotine are less harmful than regular cigarettes", "because e-cigarettes/waterpipe with nicotine are less harmful than regular cigarettes", and "because friends or family members permitted e-cigarettes/waterpipes, more than regular cigarettes" [22,23]. Students were asked to evaluate each of the 13 reasons using the following response options: "definitely yes", "probably yes", "probably no" and "definitely no".

2.3. Analysis

All the analyses were conducted by sex and subsample. Chi-square tests and the contingency coefficient of effect size were applied to analyze lifetime and current substance use. To meet the assumptions of the chi-squared test, the categories "occasionally" and "once a week" and "more than once a week" and "every day" were combined. Chi-square tests were also used to study e-cigarette contents and to analyze reasons for vaping/smoking. The data analysis categories "definitely yes" and "probably yes" were combined and considered to be an "important reason". Further, the categories "definitely no" and "probably no" were combined and were not considered to be an "important reason". Fisher's exact test was used when expected frequencies were lower than 5. All the analyses were performed using SPSS Version 23 (IBM, Armonk, NY, USA).

3. Results

The Spanish sample was composed of 236 participants (75.4% female, mean age: 20.7 years (SD = 1.6), ethnicity: 93.6% European, 1.3% Asian, 0.4% Black, 0.4 Turkish, 4.2% Other). The Turkish sample was composed of 119 participants (68.5% female, mean age: 22.5 years (SD = 1.4), ethnicity: 95.5% Turkish, 1.8% Asian, 2.7 Other). The response rates were 90.76% in the Spanish sample and 98.34% in the Turkish sample.

3.1. Lifetime Prevalence Use

Table 1 shows the lifetime prevalence of having used e-cigarettes, regular cigarettes and waterpipes. The prevalence in Turkey was higher than in Spain, for both men and women, but these differences were only statistically significant for waterpipe consumption among men. Moreover, in both subsamples (Spanish: ($X^2_{(1)}$ = 6.2; p = 0.01; Φ = 0.16; Turkey: $X^2_{(1)}$ = 5.7; p = 0.02; Φ = 0.22) significantly more men than women had used e-cigarettes. The consumption of regular cigarettes and the use of waterpipes were similar for women and in men in both samples (Cigarettes: Spain: $X^2_{(2)}$ = 0.8; p = 0.77; Turkish: $X^2_{(1)}$ = 1.5; p = 0.22. Waterpipe: Spain: $X^2_{(2)}$ = 0.1; p = 0.73; Turkish: $X^2_{(1)}$ = 2.3; p = 0.13).

Table 1. Prevalence of e-cigarette, regular cigarette and waterpipe use by country and sex, chi-square test and contingency coefficient (effect size).

Type	Male		$X^2_{(1)}$ (p)	Φ	Female		$X^2_{(1)}$ (p)
	Spain	Turkey			Spain	Turkey	
E-cigarettes	27.6%	42.9%	2.3 (0.13)	-	13.5%	21.1%	2.3 (0.13)
Cigarettes	55.2%	71.4%	2.4 (0.12)	-	57.3%	59.2%	0.08 (0.78)
Waterpipe	60.3%	80.0%	3.9 (0.05)	0.20	62.9%	65.8%	0.19 (0.66)

There was only one male in the Turkish sample who only consumed electronic cigarettes and the consumption of electronic cigarettes with regular cigarettes or with waterpipes was also rare. The consumption of regular cigarettes with waterpipes (i.e., polytobacco use) was much more common, ranging from 19% to 36% of the participants, depending on their sex and country of origin (Table 2). Polytobacco use with e-cigarettes, regular cigarettes and waterpipes was more common among men, particularly Turkish men. Participants were placed into three groups: those who did not use any of the three substances, those who only used one, and those who used two or all three. A chi-square test was performed to compare the polytobacco use of the Spanish and Turkish men ($X^2_{(2)} = 4.3$; $p = 0.12$) and women ($X^2_{(2)} = 2.8$; $p = 0.25$), but no significant differences were found. When we compared men and women in each country, there were no significant differences in the Spanish sample ($X^2_{(2)} = 1.4$; $p = 0.50$) or in the Turkish sample ($X^2_{(2)} = 3.1$; $p = 0.22$).

Table 2. Polytobacco use by substance and sex (%).

Polytobacco Type	Male		Female	
	Spain	Turkey	Spain	Turkey
No e-cigarettes, regular cigarettes or waterpipe use	24.1%	14.3%	28.7%	19.7%
Only e-cigarette use	0%	2.9%	0%	0%
Only regular cigarette use	12.1%	2.9%	8.4%	13.2%
Only waterpipe use	17.2%	11.4%	13.5%	15.8%
E-cigarettes + regular cigarettes	3.4%	0%	0%	1.3%
E-cigarettes + waterpipe	3.4%	0%	0.6%	5.3%
Waterpipe + regular cigarettes	19%	28.6%	36%	30.3%
E-cigarettes + regular cigarettes + waterpipe	20.7%	40%	12.9%	14.5%

In total, 61.4% of Spanish men, 80% of Turkish men, 69.3% of Spanish women and 63.9% of Turkish women were classified as polytobacco users, but there were no significant differences by country (Men: $X^2_{(1)} = 2.9$; $p = 0.09$; Women: $X^2_{(1)} = 0.5$; $p = 0.46$) or sex (Spanish: $X^2_{(1)} = 0.9$; $p = 0.33$; Turkish: $X^2_{(1)} = 2.4$; $p = 0.12$).

3.2. Use in the Past 30 Days

The frequency of e-cigarette consumption over the past 30 days was similar in the Turkish sample and in the Spanish sample, both in men and women (See Table 3). The proportion of daily consumers was very low, particularly in women. If we compare the consumption of men and women in the two sub-groups, there were no significant differences in the Spanish sample ($X^2_{(2)} = 3.7$; $p = 0.15$) or the Turkish sample ($X^2_{(2)} = 3.1$; $p = 0.21$).

Table 3. Frequency of e-cigarette consumption in the past 30 days by country and sex, chi-square [1] test and contingency coefficient (effect size).

Frequency	Male		Female	
	Spain	Turkey	Spain	Turkey
Never	84.5%	68.6%	90.4%	81.6%
Occasionally	8.6%	14.3%	6.2%	10.5%
Once a week	1.7%	5.7%	2.2%	3.9%
More than once a week	1.7%	5.7%	1.1%	1.3%
Every day	3.4%	5.7%	0%	2.6%
$X^2_{(2)}$ (p)	3.3 (0.19)		4.5 (0.10)	

[1] To meet the assumptions of the chi-squared test, the categories "occasionally/once a week" and "more than once a week/every day" were combined.

The frequency of regular cigarette consumption over the past 30 days was also higher in the Turkish sample, with more than 50% of Turkish men and more than one-third of Turkish women reporting that they consumed cigarettes on a daily basis. In the Spanish sample, the percentages were much lower and significant differences were found with the Turkish sample for both sexes (Table 4). If we compare the consumption of men and women within each country, there were no significant differences in the STpanish sample ($X^2_{(2)} = 0.9$; $p = 0.62$) or the Turkish sample ($X^2_{(2)} = 1.7$; $p = 0.43$).

Table 4. Regular cigarette consumption over the past 30 days by country and sex, chi-square [1] test and contingency coefficient (effect size).

Frequency	Male		Female	
	Spain	Turkey	Spain	Turkey
Never	58.6%	31.4%	57.95%	43.4%
Occasionally	15.5%	8.6%	10.7%	7.9%
Once a week	3.4%	5.7%	3.9%	1.3%
More than once a week	10.3%	2.9%	7.9%	10.5%
Every day	12.1%	51.4%	19.7%	36.8%
$X^2_{(2)}$ (p)	10.1 (0.007)		9.5 (0.009)	
Φ	0.33		0.19	

[1] To meet the assumptions of the chi-squared test, the categories "occasionally /once a week" and "more than once a week/every day" were combined.

The frequency of waterpipe consumption over the past 30 days was higher in the Turkish sample, with more than 50% of Turkish men reporting using a waterpipe every day. The differences between the two countries were statistically significant for both men and women (Table 5). If we compare the consumption of men and women within the two countries, there were no significant differences in the Spanish sample ($X^2_{(2)} = 3.1$; $p = 0.21$; Φ = 0.12), but in the Turkish sample significantly more men regularly use a waterpipe ($X^2_{(2)} = 6.1$; $p = 0.048$; Φ = 0.23).

Table 5. Waterpipe consumption over the past 30 days by country and sex, chi-square [1] test and contingency coefficient (effect size).

Frequency	Male		Female	
	Spain	Turkey	Spain	Turkey
Never	77.6%	48.6%	82.6%	60.5%
Occasionally	15.5%	40.0%	15.2%	36.8%
Once a week	3.4%	0%	1.7%	1.3%
More than once a week	3.4%	8.6%	0.6%	1.3%
Every day	0%	2.9%	0%	0%
$X^2_{(2)}$ (p)	8.5 (0.01)		14.2 (0.001)	
Φ	0.30		0.24	

[1] To meet the assumptions of the chi-squared test, the categories "occasionally/once a week" and "more than once a week/every day" were combined.

3.3. E-Cigarettes and Waterpipe Nicotine Content

Table 6 shows the percentage of e-cigarette users, according to the nicotine content. Men in both populations reported similar frequencies of nicotine in e-cigarettes, but Turkish women use e-cigarettes with nicotine more frequently than Spanish women and Spanish women use with and without nicotine more frequently.

Table 6. Percentage of e-cigarette users according to the nicotine content.

Nicotine Content	Male		Female	
	Spain	Turkey	Spain	Turkey
Without nicotine	31.3%	12.5%	26.9%	26.3%
With and without nicotine	37.5%	31.3%	61.5%	15.8%
With nicotine	31.3%	56.3%	11.5%	57.9%
$X^2_{(2)}$ (p)	2.5 (0.28)		13.0 (0.001)	
Φ	-		0.54	

Table 7 shows the percentage of waterpipe users according to the additive. Only data from the Spanish sample is available for this variable, due to a problem with the data collection. The most frequent option was to use a waterpipe with herbal shisha, but many men only use it with tobacco.

Table 7. Percentage of waterpipe users according to content.

Waterpipe Content	Male	Female
With tobacco	36.1%	12.1%
With non-tobacco or herbal shisha	37.5%	51.7%
With marijuana or hashish	0%	0.9%
With tobacco and with non-tobacco or herbal shisha	5.6%	15.5%
With tobacco and with marijuana or hashish	5.6%	2.6%
With non-tobacco or herbal shisha and with marijuana or hashish	8.3%	4.3%
With tobacco, with non-tobacco or herbal shisha or with marijuana or hashish	11.1%	12.9%

3.4. Reasons for Vaping/Smoking

Table 8 shows the percentage of participants that answered "definitely" or "probably" to each option as an important reason for using e-cigarettes. In both countries, the reason men most frequently considered important was "to experiment—to see what it is like". This reason was also identified as very important for more than 90% of Spanish women. In contrast, the most frequently selected reason among Turkish women was "because it tastes good". In general, the percentage of participants who reported each option as an important reason to use electronic cigarettes did not differ significantly between the two countries, except in the case of "to relax or relieve tension", with more Turkish men, than Spanish men ($X^2_{(1)} = 5.1$; $p = 0.02$; $\Phi = 0.38$), reporting this to be an important reason (see Table 8). Moreover, there were no significant differences in the percentage of men and women who considered each reason to be important in either country.

Table 8. Most important reasons for using e-cigarettes by country and sex, chi-square * test and contingency coefficient (effect size).

Reason	Male		$X^2_{(1)}$ (p)	Φ	Female		$X^2_{(1)}$ (p)	Φ
	Spain	Turkey			Spain	Turkey		
To experiment—to see what it is like	72.7%	66.7%	* (1)	-	93.8%	57.1%	* (0.07)	-
Because it tastes good	53.6%	60.0%	0.1 (0.83)	-	65.4%	81.3%	* (0.31)	-
Because of boredom, nothing else to do	22.2%	22.2%	* (1)	-	21.6%	33.3%	* (0.51)	-
To have a good time with my friends	31.6%	27.8%	0.1 (0.80)	-	31.4%	31.3%	0 (0.99)	-
To relax or relieve tension	20.0%	56.3%	5.1 (0.02)	0.38	16.1%	37.5%	* (0.15)	-
Because it looks cool	5.0%	22.2%	* (0.17)	-	5.4%	12.5%	* (0.58)	-
To help me quit regular cigarettes	13.3%	27.3%	* (0.35)	-	14.3%	7.1%	* (0.44)	-
To get high	0%	11.8%	* (0.49)	-	0%	0%	-	-
Because I am "hooked"—I have to have it	5.9%	22.2%	* (0.19)	-	2.8%	0%	* (0.69)	-
Because friends or family members used them	22.2%	26.7%	* (0.54)	-	17.6%	20.0%	* (0.57)	-
Because e-cigarettes without nicotine are less harmful than regular cigarettes	25.0%	35.7%	* (0.68)	-	25.0%	29.4%	* (0.75)	-
Because friends or family member allowed e-cigarettes more than regular cigarettes	0%	17.6%	* (0.10)	-	5.7%	22.2%	* (0.09)	-

* Fisher's exact test was used when the expected frequencies were lower than 5.

The item participants reported as being the most important reason to use regular cigarettes was "to relax and relieve tension" (Table 9). There were also other reasons that were considered important by more than 50% of the sample, which were: "to experiment, to see what it is like" and "have a good time with friends". Many Turkish men also reported that they used regular cigarettes "because of boredom", which was significantly higher than for Spanish men. Significantly more Turkish women, than Spanish women, reported boredom as an important reason to use regular cigarettes. In addition, more Turkish men, than Spanish men, also reported that an important reason was "because friends or family members used them". Men and women did not differ in their reasons for using regular cigarettes, with two exceptions: more Turkish men than Turkish women reported that they use regular cigarettes "because it looks cool" ($X^2_{(1)}$ = 4.7; p = 0.03; Φ = 0.25) and "because they are hooked" ($X^2_{(1)}$) = 6.7; p = 0.01; Φ = 0.30).

Table 9. Most important reasons to use regular cigarettes by subsample and sex, chi-square * test and contingency coefficient (effect size).

Reason	Male		$X^2_{(1)}$ (p)	Φ	Female		$X^2_{(1)}$ (p)	Φ
	Spain	Turkey			Spain	Turkey		
To experiment—to see what it is like	58.1%	66.7%	0.4 (0.50)	-	68.6%	61.2%	0.8 (0.37)	-
Because it tastes good	25.8%	37.0%	0.9 (0.36)	-	40.4%	37.7%	0.5 (0.50)	-
Because of boredom, nothing else to do	41.4%	74.1%	6.1 (0.01)	0.33	21.6%	33.3%	5.2 (0.02)	0.19
To have a good time with my friends	51.6%	66.7%	1.3 (0.25)	-	57.3%	69.4%	2.1 (0.15)	-
To relax or relieve tension	78.1%	88.9%	* (0.23)	-	76.0%	77.6%	0.1 (0.83)	-
Because it looks cool	31.0%	33.3%	0.03 (0.85)	-	17.6%	12.5%	0.6 (0.42)	-
To get high	14.3%	20.0%	* (0.43)	-	9.9%	20.8%	3.3 (0.07)	-
Because I am "hooked"—I have to have it	28.6%	50.0%	2.6 (0.11)	-	35.3%	20.8%	3.2 (0.07)	-
Because friends or family members used them	20.0%	46.2%	4.4 (0.04)	0.28	31.0%	38.8%	0.9 (0.35)	-

* Fisher's exact test was used when the expected frequencies were lower than 5.

The three most important reasons to use waterpipes, as reported by the participants, were: "to experiment, to see what it is like", "have a good time with friends" and "because it tastes good". More Spanish women reported that "to experiment, to see what it is like" and to "have a good time with Friends" were important reasons to use a waterpipe, but more Turkish women reported their important reasons as "to help themselves quit regular cigarettes", "because they are hooked" and "because waterpipes with nicotine are less harmful than regular cigarettes" (see Table 10). More Turkish men reported that "because friends and family members used them" as an important reason for using waterpipes, than did Spanish men. Spanish men also differed significantly from Spanish women across three reasons. More Spanish women rated the following two items to be important "to experiment, to see what it is like" ($X^2_{(1)}$ = 6.9; p = 0.01; Φ = 0.22) and "because it tastes good" ($X^2_{(1)}$ = 12.1; p = 0.001;

$\Phi = 0.29$), while more Spanish men reported an important reason to be "because they are hooked" ($X^2_{(1)} = 4.2$; $p = 0.04$; $\Phi = 0.18$). In the Turkish sample, men and women only differed significantly in one reason for using a waterpipe, with more men answering "because it looks cool" ($X^2_{(1)} = 7.8$; $p = 0.001$; $\Phi = 0.32$).

Table 10. Most important reasons to use a waterpipe (probably or definitely yes) by country and sex, chi-square * test and contingency coefficient (effect size).

Reason	Male		$X^2_{(1)}$ (p)	Φ	Female		$X^2_{(1)}$ (p)	Φ
	Spain	Turkey			Spain	Turkey		
To experiment—to see what it is like	78.9%	93.3%	* (0.17)	-	93.8%	80.0%	6.9 (0.01)	0.21
Because it tastes good	70.3%	89.3%	3.4 (0.07)	-	92.6%	84.6%	2.5 (0.12)	-
Because of boredom, nothing else to do	45.7%	53.6%	0.4 (0.54)	-	31.2%	39.2%	1.0 (0.32)	-
To have a good time with my friends	91.9%	85.7%	* (0.34)	-	93.8%	80.0%	6.8 (0.01)	0.20
To relax or relieve tension	33.3%	50.0%	1.8 (0.18)	-	32.1%	45.1%	2.5 (0.11)	-
Because it looks cool	20.0%	39.3%	2.8 (0.09)	-	15.2%	12.0%	0.3 (0.59)	-
To help me quit regular cigarettes	0%	11.1%	* (0.08)	-	2.9%	14.3%	* (0.01)	0.21
To get high	23.5%	22.2%	0.02 (0.90)	-	9.7%	14.3%	0.7 (0.40)	-
Because I am "hooked"—I have to have it	0%	7.4%	* (0.19)	-	1.0%	12.0%	* (0.01)	0.25
Because friends or family members used them	25.7%	55.6%	5.7 (0.02)	0.30	25.7%	36.0%	1.7 (0.19)	-
Because waterpipes without nicotine are less harmful than regular cigarettes	11.4%	21.4%	1.2 (0.28)	-	9.9%	22.0%	4.1 (0.04)	0.17
Because friends or family member allowed waterpipe use more than regular cigarettes	8.8%	12.0%	0.2 (0.69)	-	9.2%	19.1%	2.9 (0.10)	-

* Fisher's exact test was used when the expected frequencies were lower than 5.

Finally, the outstanding results of the present research were collected and presented in Table 11.

Table 11. Outstanding results.

1.	Lifetime prevalence of e-cigarette, cigarette and waterpipe use was high in both samples.
2.	Lifetime prevalence of waterpipe use was higher in Turkish men, than in Spanish men. In women, the prevalence was similar.
3.	The use of e-cigarettes was almost always linked to regular cigarette and waterpipe use.
4.	Daily consumption of waterpipe and regular cigarettes was higher in the Turkish sample, than in Spanish sample, but there were no differences for e-cigarette consumption.
5.	More than 50% of the Turkish participants (men and women) always use waterpipes with nicotine.
6.	The most important reason to use e-cigarettes in the Spanish sample (men and women) and for Turkish men was to experiment, to see what it is like. For Turkish women, the most important reason was because it tastes good.
7.	The most important reason to use cigarettes, in all cases, was to relax or relieve tension.
8.	The most common reasons to use waterpipes was to have a goodtime with friends, to experiment to see what it is like and because it tastes good.

4. Discussion

The first purpose of the present study was to investigate the lifetime and current use of electronic cigarettes, regular cigarettes, waterpipes and current polytobacco use among young adults, by sex and country. The data showed that lifetime e-cigarette use was higher in the Turkish sample, than in the Spanish sample. Sex differences were also found in the two samples, with more men having used e-cigarettes in their lives. Therefore, it appears that women who try e-cigarettes are more likely to become regular users than men, among the young adults in these samples.

Since 2013, electronic cigarette use has been regulated by law in Turkey and their sales are prohibited to anyone under 18 years of age [24]. Surprisingly, there was no data available about electronic cigarette use in Turkey from the Global Data Tobacco Survey [25] and, to our knowledge, no other data about e-cigarette use in Turkey has been published. The level of e-cigarette use found here among young Turkish adults shows the need for more large-scale prevalence studies in this country to investigate the use of this alternative nicotine product.

The Global Data Tobacco Survey reported the use of electronic cigarettes among the general population in Spain to be 2% (2% of men and 1.9% of women) [25]. Furthermore, the most recent national survey of Spain showed that the prevalence figures for e-cigarette use in young adults were: lifetime—15.1% of men and 10.9% of women; past 30 days—4.3% of men and 2.4% of women; and daily—1.5% of men and 1.2% of women [26]. Higher percentages were found in the present study, providing some evidence that e-cigarette use has increased in Spain and that more preventive actions must be undertaken to alert users and potential users about health risks.

In our study, lifetime regular cigarette use appeared to be higher in men than in women, in the Turkish sample, and higher in women than in men in the Spanish sample, although these differences were not statistically significant. Daily cigarette use also appeared to differ between the two countries, with more Turkish men and more Spanish women using cigarettes on a daily basis, but these differences were not statistically significant.

In line with our research findings, the WHO Global Adult Tobacco Survey showed that regular cigarette use (daily and occasional) in Turkey was more common among young men (33%) than in young women (7.4%) [27]. This sex difference was also reported in the Turkey Statistical Health Survey, where the percentage of young male daily smokers (31.4%) was significantly higher than the percentage of young females (5.7%) [28]. Anti-tobacco policies have been implemented in Turkey over the last 10 years, including tax increases and regulations, which have affected the long-term demand for cigarettes, presumably due to price sensitivity [29]. However, more preventive measures are necessary in Turkey, in particular among young men, to reduce smoking-related diseases and to reduce the rate of smoking initiation.

The most recent national Spanish survey showed that daily cigarette use in young adults was 28.5% in men and 23.2% in women, which was higher than in previous national surveys and also higher than in our study [26]. A previous study among Spanish university students also found similar daily cigarette use in females (16.9%), as in the present research, and 17.8% among males [30]. These results provide some evidence that, despite the substantial preventive efforts undertaken by the Spanish government, cigarette smoking may again be increasing among young adults. Therefore, more campaigns are needed to reduce this addictive behavior and to promote healthy lifestyles in Spain. Furthermore, interventions targeted at university students should also help them to deal with common student problems, such as stress and boredom, without the use of nicotine.

The present study found that more than 50% of the participants had used a waterpipe at some point in their life, with no sex differences. During the past 30 days, waterpipe use was more common in Turkey than in Spain, with more male users than women in Turkey, but no sex differences were found in Spain.

Previous studies in Turkey have found current waterpipe use (daily and occasional) to be more common among young men (2.5%) than in young women (1%) and that waterpipe use has declined among the general population from 2008 (men: 4%, women 0.7%) to 2012 (men: 1.1%, women: 0.5%), possibly resulting from prevention efforts such as health warnings on waterpipes [27,31]. However, these same studies also reported evidence that waterpipe smoking was increasing globally, particularly among young adults. This finding again highlights the need to continue with prevention efforts in order to maintain the decline in waterpipe use.

There is a paucity of research about waterpipe use in Spain. One study found that approximately one-third of Spanish high school students had used a waterpipe at some point in their lives, with the proportion being higher in women than in men [32]. Furthermore, another recent study reported that 13% of Spanish high school students currently (monthly or weekly) used a waterpipe [33]. These high percentages are in accordance with the present study using young adults, which demonstrates the need to include items about waterpipe use in Spanish national surveys, in order to have more complete data. Moreover, in line with the most recent National Spanish Drug Plan more preventive materials should be created to alert people about this new way of socializing in Spain and its health consequences [9].

One of the main aims of this study was to identify polytobacco use by sex and country among tobacco users. In the Turkish sample, 80% of men and 63.9% of women were polytobacco users, while in the Spanish sample, 61.4% of men and 69.3% of women were polytobacco users, although these differences (country or sex) were not statistically significant. In the same line, with previous research on Polish adolescents, dual use (regular cigarette + e-cigarette) increased over time, from 4% in 2010–2011 to 23% in 2013–2014, while exclusive regular cigarette use declined over this time (from 21% to 15%) [34]. Furthermore, research about polytobacco use among North American adolescents found that 81% of e-cigarette users also used at least one other tobacco product [35]. In a similar study among North American adolescents and young adults, 55.9% were classified as polytobacco users [36]. The results of the present study are also consistent with previous research among North American young adults that reported using at least two tobacco products, with shisha being the most common, followed by regular cigarettes and e-cigarettes [37]. The tendency toward polytobacco use is worrying, since young adults who use more tobacco products are at a greater risk for increased regular cigarette smoking and also for maintaining this polytobacco pattern of use [38].

The second purpose of the present study was to find out whether e-cigarettes and waterpipes were used with nicotine and whether there were sex and country differences. Within e-cigarettes smokers, in the Turkish sample, 56.3% of men and 57.9% of women answered that their e-cigarettes contained nicotine, while in the Spanish sample, these proportions were 31.3% of men and 11.5% of women. Our Spanish data were lower than those reported in the last National Spanish Drug survey, which found 48.4% of young adult men and 41% of young adult women smoked e-cigarettes with nicotine [26]. However, our research found that a higher proportion of the participants reported that they sometimes include nicotine in their e-cigarettes (37.5% men and 61.5% women), than was found in the most recent National Spanish Drug survey (11.5% men and 17.2% women).

Within waterpipe users, in the Spanish sample, the most frequent answer among males was that they smoked waterpipes with tobacco (36.1%), while among women the most frequent answer (57.1%) was that they smoked waterpipes with non-tobacco or herbal shisha. Approximately one-third part of men (30.6%) and women (35.3%) smoked waterpipes, combining the following: tobacco, non-tobacco or herbal shisha or marijuana/hashish. In another study among North American students, the majority of waterpipe users (90%) reported smoking tobacco, 45% marijuana, 37% herbal shisha (non-tobacco) and 18% hashish [21]. Moreover, the present research confirms that waterpipe use is a common alternative method for using nicotine. The results of the present study are concerning, since nicotine use was common, but also because of the toxic substances that have been found in waterpipe smoke, including herbal shisha. This research demonstrates the need to disseminate information about the health risks of waterpipe use among young adults [21].

The third purpose of the present study was to examine the reasons why young adults use e-cigarettes, regular cigarettes and waterpipe and whether there were any sex or country differences. The most important reason to use e-cigarettes was "to experiment, to see what is like" (Turkish sample: men 66.7% and women 57.1; Spanish sample: men 72.7% and women 93.8%), although the most important reason for Turkish women (81.3%) was "because it tastes good". No significant differences were found by sex in the reasons reported. The only exception was for the reason "Because it relieves tension", which was reported more commonly by Turkish men than Spanish men. This finding among Turkish men is in line with previous studies among North American young adults, where affect regulation was the most consistent predictor of e-cigarette use [17]. The results of our research are also in agreement with previous research about the reasons for vaping or e-cigarette use among North American adolescents. The most important reasons reported were: to experiment and because it tastes good [22], and because they are available in tasty flavors, such as mint, candy, fruit or chocolate [23].

The most commonly reported reason to consume regular cigarettes was "to relax and relieve tension" (Turkish sample: men 88.9% and women: 77.6%; Spanish sample: men 78.1% and women 76%). More than 50% of the two samples also considered the following reasons to be important: "to experiment, to see what it is like" and to "have a good time with friends". More Turkish men, than

Spanish men, and more Turkish women than Spanish women gave the reason "because of boredom". More Turkish men, than Spanish men, gave the reason "because friends or family members used them". No significant differences were found in the reasons provided by sex, with the exception of "Because it looks cool" and "because I am hooked", which were reported more by Turkish men than Turkish women. Our findings are also consistent with previous research among North American students, where high levels of regular cigarette use were associated with higher boredom relief and affect regulation motive scores [39].

The most important reasons to use waterpipes were "to experiment, to see what it is like" (Turkish sample: men 93.3% and women 80%; Spanish sample: men 78.9% and women 93.8%), "to have a good time with friends" (Turkish sample: men 85.7% and women 80.4%; Spanish sample: men 91.9% and women 93.8%) and "because it tastes good" (Turkish sample: men 89.3% and women 84.6%; Spanish sample: men 70.3% and women 92.6%). For Spanish women, the reasons "to experiment, to see what is like" and to "have a good time with friends" were more important than for Turkish women. Turkish women reported the following reasons to be more important than for Spanish women: "to help quit regular cigarettes", "because I am hooked" and "because waterpipes without nicotine are less harmful than regular cigarettes". More Turkish than Spanish men reported using waterpipes "because friends and family members used them". In the Spanish sample, men reported "because I am hooked" more often than Spanish women, but more women answered "to experiment, to see what it is like" and "because it tastes good". In the Turkish sample, more men than women reported the reason "because it looks cool". The pattern of findings in the present study are in line with the findings from a study about waterpipe use among North American adolescents, which found that adolescents strongly endorsed the following statements: if my best friend offered me a hookah, I would smoke; hookah helps young people feel more comfortable; hookah helps people relieve stress; it would be easy to quit using hookah [40]. The higher perceived social acceptability of waterpipe use among friends was also found to be related to the higher odds of having ever tried a waterpipe in North American adolescents [41]. These positive cognitions about waterpipe use, compared with regular cigarettes use, could help to explain the increased use of waterpipes in recent years. In addition, a general pattern among young adults to search for alternative ways of using tobacco has been proposed to explain waterpipe use [42].

There are limitations to this study. Firstly, this cross-sectional survey does not allow any temporal conclusions about tobacco use and the reasons examined to use these substances. This work was based on a convenience sample of university students who completed an online survey, as has been the case in previous polytobacco research in North America [17]. However, there are several possible sample and method limitations, which means the data collected here does not supersede those obtained in national surveys. Furthermore, all measures relied on self-reported behavior and may therefore be biased in some way. In particular, it is likely that the "because I am hooked" reason for smoking, one of the three measured products, has been under-reported by the participants, since being addicted to something is socially undesirable. Due to the multiple statistic tests undertaken regarding the main reasons for using regular cigarettes, e-cigarettes and waterpipes, some significant results could have been found by chance. However, the present study has to be considered a first step, so that future larger studies will be conducted which are able to analyze in depth polytobacco characteristics by country and sex.

5. Conclusions

Although there were very few differences by sex or country, the high level of polytobacco use among young adults reported in both countries (European region vs. Eastern Mediterranean region) highlights the need to develop more integrated prevention strategies. These strategies should not only include regular cigarette use, as has usually been the case, or by separating tobacco products, but must include all alternative nicotine products, such as e-cigarettes and waterpipes. This would be the way to offer a global health risk approach to nicotine use among young adults, regardless of the form of administration. Nevertheless, it is also important that the observed differences in the reasons to use these alternative tobacco products are also taken into account. Further research is also needed to examine polytobacco use in these two countries in order to better understand these new nicotine use patterns. It is suggested that future research continues to collect data about nicotine contents for waterpipes and e-cigarettes to help policy makers and to develop more accurate prevention campaigns.

Author Contributions: Conceptualization, S.F.-M. and M.J.M.S.; Data curation, M.-E.G.; Investigation, S.F.-M. and M.J.M.S.; Writing—original draft, S.F.-M. and M.J.M.S.; Writing—review and editing, S.F.-M. and M.J.M.S.

Funding: This research received no external funding.

Acknowledgments: The authors would like to thank the students from Middle East Technical University—Northern Cyprus Campus and from the Universitat de Girona for participating in this study and in particular Sabriye Gultepe and Andrea Arcas for helping to develop the online questionnaire.

Conflicts of Interest: The authors declare no conflict of interest.

References

1. World Health Organization. *Lexicon of Alcohol and Drug Terms*, 1st ed.; WHO: Geneva, Switzerland, 1994.
2. European Monitoring Center for Drugs and Drug Addiction. *Polydrug Use: Patterns and Responses*, 1st ed.; Publications Office of the European Union: Luxembourg, 2009.
3. European Monitoring Center for Drugs and Drugs Addiction. *European Drug Report: Trends and Developments 2019*, 1st ed.; Office of the European Union: Luxembourg, 2019.
4. Font-Mayolas, S.; Hernández-Serrano, O.; Gras, M.E.; Sullman, M.J.M. Types of polydrug use among Spanish students in health sciences. *J. Addict. Nurs.* **2019**, *30*, 108–113. [CrossRef] [PubMed]
5. Bombard, J.M.; Rock, V.; Pederson, L.L.; Asman, K. Monitoring polytobacco use among adolescents. Do cigarette smokers use other forms of tobacco? *Nicotine Tob. Res.* **2008**, *10*, 1581–1589. [CrossRef] [PubMed]
6. Fix, B.V.; O'Connor, R.J.; Vogl, L.; Smith, D.; Bansal-Travers, M.; Conway, K.P.; Ambrose, B.; Yang, L.; Hyland, A. Patterns and correlates of polytobacco use in the United States over a decade: NSDUH 2002-2011. *Addict. Behav.* **2014**, *39*, 768–781. [CrossRef] [PubMed]
7. Haardörfer, R.; Berg, C.J.; Lewis, M.; Payne, J.; Pillai, D.; McDonald, B.; Windle, M. Polytobacco, marijuana, and alcohol use patterns in college students: A latent class analysis. *Addict. Behav.* **2016**, *59*, 58–64. [CrossRef]
8. Martinasek, M.P.; McDermott, R.J.; Martini, L. Waterpipe (hookah) tobacco smoking among youth. *Curr. Probl. Pediatr. Adolesc. Health Care* **2011**, *41*, 34–57. [CrossRef] [PubMed]
9. Ministry of Health, Social Services and Equality. *Plan Nacional Sobre Drogas. Memoria 2017*, 1st ed.; MHSSE: Madrid, Spain, 2017.
10. Case, K.R.; Creamer, M.R.; Cooper, M.R.; Loukas, A.; Perry, C.L. Hookah use as a predictor of other tobacco product use: A longitudinal analysis of Texas college students. *Addict. Behav.* **2018**, *87*, 131–137. [CrossRef]
11. Akl, E.A.; Gaddam, S.; Gunukula, S.K.; Honeine, R.; Jaoude, P.A.; Irani, J. The effects of waterpipe tobacco smoking on health outcome: A systematic review. *Int. J. Epidemiol.* **2010**, *39*, 834–857. [CrossRef]
12. Waziry, R.; Jawad, M.; Ballout, R.A.; Al Akel, M.; Akl, E.A. The effects of warerpipe tobacco smoking on health outcomes: An updated systematic review and meta-analysis. *Int. J. Epidemiol.* **2017**, *46*, 32–43.
13. WHO Study Group on Tobacco Product Regulation (TobReg). Advisory Note: Waterpipe Tobacco Smoking: Health Effects, Research Needs and Recommended Actions by Regulators. Available online: http://apps.who.int/iris/bitstream/10665/161991/1/9789241508469_eng.pdf?ua=1&ua=1 (accessed on 14 September 2019).
14. Goniewicz, M.L.; Knysak, J.; Michal, G.; Gawron, M.; Kosmider, L.; Sobczak, A.; Kurek, J.; Prokopowicz, A.; Jablonska-Czapla, M.; Rosik-Dulewska, C.; et al. Levels of selected carcinogens and toxicants in vapour from electronic cigarettes. *Tob. Control* **2014**, *23*, 133–139. [CrossRef]
15. Bombard, J.M.; Pederson, L.L.; Koval, J.J.; O'Hegarty, M.O. How are lifetime polytobacco users different than current cigarette-only users? Results from a Canadian young adult population. *Addict. Behav.* **2009**, *34*, 1069–1072. [CrossRef]
16. Bertoni, N.; Szklo, A.; De Boni, R.; Coutinho, C.; Vasconcellos, M.; Silva, P.N.; de Almeida, L.M.; Bastos, F.I. Electronic cigarettes and narguile users in Brazil: Do they differ from cigarette smokers? *Addict. Behav.* **2019**, *98*, 106007. [CrossRef] [PubMed]

17. Doran, N.; Brikmanis, K. Expectancies for and use of-ecigarettes and hookah among young adults. *Addict. Behav.* **2016**, *51*, 131–135. [CrossRef] [PubMed]
18. Doran, N.; Trim, R.S. Correlates of other tobacco use in a community sample of young adults. *Addict. Behav.* **2015**, *51*, 131–135. [CrossRef] [PubMed]
19. Lopez, A.A.; Eissenberg, T.; Jaafar, M.; Afifi, R. Now is the time to advocate for interventions designed specifically to prevent and control waterpipe tobacco smoking. *Addict. Behav.* **2017**, *66*, 41–47. [CrossRef] [PubMed]
20. Ministry of Health, Social Services and Equality. *Encuesta Sobre Uso de Drogas en Estudiantes de Secundaria en España*, 1st ed.; MHSSE: Madrid, Spain, 2017.
21. Sutfin, E.L.; Song, E.Y.; Reboussin, B.A.; Wolfson, M. What are young adult smoking in their hookahs? A latent class analysis of substances smoked. *Addict. Behav.* **2014**, *39*, 1191–1196. [CrossRef]
22. Evans-Polce, R.J.; Patrick, M.E.; Lanza, S.T.; Miech, R.A.; O'Malley, P.M.; Johnston, L.D. Reasons for vaping among U.S. 12th Graders. *J. Adolesc. Health* **2018**, *62*, 457–462. [CrossRef]
23. Tsai, J.; Walton, K.; Coleman, B.N.; Sharapova, S.R.; Johnson, S.E.; Kenedy, S.M.; Caraballo, R.S. Reasons for electronic cigarette use among middle and high school students—National youth tobacco survey, United States, 2016. *MMWR* **2018**, *67*, 196–200. [CrossRef]
24. Nayir, E.; Karacabey, B.; Kirca, O.; Ozdogan, M. Electronic cigarettes (e-cigarette). *J. Oncol. Sci.* **2016**, *2*, 16–20. [CrossRef]
25. Agaku, I.T.; Filippidis, F.T.; Vardavas, C.I.; Odukoya, O.O.; Awopegba, A.J.; Ayo-Yusuf, O.A.; Connolly, G.N. Poly-tobacco use among adults in 44 countries during 2008-2012: Evidence for an integrative and comprehensive approach in tobacco control. *Drug Alcohol Depend.* **2014**, *139*, 60–70. [CrossRef]
26. Ministry of Health, Social Services and Equality. *Encuesta Sobre Alcohol y Otras Drogas en España (EDADES) 2017*, 1st ed.; MHSSE: Madrid, Spain, 2017.
27. Republic of Turkey Ministry of Health. *Global Adult Tobacco Survey 2012 Report*, 1st ed.; Publication 948; RTMH: Ankara, Turkey, 2014.
28. Köse, E.; Ózcebe, H. Tobacco epidemic keeps spreading among Turkish youth. *Eurasian J. Pulmonol.* **2017**, *64*, 217–222. [CrossRef]
29. Cetin, T. The effect of taxation and regulation on cigarette smoking: Fresh evidence from Turkey. *Health Policy* **2017**, *121*, 1288–1295. [CrossRef] [PubMed]
30. Hernández-Serrano, O.; Font-Mayolas, S.; Gras, M.E. Polydrug use and its relationship with the familiar and social context amongst yong college students. *Adicciones* **2015**, *27*, 205–213. [CrossRef] [PubMed]
31. Erdöl, C.; Ergüder, T.; Morton, J.; Palipudi, K.; Gupta, P.; Asma, S. Waterpipe tobacco smoking in Turkey: Policy, implications and trends from the Global Adult Tobacco Survey (GATS). *Int. J. Environ. Public Health* **2015**, *12*, 15559–15566. [CrossRef] [PubMed]
32. Jorge-Araujo, P.; Torres-García, M.; Saavedra-Santana, P.; Navarro-Rodríguez, C. Waterpipe tobacco consumption in secondary education and high school in students from the province of Las Palmas. *Health Addict.* **2017**, *17*, 121–131.
33. Sáenz-Lussagnet, J.M.; Rico-Villademoros, F.; Luque-Romero, L.G. Waterpipe and cigarette smoking among adolescents in Seville (Spain): Prevalence and potential determinants. *Adicciones* **2019**, *31*, 170–173.
34. Smith, D.M.; Gawron, M.; Balwicki, L.; Sobczak, A.; Matynia, M.; Goniewicz, M.J. Exclusive versus dual use of tobacco and electronic cigarettes among adolescents in Poland, 2010–2016. *Addict. Behav.* **2019**, *90*, 341–348. [CrossRef]
35. Lee, Y.O.; Pepper, J.K.; MacMonegle, A.J.; Nonnemaker, J.M.; Duke, J.C.; Porter, L. Examining youth dual and polytobacco use with e-cigarettes. *Int. J. Environ. Public Health* **2018**, *15*, 699. [CrossRef]
36. King, J.L.; Reboussin, D.; Cornacchione, J.; Wiseman, K.D.; Wagoner, K.G.; Sutfin, E.L. Polytobacco use among a nationally representative sample of adolescent and young adult e-cigarette users. *J. Adolesc. Health* **2018**, *67*, 407–412. [CrossRef]
37. Leavens, E.L.S.; Meier, E.; Brett, E.I.; Stevens, E.M.; Tackett, A.P.; Villanti, A.C.; Wagener, T.L. Polytobacco use and risk perceptions among young adults: The potential role of habituation to risk. *Addict. Behav.* **2019**, *90*, 278–284. [CrossRef]
38. Petersen, A.; Myers, M.G.; Tully, L.; Brikmanis, K.; Doran, N. Polytobacco use among young adult smokers: Prospective association with cigarette consumption. *Tob. Control* **2018**, 1–6. [CrossRef]

39. Wong, E.C.; Haardörfer, R.; Windle, M.; Berg, C.J. Distinct motives for use among polytobacco versus cigarette only users and among single tobacco product users. *Nicotine Tob. Res.* **2018**, *20*, 117–123. [CrossRef] [PubMed]
40. Barnett, T.E.; Livingston, M.D. Hookah use among adolescents: Differential cognitions about hookah and cigarettes. *Addict. Behav.* **2017**, *75*, 75–78. [CrossRef] [PubMed]
41. Flitzpatrick, M.; Johnson, A.C.; Tercyak, K.P.; Hawkins, K.B.; Villanti, A.C.; Mays, D. Adolescent beliefs about hookah and hookah tobacco use ad implication for preventing use. *Prev. Chronic Dis.* **2019**, *16*, 1–11.
42. Castaneda, G.; Barnett, T.E.; Soule, E.K.; Young, M.E. Hookah smoking behavior initiation in the context of Millenials. *Public Health* **2016**, *137*, 124–130. [CrossRef] [PubMed]

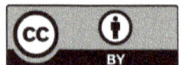

© 2019 by the authors. Licensee MDPI, Basel, Switzerland. This article is an open access article distributed under the terms and conditions of the Creative Commons Attribution (CC BY) license (http://creativecommons.org/licenses/by/4.0/).

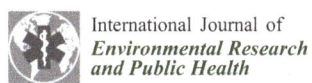

Article

Understanding the Relationship between Predictors of Alcohol Consumption in Pregnancy: Towards Effective Prevention of FASD

Isabel Corrales-Gutierrez [1,2], Ramon Mendoza [3,4,5], Diego Gomez-Baya [3,4,]* and Fatima Leon-Larios [6]

1. Foetal Medicine Unit, University Hospital Virgen Macarena, C.P. 41009 Seville, Spain; icorrales@us.es
2. Department of Surgery, University of Seville, 41009 Seville, Spain
3. Department of Social, Developmental and Educational Psychology, University of Huelva, 21007 Huelva, Spain; ramon@dpsi.uhu.es
4. Research Group on Health Promotion and Development of Lifestyle across Lifespan, University of Huelva, 21007 Huelva, Spain
5. Center for Research in Contemporary Thought and Innovation for Social Development (COIDESO), 21007 Huelva, Spain
6. Nursing Department, Faculty of Nursing, Physiotherapy and Podiatry, University of Seville, 41009 Seville, Spain; fatimaleon@us.es
* Correspondence: diego.gomez@dpee.uhu.es; Tel.: +34-959219213

Received: 29 December 2019; Accepted: 18 February 2020; Published: 21 February 2020

Abstract: Background: Prenatal alcohol exposure can produce serious changes in neurodevelopment that last a lifetime, as well as a wide range of congenital abnormalities, and is the main non-hereditary, avoidable cause of intellectual disability in developed countries. It is therefore crucial to understand the determinants of alcohol consumption during pregnancy. This study is aimed at determining the factors that predict it, as well as the interactions between them. Methods: A cross-sectional study was carried out using a random sample of 426 pregnant women being treated at the outpatient clinic of a public university hospital in Seville (Spain), when they were in their twentieth week of pregnancy. A custom-designed questionnaire was used for data collection and applied in the course of an interview administered by trained health professionals. The data collected were analyzed using hierarchical regression, moderation analysis, and a structural equations model. Results: Alcohol consumption prior to pregnancy proved to be the most powerful predictor of alcohol intake during pregnancy. Other particularly significant predictors were the percentage of professionals who gave correct advice to the expectant mother—not to consume any alcohol during pregnancy—and perception of the risk from drinking wine during pregnancy. The number of pregnancies correlates positively with alcohol intake during pregnancy, while the expectant mother's level of education correlates negatively. Conclusions: Identifying these predictive factors will allow the design of more effective fetal alcohol spectrum disorder (FASD) prevention strategies.

Keywords: prevention; alcohol consumption; pregnancy; FASD; lifestyle; public health; Spain

---

1. Introduction

Currently, there is extensive evidence of the teratogenic effects of prenatal alcohol exposure, which can translate into a broad spectrum of abnormalities that make up what is known as fetal alcohol spectrum disorder (FASD) [1,2]. The damage caused to the forming nervous system is permanent and has a number of consequences for the biological development of the fetus as a whole, as well as for subsequent neurocognitive and social development in childhood and the other stages in lifespan [3]. FASD therefore represents a major health and socio-educational problem, since it is the main non-hereditary, avoidable cause of learning difficulties in developed countries, with serious consequences for new-born babies that will last their entire lives [4–6].

It is uncertain how prevalent alcohol consumption during pregnancy is, due to the tendency for it to be underestimated when it is assessed using scales, and as a result of the lack of studies with biomarkers that allow it to be estimated reliably. However, there are worrying data available that tell us that alcohol consumption is a very widespread practice among expectant mothers (particularly in Europe, North America, Australia, and in countries such as South Africa). Its incidence worldwide has been estimated at 9.8% [7]. In a study carried out on expectant and new mothers found online from eleven European countries, 15.8% of them stated that they consumed alcohol during pregnancy, with the United Kingdom (28.5%) and Russia (26.5%) being the countries with the highest estimated level of prevalence in this study [8]. In parallel to consumption, the countries that have the highest estimated prevalence of FASD (19.8 per 1000 population) are those that belong to the European region of the WHO [9]. All of this makes FASD a global public health problem, requiring effective strategies for prevention and early diagnosis, and representing a crucial challenge for healthcare personnel in general, and obstetricians and midwives in particular.

Health professionals play a very important role in providing preventive advice regarding healthy lifestyles in the periconceptional period, during pregnancy, and postnatally. However, there are signs that large sections of healthcare professionals (general practitioners (GPs), obstetricians, and midwives) are not doing their job fully and properly in this regard. The health advice that pregnant women receive about the risks inherent in consuming alcohol during pregnancy frequently proves contradictory, or else it does not reach those with a lower level of education effectively [10]. A number of studies suggest that not having received any specific training in this area could explain why not all professionals routinely inquire about alcohol consumption when caring for pregnant women, or do not always provide appropriate information on the subject [11,12].

Another factor which might explain this is the ambivalence of the official guidelines themselves in this area, or their inconsistency from one country to another, and over time. A review of the Australian and American guidelines related to alcohol consumption during pregnancy, carried out by Whitehall in 2006 [13], highlighted the fact that there was a certain permissiveness shown by the health authorities regarding alcohol consumption during pregnancy. They even failed to recommend abstention, arguing that it might cause disproportionate anxiety and therefore prove even more harmful than alcohol consumption. At the same time, another review of the policies and guidelines on alcohol consumption during pregnancy in English-speaking countries [14] showed that these varied from country to country and within the countries themselves. With the passing of time, since it has not been possible to establish that there are safe levels of alcohol consumption during pregnancy, and at the same time, since there is increasing evidence that low levels of alcohol consumption can lead to risks to fetal development [15], there are many countries where official health guidelines on pregnancy recommend abstaining completely from drinking alcohol during this time. Thus, since 2002, France has recommended total abstention from alcoholic beverages during pregnancy [16]. National public health bodies in Australia [17], Denmark [18], and Norway [19] have made equivalent recommendations. At the same time, in Scotland, since 2012, the Chief Medical Officer has advised that "pregnant women and those trying to conceive should avoid alcohol" [20]. Equally, in the USA, the Message to Women from the U.S. Surgeon General stated "No amount of alcohol consumption can be considered safe during pregnancy" [21]. At the same time, the American Academy of Pediatrics recommends that health professionals promote total avoidance of alcohol consumption throughout pregnancy, in line with the principle of precaution [4]. In Canada, the 2010 consensus guidelines from the Society of Obstetricians and Gynaecologists of Canada support alcohol abstention during pregnancy [22].

In order to be able to develop effective FASD prevention, the starting point must be a good understanding of the current situation of the problem. It is particularly crucial to know about the factors that cause or encourage expectant mothers to consume alcohol during pregnancy.

There are some studies which aim to identify the factors that predict alcohol consumption during pregnancy. Several of them have concluded that the most important factor is the frequent consumption of alcohol prior to pregnancy [23–27]. Bearing this in mind, it is particularly worrying that in countries such as Spain, at present, two thirds of women of child-bearing age consume alcohol. According to the Spanish National Health Survey of 2017 [28], only 36.96% of women aged 15–24 years of age and 23.78% aged between 25 and 34 identified themselves as non-drinkers. These data present us with a potential problem in the years to come—an increased incidence of FASD—unless effective healthcare provided during the periconceptional period helps them to stop consuming alcohol.

Other predictive factors identified in some studies are having been the target of violence [25], high socioeconomic status, an unplanned pregnancy, and late childbearing age [29]. Similarly, smoking or using other drugs prior to becoming pregnant prove to be predictors of alcohol consumption during pregnancy [26,30,31].

Research to date into the factors that predict alcohol consumption during pregnancy is limited and some yield contradictory results. There are also some potential predictors that have scarcely been explored, such as obstetric history, the partner's alcohol consumption, health advice received regarding alcohol consumption during pregnancy, and the perception of damage resulting from prenatal exposure to alcohol. These factors, in real life, presumably do not act in isolation, but rather interact with one another. To our knowledge, the interaction between a wide range of predictive factors of alcohol consumption during pregnancy has not been studied to date. It is also particularly important to identify these predictors and the interactions between them in those regions of the world where there is a combination of a high rate of alcohol consumption among women of childbearing age and limited implementation of healthcare programs aimed at FASD prevention. The case of Spain, just like that of other European countries, may be particularly illustrative for all regions of the world where these circumstances exist.

Therefore, our study, conducted using a sample of expectant mothers who attended a routine pregnancy check-up in a city in the south of Europe, aimed to determine a wide range of factors that predict alcohol consumption during pregnancy and to identify the relative weight of each of them. Additionally, the study was also designed to assess the degree of interaction between different factors (sociodemographic factors, obstetric history, the partner's alcohol consumption, health advice received, and beliefs about the possible risks) and how much they moderate the relationship between previous consumption and alcohol intake during pregnancy.

2. Participants and Methods

2.1. Study Design

A cross-sectional study was carried out, through interviews, on a representative sample of the pregnant women treated in a publicly managed university hospital in Seville (Spain). The sample was randomly selected from women who attended the morphology ultrasound clinic, located in the outpatient area of the hospital, in their 20th week of pregnancy, during a five-month period in 2016.

2.2. Data Collection and Participants

The population of expectant mothers in the twentieth week of pregnancy in the health area of this university hospital during the period when the data were collected was 1664. The sample selection criteria were set as an interview with one out of every two pregnant women, to be chosen at random, i.e., 832 pregnant women. Of these, 426 agreed to be interviewed. The minimum desired sample size was 400 participants. All of them had the same gestational age, and in this regard, it was a homogeneous sample and one that was representative of the population of pregnant women treated by the aforementioned public hospital. For the collection of data, face-to-face interviews were conducted, carried out by health professionals who had previously been instructed on how to do so.

The questionnaire was custom designed by the research group and was delivered under conditions that ensured the anonymity of those interviewed and the confidentiality of the information collected.

The eligibility criteria for inclusion in the study were: Pregnant women of 16 years of age or older, who speak and read Spanish fluently, who accepted and signed the informed consent for inclusion in the study. Further characteristics of the sample are described elsewhere [32].

2.3. Ethics

Before the study was carried out, both its protocol and the questionnaire prepared by the research group were approved by the Clinical Research Ethics Committee of the University Hospital Virgen Macarena (Research code: ICG15/Internal code: 0254N-15).

As a prerequisite for conducting the interview, pregnant women were given oral and written information about the study and an informed consent form, which they had to complete and sign voluntarily if they wanted to be part of the study, delivering one copy to the research team and keeping the other. This documentation reflected all the information related to the objective of the study, as well as the guarantees of confidentiality, privacy, and preservation of anonymity in the responses. The participants gave their informed consent by signing and returning this form. The Helsinki declaration of 1975 and its subsequent amendments were respected.

2.4. Questionnaire

The instrument used for the collection of information was a questionnaire prepared and designed ad hoc for the study by the team of researchers who conceived and carried out this research project. Each of the completed questionnaires was given a code that preserved the anonymity of the users. The members of the research group included health professionals (a GP, two from the field of obstetrics, in particular—an obstetrician and a midwife—and a neonatologist), as well as professionals from the fields of psychology and sociology. The experience of all of them, as well as their knowledge in the field as a result of their research background, made it possible to prepare the customized questionnaire for the population to which it was addressed. Furthermore, a preliminary pilot was carried out in order to verify understanding of the questions, as well as the possibility of adding or removing categories in the answers to the multiple-choice questions. The questions regarding consumption patterns were taken from the Alcohol Use Disorders Identification Test (AUDIT) [33].

Most of the questions in the questionnaire provided the possibility of answering with several predetermined options; however, one of them was "other", which allowed the interviewer to note down all answers provided spontaneously by the pregnant women that were not in line with the categories established. Subsequently, the research group transcribed these answers to categorize them into the options that had been established beforehand, or put them into a new category, thus preventing information from being lost. In addition to these multiple-choice questions, there were also open-ended questions in the questionnaire that were recorded by taking notes. After the data were collected, categories were created for these answers based on a thematic analysis of them.

The questionnaire's content covers the following groups of variables:

(a) Sociodemographic variables: Age, educational level (categorized into three groups from lowest to highest level: (1) Low level of studies, e.g., primary education; (2) medium level of studies, e.g., compulsory secondary education, professional training; (3) university studies and employment status (categorized from the best to the worst employment status in five groups: Full-time employment, part-time employment, unemployed, housewife—as a self-defined employment status—and other employment statuses, such as: Student, on sick leave, under legal working age).
(b) Obstetric variables: Number of pregnancies, including the current one, and pregnancy planning.
(c) Risk awareness of alcohol consumption during pregnancy (categorized as: (1) Risk(s) mentioned; (2) says she doesn't know but gives an opinion; (3) she doesn't know; (4) other answer, and the

perceived duration of damage resulting from alcohol consumption during pregnancy (categorized as seven possible answers: (1) During pregnancy; (2) during childhood; (3) first years; (4) many years; (5) lifelong; (6) she doesn't know; (7) other). The categorization of answers was performed following the piloting of the study, in which these same questions were asked, allowing those responding to provide open answers, which were subsequently categorized. Furthermore, the "other" answer option was provided, as described above.

(d) Variables related to health professionals: The numbers of health professionals who provided information and the percentage of professionals who provided correct information (recommendation not to drink any alcohol during pregnancy).

(e) Variables related to the risk perception of consuming alcohol during pregnancy for specific types of drinks (beer, wine), in terms of the amount and frequency of consumption for each of them, with five response categories: "Any amount during pregnancy is harmful", "consuming alcohol less than once a month is not harmful", "consuming alcohol less than once a week is not harmful", "drinking a small amount every day is not harmful", "drinking as much and as often as a person wants to is not harmful". These categories were established after the answers obtained in the study pilot were studied. The "other" answer option was also included.

(f) Average daily alcohol consumption during pregnancy (in grams of pure alcohol) and average daily alcohol consumption before pregnancy (also in grams of pure alcohol). In both cases, the average daily number of grams was estimated from questions on the AUDIT scale [33], which ask about the frequency and amount of consumption of different types of drinks. Days of non-consumption were included in both calculations.

2.5. Data Analysis

First, a hierarchical regression analysis was conducted in order to examine the explained variance of alcohol consumption during pregnancy. In the first step, demographics (i.e., age, educational level, and employment status) were introduced in the regression equation, while obstetric history was added in the second (i.e., number of pregnancies and pregnancy planning). In the third and fourth steps, previous alcohol consumption and the partner's alcohol consumption were included. In the fifth and sixth steps of the regression analysis, advice received from health professionals (i.e., the number of health professionals who gave advice and the percentage of health professionals who provided the correct advice) and beliefs about risks (i.e., risk awareness of alcohol consumption during pregnancy, perceived duration of the damage caused by prenatal alcohol exposure, and the risk perception of drinking beer or wine during pregnancy) were included to explain alcohol consumption during pregnancy. R^2 were calculated at each step including subsequent variables in the analysis, as well as the change in F. Additionally, t and β coefficients were examined for each indicator. These analyses were carried out with SPSS 21.0 (IBM Corp, New York, NY, USA, 2012).

Second, moderation analyses were conducted to explore how the previous indicators (i.e., demographics, obstetric history, the partner's alcohol consumption, advice received from health professionals, and beliefs about risks) moderate the relationship between previous alcohol consumption and consumption during pregnancy. These analyses were carried out following the recommendations described by Hayes [34], based on regression analyses. The effects described in this model represent causal assumptions, because there is no causation verification without variable manipulation. Thus, only associations among variables may be concluded. Standardized coefficients were calculated to estimate the effect of one variable (assumed to be the independent variable) on another variable (assumed to be the criterion variable), and the moderation was analyzed as the interaction between the independent variable and the moderator to explain the dependent variable. Process v3.3 macro for SPSS was used, by specifically applying the model number 1, which performs a total of 1000 bootstrap samples for bias-corrected bootstrap confidence intervals. Huber-White heteroscedasticity-consistent inference was carried out.

Third, structural equation modelling was performed to integrate the effects of demographics, obstetric history, self-reported previous alcohol consumption, the partner's alcohol consumption, advice received from health professionals, and beliefs about risks, on self-reported alcohol consumption during pregnancy, as well as the relationships between those indicators. χ^2, Comparative Fit Index (CFI), and Root Mean Square Error of Approximation (RMSEA) were analyzed as overall data fit indexes. Lagrange multipliers and Wald tests were sequentially performed for model modifications to improve overall fit. R^2 was calculated to analyze the explained variance, and standardized solutions were examined. This model was tested with EQS 6.3 (Multivariate Software Inc., Temple City, CA, USA, 2017), following the recommendations by Byrne [35].

3. Results

3.1. Descriptive Characteristics of the Sample

A total of 832 pregnant women randomly selected in accordance with the procedure described above were invited to participate. Of them, 426 (51.2%) accepted. The total number of pregnant women who attended the morphological ultrasound clinic during the period in which the study was performed (5 months in 2016) was 1664. Most of the participants were Spanish (92.2%). The average age was 31.9 years (SD = 5.3). Information concerning demographic and obstetric variables was described in a previous work [32].

Table 1 displays the primary information from the different variables on which data were collected.

Table 1. Descriptive statistics of study variables.

Partner's Alcohol Consumption (%)	Never = 21.4 Once a month or less = 19.5 Twice to four times a month = 29.5 Twice to three times a week = 13.3 Four or more times a week = 15.5 No partner = 0.7
Number of health professionals who provided information (%)	Zero = 43.0 One = 26.5 Two = 14.1 Three = 16.4
% of health professionals who provided correct advice	None = 19.8 A third = 0.4 Half = 2.1 Two thirds = 1.6 All = 76.1
Risk awareness of alcohol consumption during pregnancy	Risk(s) mentioned = 59.5 She doesn't know but gives opinion = 12.7 She doesn't know = 27.1 No risk = 0.7
Perceived duration of damage	During pregnancy = 2.4 Childbirth = 3.8 First years = 9.3 Many years = 5.2 Lifelong = 48.1 She doesn't know = 27.5 Other = 3.8
Risk perception of drinking beer during pregnancy	Any amount is harmful = 31.5 Less than once a month is not harmful = 27.6 Less than once a week is not harmful = 25.3 A small amount every day is not harmful = 14.8 It is not harmful, regardless of the amount = 0.8

Table 1. Cont.

Risk perception of drinking wine during pregnancy	Any amount is harmful = 38.4 Less than once a month is not harmful = 30.6 Less than once a week is not harmful = 24.2 A small amount/day is not harmful = 5.9 It is not harmful, regardless of the amount = 0.9
Average daily alcohol consumption before pregnancy (grams)	M = 4.68, SD = 10.30
Average daily alcohol consumption during pregnancy (grams)	M = 0.38, SD = 1.55

3.2. Regression Analysis to Explain Alcohol Consumption during Pregnancy

Table 2 presents the results of the hierarchical regression analysis to explain self-reported alcohol consumption during pregnancy. In the first step, both educational level and employment status showed negative effects, such that lower alcohol consumption was detected in women with a higher educational level and among those self-labelled as "housewives". In the second step, obstetric history showed a significant effect, with more alcohol consumption in women who had more pregnancies. In the third step, previous alcohol consumption had a remarkable positive effect. Those women who reported higher previous alcohol consumption also indicated higher alcohol consumption during pregnancy. In the fourth step, the partner's alcohol consumption did not have a significant effect. In the fifth, a notable negative effect was observed for the percentage of professionals who provided correct advice. Thus, a lower percentage of professionals providing correct advice—not to consume any alcohol at all during pregnancy—is related to higher self-reported alcohol consumption. Lastly, in the sixth step, beliefs about risks were added, obtaining a final explained variance of 27%. Higher alcohol consumption during pregnancy was observed in those women who reported lower risk perception for wine.

Table 2. Hierarchical regression analysis of demographics, obstetric history, previous alcohol consumption, the partner's alcohol consumption, advice received from health professionals, and beliefs about risks, as correlates of alcohol consumption during pregnancy.

Title	R^2	ΔF	F	t	β
Step 1	0.04	5.24 **	5.24 **		
Age				−0.67	−0.04
Educational Level				−2.85	−0.14 **
Employment status				−3.91	−0.18 ***
Step 2	0.05	2.07	4.00 **		
Number of pregnancies				2.91	0.13 **
Pregnancy planning				−1.04	−0.05
Step 3	0.17	62.64 ***	14.25 ***		
Self-reported previous alcohol consumption				7.25	0.32 ***
Step 4	0.17	1.13	12.38 ***		
Partner's alcohol consumption				1.12	0.05
Step 5	0.24	19.76 ***	14.89 ***		
Number of health professionals who provided advice				0.33	0.02
% who provided correct information				−5.29	−0.26 ***
Step 6	0.27	4.28 **	11.95 ***		
Risk awareness of alcohol consumption during pregnancy				−1.86	−0.08
Perceived duration of damage				0.02	0.01
Perceived risk of drinking beer during pregnancy				−1.85	−0.17
Perceived risk of drinking wine during pregnancy				3.18	0.29 **

*** $p < 0.001$; ** $p < 0.01$.

3.3. Moderation Analysis in the Relationship between Previous Alcohol Consumption and Consumption during Pregnancy

Table 3 shows the results of the regression analyses to examine moderations in the relationships between previous and current alcohol consumption. Higher alcohol consumption during pregnancy was observed in women who reported higher previous consumption and had a low level of education. With regard to obstetric history, higher consumption during pregnancy was observed in women with greater previous consumption and more experience of pregnancies. Furthermore, higher consumption was also observed in women with higher previous consumption and those who reported a lower degree of correct advice received from health professionals. Lastly, risk perception regarding beer and wine also moderated that relationship. Higher alcohol consumption during pregnancy was observed in women with higher previous consumption and lower risk perception for the two types of alcoholic drinks studied.

Table 3. Regression analyses of the moderations by demographics, obstetric history, the partner's alcohol consumption, advice received from health professionals, and beliefs about risks, in the relationships between previous and current alcohol consumption.

"Previous Alcohol Consumption" x:	R^2	F	t	β
Age	0.01	0.40	−0.63	−0.06
Educational Level	0.03	6.69 *	−2.59	−0.19 *
Employment status	0.01	1.00	1.00	0.07
Number of pregnancies	0.02	4.69 *	2.16	0.16 *
Pregnancy planning	0.01	0.03	−0.18	−0.01
Partner's alcohol consumption	0.01	1.36	−1.17	−0.08
Number of health professionals who provided information	0.02	9.75 **	−3.12	−0.16 **
% of health professionals who provided correct information	0.10	31.94 ***	−5.65	−0.35 ***
Risk awareness of alcohol consumption during pregnancy	0.01	3.14	−1.77	−0.11
Perceived duration of the damage	0.01	2.52	1.59	0.14
Risk perception of drinking beer during pregnancy	0.02	4.43 *	2.11	0.14 *
Risk perception of drinking wine during pregnancy	0.02	4.66 *	2.16	0.15 *

Note. Dependent variable: Alcohol consumption during pregnancy. *** $p < 0.001$; ** $p < 0.01$; * $p < 0.05$.

3.4. Structural Equation Model

Lastly, the relationships between the study variables were integrated in a structural equation model. After conducting Lagrange multipliers and Wald tests, the final model reached a good overall data fit, $\chi^2(63, N = 426) = 118.17$, $p < 0.001$, $\chi^2/df = 1.88$, CFI = 0.95, RMSEA = 0.05, 90% CI RMSEA = 0.03–0.06. Table 4 describes the effects and associations included in the model, which all reached statistical significance ($p < 0.05$).

First, regarding alcohol consumption during pregnancy, the model showed negative effects for risk awareness of alcohol consumption during pregnancy, the percentage of health professionals who provided correct advice, educational level and employment status, with higher consumption among those women with better employment status, and positive effects for risk perception of drinking wine during pregnancy, previous alcohol consumption, and number of pregnancies. This equation presented a $R^2 = 0.25$ (MSE = 0.87), with the strongest effects for the percentage of health professionals who provided correct advice and previous alcohol consumption. Second, with regard to risk perception of drinking beer during pregnancy ($R^2 = 0.05$, MSE = 0.97) and wine ($R^2 = 0.01$, MSE = 0.99), previous alcohol consumption was positively related. Moreover, age and the number of health professionals who provided information were negatively related to risk perception of drinking beer during pregnancy.

Furthermore, some associations were also significant in the model. First, perceived risks of wine and beer were found to be positively interrelated. Moreover, beliefs about the duration of the damage and risk awareness of alcohol consumption during pregnancy were also positively associated. Second, the partner's alcohol consumption was positively associated with previous consumption and age, and negatively with beliefs about the duration of the damage. Third, the number of pregnancies was negatively related to previous alcohol consumption. Moreover, pregnancy planning was positively associated with age and educational level.

Table 4. Significant effects and associations included in the structural equation model.

Direct Effects	
Effects on alcohol consumption during pregnancy -Risk awareness: −0.09 -Risk perception of drinking wine during pregnancy: 0.14 -Previous alcohol consumption: 0.33 -% who correctly informed: −0.25 -Educational level: −0.14 -Employment status: −0.18 -Number of pregnancies: 0.13	*Effects on risk perception regarding beer* -Previous alcohol consumption: 0.10 -Number of health professionals who provided information: −0.05 -Age: −0.20 *Effects on risk perception regarding wine* -Previous alcohol consumption: 0.08
Associations	
Between variables: -Partner's alcohol consumption/previous consumption: 0.13 -Number of pregnancies/previous consumption: −0.17 -Number of health professionals who provided information/% who provided correct information: 0.37 -Employment status/% who correctly informed: −0.18 -Partner's alcohol consumption/age: 0.12 -Partner's alcohol consumption/perceived duration of the damage: −0.13 -Previous consumption/% who correctly informed: −0.12 -Age/educational level: 0.40 -Age/employment status: −0.23 -Number of pregnancies/age: 0.25 -Pregnancy planning/age: 0.25 -Employment status/educational level: −0.21 -Pregnancy planning/educational level: 0.20 *Between measurement errors of the variables:* -Duration of damage/risk awareness of alcohol consumption during pregnancy: 0.32 -Risk perception regarding wine/risk perception regarding beer: 0.88	

4. Discussion

The aim of this study was to analyze a wide range of potential predictors of alcohol consumption during pregnancy, with a view of identifying the specific weight of each of them, as well as the interactions between them. We thus intended to address the fragmented vision offered by studies conducted on this subject in general to date [8,24,31]. In order to examine the role of different factors as predictors of alcohol consumption during pregnancy, a random and representative sample of pregnant women receiving care in the outpatient clinics of a public hospital in a southern European city (Seville, Spain) was interviewed in the 20th week of pregnancy.

As in other previous studies [23–27], alcohol consumption prior to pregnancy was identified as the most powerful predictor of alcoholic beverage intake during pregnancy. This finding suggests, in short, that an expectant mother's previous lifestyle tends to continue during her pregnancy, particularly in terms of products that can lead to dependence and whose consumption is socially accepted in societies like Spain, such as alcoholic beverages. In this country, the average maternal age at delivery of the first child is particularly high (31.02 years of age in 2018, [36]), and the average age to start drinking alcoholic beverages is notably low (14.1 years of age among those female students who have ever drunk alcohol, [37]), and, as such, many women will have been drinking alcohol regularly for almost 20 years before their first pregnancy. It is not easy to drastically change behavior that is deeply rooted in lifestyles and has strong social support. It should not be forgotten, furthermore, that many pregnancies are unplanned (44% worldwide [38]; 25.4% in the sample used in this study) and that alcohol may be having a teratogenic effect on the embryo before the woman is aware she is pregnant, precisely in the period of prenatal development that is most sensitive to the action of teratogens (organogenesis).

A review carried out by Stephenson et al. highlights that the state of health of the expectant mother, as well as her lifestyle during the perigestational period, has an influence on the perinatal results of the new-born baby. It therefore proves very important to promote healthy lifestyles among women of child-bearing age, and more specifically, among those who are trying to conceive, by providing preconception care [39]. According to another retrospective study, developed by Goossens et al., the adoption of these healthy lifestyles before pregnancy is more likely in nulliparous women and in those with a previous miscarriage. At the same time, women who have had previous pregnancies, as well as those who are of a lower socio-economic level are less likely to change their lifestyles and make them healthier [40]. It is therefore necessary to combine general strategies for promoting healthy lifestyles among women of child-bearing age with others aimed specifically at each sector of these women, in such a way that makes it easier for all of them to choose the healthiest options in their daily lives.

The structural equations model created also concludes that another important predictive factor, although with less weight than the previous one, is health advice received from health professionals and, more specifically, the percentage of health professionals who have provided pregnant women with the correct advice: To abstain completely from consuming alcoholic beverages during pregnancy. This is a new finding and one that had not been previously identified in the research in this field. This result suggests that the performance of health professionals who treat pregnant women (GPs, obstetricians, midwives) may have a significant influence on their lifestyle, and specifically, on their alcohol consumption. This is consistent with the results of previous studies which corroborated the thinking that adequate health advice from professionals who care for pregnant women first-hand tends to reduce or stop alcohol consumption during pregnancy [41,42].

However, several studies carried out in the United Kingdom [43], Australia [44], and Spain [10] conclude that health advice on alcohol consumption provided to pregnant women is often contradictory and inconsistent. What the result of our study suggests is that providing pregnant women with correct advice on the issue—clearly explaining the appropriateness of not consuming any alcohol during pregnancy—proves to be crucial, as well as consistency of information in this regard among the different health professionals who care for pregnant women or women of childbearing age.

Although the predictive factors described above are those that have greater specific weight in the model developed in our work, other factors that may be relevant are also identified. Thus, the model establishes that pregnant women with better employment status (in the sense of having a full-time job) are more likely to consume alcohol than those with a part-time job or those who are unemployed. It is possible that the explanation for this lies in the likely higher level of income of the former compared to the latter. The greater their purchasing power, the more alcoholic beverages become financially accessible. A number of studies on correlates of alcohol consumption during pregnancy carried out in Ireland and Australia have concluded that high socioeconomic status (or a high income level) is associated with greater alcohol consumption during pregnancy [29,45,46]. At the same time, a study carried out in the USA also concluded that estimated level of income is positively related to drinking alcohol during pregnancy [23]. In a review of predictors of alcohol consumption during pregnancy, it was found that higher income or higher social class was found to be a predictor of drinking during pregnancy in four out of five studies that assessed this factor [25]. It has also been established that certain social situations (business dinners, etiquette ...) can encourage alcohol consumption, which is a pressure that might also affect pregnant women [47].

Educational level is identified as a predictor of relevant significance in this study, with a weight equivalent to that of the number of pregnancies. The model establishes that the higher the educational level, the lower the consumption of alcohol tends to be during pregnancy. This could be interpreted as meaning that women with a higher level of education are more easily able to seek and incorporate quality information in this field. However, this result is different from that found in a study carried out with pregnant women from 15 European countries, selected through websites, in which it was detected that pregnant women and new mothers of a higher educational level are those who state in a greater proportion that they consume or have consumed alcohol during pregnancy [48]. It is possible that the relationship between the level of education and alcohol consumption during pregnancy varies depending on the country, and also, depending on the way in which the sample of pregnant women is selected, or depending on the procedure used to estimate alcohol consumption.

The model shows that a higher number of previous pregnancies has a positive effect on alcohol consumption during pregnancy. This may have a plausible explanation, since the experience of a higher number of pregnancies in pregnant women who have presumably consumed alcohol without visible negative effects in the perinatal results, can result in consumption in later pregnancies, due to decreasing the perceived risk with respect to the harmful effect of alcohol. This interpretation was described in Testa's 1996 article [49], and later by Raymond [43], whose study suggests that pregnant women are influenced by experiences in their previous pregnancies with respect to alcohol consumption. If this consumption has not had a pernicious effect on her or on the fetus, this may make it easier for the pregnant woman to be more permissive in terms of intake.

The model identifies the perceived risk of drinking wine while pregnant as another predictor of alcohol consumption during pregnancy, in the sense that might be expected: The lower the perceived risk, the greater the consumption (estimated in grams of pure alcohol). Studies carried out in Australia [50], France [16], and Spain [32] found that low perception of the risks posed by consuming wine while pregnant dominates among expectant mothers. In Spain (and perhaps in other social contexts where low perception of the potential teratogenic effects of this alcoholic beverage dominates), it is precisely those expectant mothers who are most aware of the adverse effects on the fetus who present lower alcohol consumption during pregnancy.

Interactions between the predictors, laid out in the Results section, appear generally logical and may have clear implications for prevention. Thus, for example, it was found that the effect of alcohol consumption before pregnancy on consumption during the actual pregnancy is particularly intense when the expectant mother has a low level of education. Therefore, according to these results, those women with the lowest level of education would constitute a high-priority sector for interventions aimed at preventing FASD, probably requiring communication strategies (both within and outside the healthcare system) that are specially adapted to their socio-educational characteristics. It can also be observed that alcohol consumption by the partner and alcohol consumption before pregnancy are interrelated, which suggests that preventive interventions should not be aimed solely at expectant mothers and women before they become pregnant, but also at their partners.

As intervention suggestions resulting from the analysis of these predictive factors, we can highlight the need for health professionals to warn pregnant women of the deleterious effect of alcohol in pregnancy, conveying in clear and understandable terms the message that abstaining from alcohol consumption is the only safe practice. In turn, for health professionals to adequately assess the alcohol consumption habits of pregnant women (or women of a childbearing age in general) and develop with them culturally adapted and effective communication strategies, the implementation of suitable continued training is required, as well as the development of institutional programs in the health system that facilitate and promote the full exercising of their role in the prevention of FASD. In this field, the experience of countries that have made a greater effort in preventing FASD to date, such as Australia, Canada, the United States, and New Zealand, among others [51–53], should be taken into account in particular.

Finally, we should not forget that a pregnant woman is influenced by social perceptions about alcoholic beverages, as well as whatever interpretation she might have made of her own personal experiences of drinking alcoholic beverages, if she has had any. A popular perception of alcohol which has become more widespread over the last few decades is the idea that the regular consumption of moderate quantities of alcoholic beverages (wine in particular) can prove to be a cardiovascular protector. This belief serves to support another: Adults are recommended to drink low doses of alcohol regularly. Today, it is clear that both ideas are lacking in any solid foundation. According to Naimi et al. (2017), to date, there has been no randomized clinical trial of low-volume alcohol consumption that has assessed any mortality outcome. Everything we know about the impact on health of drinking low doses of alcohol is based on observational studies which, in general, suffer from serious selection biases, as detailed by these authors, which constitutes in their opinion a reason to suggest that the existing research may systematically overestimate the protective effects of "moderate" alcohol consumption [54]. At the same time, the Global Burden of Disease Study 2016, carried out using data from 195 countries and territories in the period 1990-2016, concluded that the level of alcohol consumption that minimized harm across health outcomes was zero standard drinks per week [55]. This could be expressed in other terms: No level of alcohol consumption improves health [56]. It proves easier to provide pregnant women and the people around them with correct information about the risks of drinking alcoholic beverages during pregnancy in a social context which is neutral to alcohol consumption than in one where ideas in favor of drinking are widespread. If it is explained to the population as a whole in appropriate terms by the healthcare system that there is no solid scientific basis to support the idea that moderate alcohol consumption is beneficial for health, this will contribute to reducing the enormous burden of health, social and education problems resulting from alcohol consumption, including FASD.

The study performed has both strengths and limitations. Among its strengths, it should be noted that the sample was randomly selected among all pregnant women who attended a programmed control clinic in the same week of pregnancy (week 20). Furthermore, the interviews were conducted in person (face to face) by health staff trained specifically in this area. Data analysis includes the use of a structural equations model and other confirmatory multivariate techniques. On the other hand, one limitation that can be highlighted is that, since the study is cross-sectional, it is not possible to establish inferences of causal relationships between variables. Furthermore, all immigrant pregnant women who could not take part in the interview because they had limited fluency in Spanish were excluded from the sample, due to the absence of auxiliary translation services. The participation rate was 51.2%, which does not exclude the likelihood of selection bias. Alcohol consumption was evaluated only through self-reported data, and not through biomarker analysis too. A validated scale was not used to assess the degree of planning of the pregnancy.

5. Conclusions

Among the conclusions derived from this study, we can establish that alcohol consumption prior to pregnancy is a predictor that has a powerful direct relationship with alcohol during pregnancy. Second, the percentage of health professionals who adequately inform pregnant women about the harmful effects of alcohol consumption in pregnancy has a powerful inverse relationship with alcohol intake during pregnancy. Furthermore, previous alcohol consumption during pregnancy is especially related to this consumption being maintained during pregnancy among expectant mothers with low educational levels.

Author Contributions: I.C.-G., F.L.-L., D.G.-B. and R.M. conceived and designed the study. I.C.-G., F.L.-L. and R.M. coordinated the data collection. D.G.-B. was responsible for the data analysis. All authors interpreted the results, drafted, reviewed and approved the final version of the article. All authors have read and agreed to the published version of the manuscript.

Funding: This research was funded by the Research Group on Health Promotion and Development of Lifestyle across a LifeSpan (University of Huelva) with funding received from the Scientific Policy Strategy of the University of Huelva and the Andalusian Plan for Research, Development and Innovation(PAIDI).

Acknowledgments: The authors acknowledge E. Morales-Marente, M.S. Palacios and C. Rodriguez-Reinado (University of Huelva) O. García-Algar (Hospital Clinic, Barcelona), and Rocío Medero (Hospital N.S. Valme, Andalusian Health Service) for their contributions to the design and development of this study as research team members.

Conflicts of Interest: The authors declare no conflict of interest.

References

1. Pruett, D.; Waterman, E.H.; Caughey, A.B. Fetal Alcohol Exposure. *Obstet. Gynecol. Surv.* **2013**, *68*, 62–69. [CrossRef] [PubMed]
2. Caputo, C.; Wood, E.; Jabbour, L. Impact of fetal alcohol exposure on body systems: A systematic review. *Birth Defects Res. Embryo Today* **2016**, *108*, 174–180. [CrossRef] [PubMed]
3. Wozniak, J.R.; Riley, E.P.; Charness, M.E. Clinical presentation, diagnosis, and management of fetal alcohol spectrum disorder. *Lancet Neurol.* **2019**, *18*, 760–770. [CrossRef]
4. Williams, J.F.; Smith, V.C. Fetal Alcohol Spectrum Disorders. *Pediatrics* **2015**, *136*, 1395–1406. [CrossRef] [PubMed]
5. Cook, J.L.; Green, C.R.; Lilley, C.M.; Anderson, S.M.; Baldwin, M.E.; Chudley, A.E.; Conry, J.L.; LeBlanc, N.; Loock, C.A.; Lutke, J.; et al. Fetal alcohol spectrum disorder: A guideline for diagnosis across the lifespan. *CMAJ* **2015**, *188*, 191–197. [CrossRef] [PubMed]
6. Popova, S.; Lange, S.; Shield, K.; Mihic, A.; Chudley, A.E.; Mukherjee, R.A.; Bekmuradov, D.; Rehm, J. Comorbidity of fetal alcohol spectrum disorder: A systematic review and meta-analysis. *Lancet* **2016**, *387*, 978–987. [CrossRef]
7. Popova, S.; Lange, S.; Probst, C.; Gmel, G.; Rehm, J. Estimation of national, regional, and global prevalence of alcohol use during pregnancy and fetal alcohol syndrome: A systematic review and meta-analysis. *Lancet Glob. Health* **2017**, *5*, 290–299. [CrossRef]
8. Mårdby, A.C.; Lupattelli, A.; Hensing, G.; Nordeng, H. Consumption of alcohol during pregnancy—A multinational European study. *Women Birth* **2017**, *30*, 207–213. [CrossRef]
9. Lange, S.; Probst, C.; Gmel, G.; Rehm, J.; Burd, L.; Popova, S. Global Prevalence of Fetal Alcohol Spectrum Disorder Among Children and Youth. *JAMA Pediatr.* **2017**, *171*, 948–956. [CrossRef]
10. Mendoza, R.; Morales-Marente, E.; Palacios, M.; Rodríguez-Reinado, C.; Corrales-Gutiérrez, I.; García-Algar, Ó. Health advice on alcohol consumption in pregnant women in Seville (Spain). *Gac. Sanit.* **2019**. [CrossRef]
11. Payne, J.; Elliott, E.; D'Antoine, H.; O'Leary, C.; Mahony, A.; Haan, E.; Bower, C. Health professionals' knowledge, practice and opinions about fetal alcohol syndrome and alcohol consumption in pregnancy. *Aust. N. Z. J. Public Health* **2005**, *29*, 558–564. [CrossRef] [PubMed]
12. Payne, J.M.; Watkins, R.E.; Jones, H.M.; Reibel, T.; Mutch, R.; Wilkins, A.; Whitlock, J.; Bower, C. Midwives' knowledge, attitudes and practice about alcohol exposure and the risk of fetal alcohol spectrum disorder. *BMC Pregnancy Childbirth* **2014**, *14*, 337. [CrossRef] [PubMed]
13. Whitehall, J.S. National guidelines on alcohol use during pregnancy: A dissenting opinion. *Med. J. Aust.* **2007**, *186*, 35–37. [CrossRef] [PubMed]
14. O'Leary, C.M.; Heuzenroeder, L.; Elliot, E.J.; Bower, C. A review of policies on alcohol use during pregnancy in Australia and other English-speaking countries, 2016. *Med. J. Aust.* **2007**, *186*, 466–471. [CrossRef]
15. Montag, A.; Brodine, S.K.; Alcaraz, J.E.; Clapp, J.D.; Allison, M.A.; Calac, D.J.; Hull, A.D.; Gorman, J.R.; Jones, K.L.; Chambers, C.D. Preventing Alcohol-ExposedPregnancyAmongan American Indian/Alaska NativePopulation: Effect of a Screening, BriefIntervention, and Referral to TreatmentIntervention. *Alcohol Clin. Exp. Res.* **2015**, *39*, 126–135. [CrossRef] [PubMed]
16. Dumas, A.; Toutain, S.; Hill, C.; Simmat-Durand, L. Warning about drinking during pregnancy: Lessons from the French experience. *Reprod. Health* **2018**, *15*, 20. [CrossRef] [PubMed]
17. National Health and Medical Research Council. *Australian Guidelines to Reduce Health Risks from Drinking Alcohol*; Commonwealth of Australia: Canberra, Australia, 2009.
18. Kesmodel, U.; Kesmodel, P. Alcohol in pregnancy: Attitudes, knowledge, and information Practice among midwives in Denmark 2000 to 2009. *Alcoholism* **2011**, *35*, 2226–2230. [CrossRef]
19. Norwegian Health Service web. Alcohol and Pregnancy in Norway. Available online: https://helsenorge.no/other-languages/english/alcohol-and-pregnancy (accessed on 5 February 2020).
20. NHS. Scottish Guidelines. *Alcohol and Pregnancy. No Alcohol, No Risk.* Available online: https://www.nhsaaa.net/media/5701/alcohol-pregnancy-a5-booklet-final.pdf (accessed on 5 February 2020).
21. American Academy of Pediatrics. Advisory on Alcohol Use in Pregnancy. Available online: https://www.cdc.gov/ncbddd/fasd/documents/sg-advisory-508.pdf (accessed on 5 February 2020).
22. Carson, G.; Cox, L.V.; Crane, J.; Croteau, P.; Graves, L.; Kluka, S. Society of Obstetricians of Canada. Alcohol use and pregnancy consensus clinical Guidelines. *J. Obstet. Gynaecol. Can.* **2010**, *32*, S1–S31. [CrossRef]

23. Chang, G.; McNamara, T.K.; Orav, E.J.; Wilkins-Haug, L. Alcohol use by pregnant women: Partners, knowledge, and other predictors. *J. Stud. Alcohol* **2006**, *67*, 245–251. [CrossRef]
24. Palma, S.; Pardo-Crespo, R.; Mariscal, M.; Perez-Iglesias, R.; Llorca, J.; Delgado-Rodriguez, M. Weekday but not weekend alcohol consumption before pregnancy influences alcohol cessation during pregnancy. *Eur. J. Public Health* **2007**, *17*, 394–399. [CrossRef]
25. Skagerström, J.; Chang, G.; Nilsen, P. Predictors of Drinking During Pregnancy: A Systematic Review. *J. Womens Health* **2011**, *20*, 901–913. [CrossRef] [PubMed]
26. Mallard, S.R.; Connor, J.L.; Houghton, L.A. Maternal factors associated with heavy periconceptional alcohol intake and drinking following pregnancy recognition: A post-partum survey of New Zealand women. *Drug Alcohol Rev.* **2013**, *32*, 389–397. [CrossRef] [PubMed]
27. Zammit, S.L.; Skouteris, H.; Wertheim, E.H.; Paxton, S.J.; Milgrom, J. Pregnant Women's Alcohol Consumption: The Predictive Utility of Intention to Drink and Prepregnancy Drinking Behavior. *J. Womens Health* **2008**, *17*, 1513–1522. [CrossRef] [PubMed]
28. Ministerio de Sanidad, Consumo y Bienestar Social—Portal Estadístico del SNS—Encuesta Nacional de Salud de España 2017 Mscbs.gob.es. 2019. Available online: http://www.mscbs.gob.es/estadEstudios/estadisticas/encuestaNacional/encuesta2017.htm (accessed on 16 December 2019).
29. McCormack, C.; Hutchinson, D.; Burns, L.; Wilson, J.; Elliott, E.; Allsop, S.; Najman, J.; Jacobs, S.; Rossen, L.; Olsson, C.; et al. Prenatal Alcohol Consumption Between Conception and Recognition of Pregnancy. *Alcohol Clin. Exp. Res.* **2017**, *41*, 369–378. [CrossRef] [PubMed]
30. Murphy, D.J.; Mullally, A.; Cleary, B.J.; Fahey, T.; Barry, J. Behavioural change in relation to alcohol exposure in early pregnancy and impact on perinatal outcomes—A prospective cohort study. *BMC Pregnancy Childbirth* **2013**, *13*, 8. [CrossRef] [PubMed]
31. O'Keeffe, L.M.; Kearney, P.M.; McCarthy, F.P.; Khashan, A.S.; Greene, R.A.; North, R.A.; Poston, L.; McCowan, L.M.; Baker, P.N.; Dekker, G.A.; et al. Prevalence and predictors of alcohol use during pregnancy: Findings from international multicentre cohort studies. *BMJ Open* **2015**, *5*, e006323. [CrossRef] [PubMed]
32. Corrales-Gutierrez, I.; Mendoza, R.; Gomez-Baya, D.; Leon-Larios, F. Pregnant Women's Risk Perception of the Teratogenic Effects of Alcohol Consumption in Pregnancy. *J Clin. Med.* **2019**, *8*, 907. [CrossRef]
33. Babor, T.F.; Higgins-Biddle, J.C.; Saunders, J.B.; Monteiro, M.G. *The Alcohol Use Disorders. Identification Test. Guidelines for Use in Primary Care*, 2nd ed.; World Health Organization: Geneva, Switzerland, 2001; p. 17. [CrossRef]
34. Hayes, A.; Rockwood, N. Regression-based statistical mediation and moderation analysis in clinical research: Observations, recommendations, and implementation. *Behav. Res. Ther.* **2017**, *98*, 39–57. [CrossRef]
35. Byrne, B.M. *Structural Equation Modeling with EQS*, 2nd ed.; Routledge: New York, NY, USA, 2013.
36. Instituto Nacional de estadística. España en cifras. INE. 2018. Available online: https://www.ine.es/prodyser/espa_cifras/2018/3/ (accessed on 25 December 2019).
37. Ministerio de Sanidad, Consumo y Bienestar Social—Portal Estadístico del SNS. La Encuesta sobre uso de drogas en Enseñanzas Secundarias en España, ESTUDES 2018 Mscbs.gob.es. 2019. Available online: http://www.pnsd.mscbs.gob.es/profesionales/sistemasInformacion/sistemaInformacion/encuestas_ESTUDES.htm (accessed on 25 December 2019).
38. Bearak, J.; Popinchalk, A.; Alkema, L.; Sedgh, G. Global, regional, and subregional trends in unintended pregnancy and its outcomes from 1990 to 2014: Estimates from a Bayesian hierarchical model. *Lancet Glob. Health* **2018**, *6*, 380–389. [CrossRef]
39. Stephenson, J.; Heslehurst, N.; Hall, J.; Schoenaker, D.A.; Hutchinson, J.; Cade, J.E.; Poston, L.; Barrett, G.; Crozier, S.R.; Barker, M.; et al. Before the beginning: Nutrition and lifestyle in the preconception period and its importance for future health. *Lancet* **2018**, *391*, 1830–1841. [CrossRef]
40. Goossens, J.; Beeckman, D.; Van Hecke, A.; Delbaere, I.; Verhaeghe, S. Preconception lifestyle changes in women with planned pregnancies. *Midwifery* **2018**, *56*, 112–120. [CrossRef] [PubMed]
41. Nilsen, P. Brief alcohol intervention to prevent drinking during pregnancy: An overview of research findings. *Curr. Opin. Obstet. Gynecol.* **2009**, *21*, 496–500. [CrossRef] [PubMed]
42. O'Connor, M.J.; Whaley, S.E. Brief Intervention for Alcohol Use by Pregnant Women. *Am. J. Public Health* **2007**, *97*, 252–258. [CrossRef] [PubMed]
43. Raymond, N.; Beer, C.; Glazebrook, C.; Sayal, K. Pregnant women's attitudes towards alcohol consumption. *BMC Public Health* **2009**, *9*, 175. [CrossRef] [PubMed]

44. Anderson, A.E.; Hure, A.J.; Kay-Lambkin, F.J.; Loxton, D.J. Women's perceptions of information about alcohol use during pregnancy: A qualitative study. *BMC Public Health* **2014**, *14*, 1048. [CrossRef] [PubMed]
45. Murphy, D.J.; Dunney, C.; Mullally, A.; Adnan, N.; Fahey, T.; Barry, J. A prospective cohort study of alcohol exposure in early and late pregnancy within an urban population in Ireland. *Int. J. Environ. Res. Public Health* **2014**, *11*, 2049–2063. [CrossRef]
46. Muggli, E.; O'Leary, C.; Donath, S.; Orsini, F.; Forster, D.; Anderson, P.J.; Lewis, S.; Nagle, C.; Craig, J.M.; Elliott, E.; et al. "Did you ever drink more?" A detailed description of pregnant women's drinking patterns. *BMC Public Health* **2016**, *2*, 683. [CrossRef]
47. Tan, C.H.; Denny, C.H.; Cheal, N.E.; Sniezek, J.E.; Kanny, D. Alcohol use and binge drinking among women of childbearing age—United States, 2011–2013. *MMWR Morb. Mortal. Wkly. Rep.* **2015**, *25*, 1042–1046. [CrossRef]
48. Mårdby, A.C.; Lupattelli, A.; Hensing, G.; Smedberg, J.; Nordeng, H. Factors associated with alcohol consumption during pregnancy—A cross-sectional study in 15 European countries. *Eur. J. Public Health* **2014**, *24*. [CrossRef]
49. Testa, M.; Reifman, A. Individual differences in perceived riskiness of drinking in pregnancy: Antecedents and consequences. *J. Stud. Alcohol* **1996**, *57*, 360–367. [CrossRef]
50. Crawford-Williams, F.; Steen, M.; Esterman, A.; Fielder, A.; Mikocka-Walus, A. "My midwife said that having a glass of red wine was actually better for the baby": A focus group study of women and their partner's knowledge and experiences relating to alcohol consumption in pregnancy. *BMC Pregnancy Childbirth* **2015**, *15*, 79. [CrossRef] [PubMed]
51. Fitzpatrick, J.P.; Oscar, J.; Carter, M.; Elliott, E.J.; Latimer, J.; Wright, E.; Boulton, J. The Marulu Strategy 2008–2012: Overcoming Fetal Alcohol Spectrum Disorder (FASD) in the Fitzroy Valley. *Aust. N. Z. J. Public Health* **2017**, *41*, 467–473. [CrossRef] [PubMed]
52. Hanson, J.D.; Ingersoll, K.; Pourier, S. Development and Implementation of CHOICES Group to Reduce Drinking, Improve Contraception, and Prevent Alcohol-Exposed Pregnancies in American Indian Women. *J. Subst. Abuse Treat.* **2015**, *59*, 45–51. [CrossRef] [PubMed]
53. Symons, M.; Pedruzzi, R.A.; Bruce, K.; Milne, E. A systematic review of prevention interventions to reduce prenatal alcohol exposure and fetal alcohol spectrum disorder in indigenous communities. *BMC Public Health* **2018**, *18*, 1227. [CrossRef] [PubMed]
54. Naimi, T.S.; Stockwell, T.; Zhao, J.; Xuan, Z.; Dangardt, F.; Saitz, R.; Liang, W.; Chikritzhs, T. Selection biases in observational studies affect associations between 'moderate' alcohol consumption and mortality. *Addiction* **2017**, *112*, 207–214. [CrossRef]
55. GBD 2016 Alcohol Collaborators. Alcohol use and burden for 195 countries and territories, 1990–2016: A systematic analysis for the Global Burden of Disease Study 2016. *Lancet* **2018**. [CrossRef]
56. Burton, R.; Sheron, N. No level of alcohol consumption improves health. *Lancet* **2018**. [CrossRef]

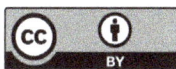

© 2020 by the authors. Licensee MDPI, Basel, Switzerland. This article is an open access article distributed under the terms and conditions of the Creative Commons Attribution (CC BY) license (http://creativecommons.org/licenses/by/4.0/).

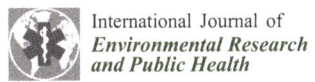

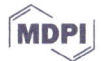

Article

Effect of Sex on the Association Between Nonmedical Use of Opioids and Sleep Disturbance Among Chinese Adolescents: A Cross-Sectional Study

Di Xiao [1,2,3], Lan Guo [1], Meijun Zhao [1], Sheng Zhang [1], Wenyan Li [1], Wei-Hong Zhang [2,4,*,†] and Ciyong Lu [1,3,*,†]

1. Department of Medical Statistics and Epidemiology, School of Public Health, Sun Yat-sen University, Guangzhou 510080, China; Di.Xiao@UGent.be (D.X.); guolan3@mail.sysu.edu.cn (L.G.); zhaomj5@mail2.sysu.edu.cn (M.Z.); zhangsh46@mail2.sysu.edu.cn (S.Z.); liwy23@mail2.sysu.edu.cn (W.L.)
2. International Centre for Reproductive Health (ICRH), Department of Public Health and Primary Care, Ghent University, 9000 Gent, Belgium
3. Guangdong Provincial Key Laboratory of Food, Nutrition and Health, Sun Yat-sen University, Guangzhou 510080, China
4. Research Laboratory for Human Reproduction, Faculty of Medicine, Université Libre de Bruxelles (ULB), 1050 Bruxelles, Belgium
* Correspondence: weihong.zhang@ugent.be (W.-H.Z.); luciyong@mail.sysu.edu.cn (C.L.); Tel.: +86-20-8733-2477 (C.L.)
† These authors contributed equally to this work.

Received: 16 October 2019; Accepted: 5 November 2019; Published: 7 November 2019

Abstract: Sleep disturbance and non-medical prescription opioid use (NMPOU) are currently growing public health concerns, and sex differences may result in differential exposure to frequency of NMPOU or sleep disturbance. This study aimed to explore the association between the frequency of lifetime or past-year NMPOU and sleep disturbance and to evaluate whether there was any sex difference in this association among Chinese adolescents. A cross-sectional study was performed in seven randomly selected Chinese provinces through the 2015 School-Based Chinese Adolescents Health Survey. A total of 159,640 adolescents were invited to participate and among them, 148,687 adolescents' questionnaires were completed and qualified for this study (response rate: 93.14%). All analyses were performed for boys and girls separately. There were significant sex differences in the prevalence of lifetime or past-year opioid misuse and sleep disturbance ($p < 0.05$). Among girls, frequent lifetime NMPOU (adjusted odds ratio [aOR] = 2.09, 95% CI = 1.80–2.44) and past-year NMPOU (aOR = 2.16, 95% CI = 1.68–2.77) were positively associated with sleep disturbance. Among boys, these associations were also statistically significant, while the magnitudes of associations between frequent lifetime NMPOU or past-year NMPOU and sleep disturbance were greater in girls than those in boys. There is a significant sex difference in the prevalence of lifetime or past-year NMPOU and sleep disturbance. Furthermore, exposure to more frequent lifetime or past-year NMPOU is associated with a greater risk of sleep disturbance, especially among girls. Taking into account the sex difference for lifetime or past-year NMPOU may help to decrease the risk of sleep disturbance.

Keywords: non-medical prescription opioid use; sleep disturbance; sex differences; adolescents

1. Introduction

Sleep plays an important role in the development and maintenance of physical and mental health, especially in adolescents [1,2]. Evidence shows that sleep disruption is highly prevalent among adolescents [3]. Research in western countries has shown that approximately 25%–40% of adolescents have sleep disorders [4,5]. In China, it was estimated that the prevalence rate of sleep disturbance among adolescents ranged from 18.0% to 39.6% [6–8]. Recent studies have shown that sleep problems were associated with serious behavioral problems [9], depression [10], Attention-Deficit/Hyperactivity Disorder (ADHD) [11], poor school performance [12], and suicide [13] among children and adolescents. Sleep disturbance among adolescents has become a major international health concern.

The rise in non-medical prescription opioid use (NMPOU) is an emerging public health problem in adolescents [14]. Over the past two decades, the prevalence of prescription opioid misuse has increased more than threefold in the United States [15]. Most recent evidence from the National Survey on Drug Use and Health (NSDUH) showed that 3.5% of adolescents aged 12 to 17 engaged in NMPOU in the past year [16]. Moreover, based on the data from the 2014 NSDUH, 7.3% of responding adolescents aged 12–17 reported NMPOU during their lifetime [17]. A survey in China also found that NMPOU was prevalent among Chinese adolescents, and the prevalence of the lifetime NMPOU use was 7.7% [18]. In China, the most commonly used medicine was licorice tablets with morphine, cough syrup with codeine, diphenoxylate, and tramadol [6]. Further, Guo et al. [19] reported that "to relax or relieve tension" was the most prevalent reason for nonmedical use of opioids among adolescents. The misuse of prescription opioids can lead to numerous adverse consequences, such as sexual behavior [20], heroin use [21], drug injection [21], depression [22], and suicidal behavior [23]. Evidence has shown that opioids can increase wakefulness and decrease total sleep time [24], delta sleep [25], sleep efficiency [25], and rapid eye movement (REM) sleep [26]. Walker et al. [27] reported a dose-dependent relationship between chronic opioid use and sleep disorders. Although there have been indications that past-month NMPOU could predict poor sleep [6], there is a dearth of studies addressing the potential association between the frequency of lifetime or past-year NMPOU and sleep disturbance in adolescents.

Sex differences may lead to differential exposure to prescription drug misuse or sleep disturbance. The prevalence of NMPOU in boys is reportedly greater than in girls [28,29], and girls complain more about their sleep than boys [30]. Research found that boys may have a stronger need for sensation-seeking than girls [31], and seeking pleasure and release of tension were the most common reasons for substance use [32,33]. Moreover, differences in the process of physiological changes related to puberty may lead to the sex differences in sleep disorders [34]. Whether the effects of lifetime or past-year NMPOU on sleep disturbance are similar or different for boys and girls is not clear and little attention has been paid to sex differences across these associations. Understanding the relationship between NMPOU and sleep disturbance among adolescents, as well as identifying the mechanisms that underlie potential sex differences may provide valuable insights and facilitate the design of sex-sensitive sleep disturbance preventive programs.

Therefore, to address the above questions, a large national study in China was conducted to assess the prevalence of lifetime NMPOU, past-year NMPOU, and sleep disturbance among Chinese adolescents; to explore the independent associations between the frequency of lifetime and past-year NMPOU with sleep disturbance; and to investigate whether there are sex differences within the associations.

2. Materials and Methods

2.1. Study Design

The cross-sectional data of the current study were collected from the 2015 School-based Chinese Adolescents Health Survey (SCAHS) [18,35]. SCAHS is an ongoing survey of health-related behaviors in 7th–12th grades students in China, which has been conducted every two years since 2007. The 2015 SCAHS is the most recent version [18].

2.2. Data Collection and Sample

Data collection procedures have been described in detail elsewhere [36]. Briefly, adolescents were selected using a multistage, stratified cluster sampling method. In stage 1, based on geographic location, a total of seven large provinces in China were selected. Each province was divided into three stratifications according to the Gross Domestic Product (GDP: high, medium, and low), then two cities were selected randomly from each stratus. In stage 2, from each representative city, the schools were classified according to three categories, including junior high school (grades 7–9), senior high school (grades 10–12), and vocational school (grades 10–12). We randomly selected 6 to 7 junior high schools, 4 to 5 senior high schools, and 2 to 3 vocational schools from each city. In stage 3, we randomly selected two classes from each grade and we investigated all the available students in these classes. Finally, a total of 159,640 adolescents were invited to participate in our survey, and 148,687 Chinese students completed the questionnaires (response rate: 93.14%). To avoid any potential information bias, a Chinese-language self-administered questionnaire was completed by each student within one class period with the supervision of research assistants. To protect the privacy of the students, the questionnaire was completed anonymously and without a teacher present.

2.3. Measures

2.3.1. Dependent Variable

Sleep quality and disturbances over the past month were assessed by the Chinese version of the Pittsburgh Sleep Quality Index (PSQI). The Chinese version of the PSQI has been validated [37] and has been extensively used [8,38] with Chinese adolescents. The survey assessed the 19-item PSQI, which consists of seven components containing subjective sleep quality, sleep latency, sleep duration, habitual sleep efficiency, sleep disturbance, use of sleep medications, and daytime dysfunction. The sum of the scores for these seven components yields one global score with a range from 0 to 21, with higher scores indicating a higher level of sleep disturbance [37]. In China, a PSQI global score that is greater than 7 points indicates poor sleep quality, which is collectively known as sleep disturbance [7].

2.3.2. Independent Variable

In the present study, four opioid drugs were investigated: cough syrup compounded with codeine, compounded licorice tablets (opium), tramadol hydrochloride, and diphenoxylate. Lifetime NMPOU was measured by the following question: "Have you ever used the following list of prescription opioid drugs even once, when you were not sick or just for the intended purpose to experiment or to get high without a doctor's prescription?" The question was followed by a list of the above prescription opioid drugs, with responses coded as "never = 0", "once or twice" = 1, and "at least three times" = 2. If the answer was "once or twice" or "at least three times", we then asked about the student's past-year NMPOU. Students who reported "never" were classified as abstainers, those who admitted once or twice were classified as experimenters, and those students who answered at least three times were classified as frequent users [19].

2.3.3. Other Variables

The demographic variables included age, sex (boy = 1 and girl = 2), grade, academic pressure, academic achievement, classmate relationships, relationships with teachers, bullying experience, current smoking, and current drinking. Academic pressure and academic achievement were assessed by asking about the student's self-rating of his or her academic pressure or achievement relative to that of his or her classmates (responses were coded as "below average", "average", or "above average"). Relationships with teachers and classmate relationships were measured according to the students' self-rating of their relationships with their teachers and classmates (categorized into "good = 1", "average = 2", and "poor = 3").

Bullying experience was measured with the Olweus Bully/Victim Questionnaire. The respondents were asked about the following question: "How often have you been bullied (kicked, intentionally excluded from participating, made fun of with sexual jokes, etc.) at school in the past 30 days?" [39]. The response options were (1) "never", (2) "sometimes or rarely (one or two times)", or (3) "often (more than three times)". Students who selected a frequency of "often" in the past 30 days were defined as being bullied [40].

Current smoking was investigated by asking students the following question: "How many days did you smoke cigarettes during the past 30 days?" Responses were defined as current smokers when the selected answers indicated 1 or more days [41]. Current drinking was assessed with the following question: "During the past 30 days, on how many days did you drink alcohol?" Responses were defined as current drinkers when the selected answers indicated 1 or more days [42].

2.4. Ethical Considerations

The Sun Yat-Sen University School of Public Health Institutional Review Board approved this study (L2014076). Then, a written informed consent form was obtained from each school and one of the parents (or legal guardians) of each participating adolescent after the study procedures had been fully described.

2.5. Statistical Analysis

SAS 9.4 (SAS Institute, Inc., Cary, NC, USA) was used to perform all statistical analyses. Firstly, to describe the sample characteristics, the prevalence of lifetime or past-year NMPOU, and sleep disturbance, descriptive analyses that were stratified by sex were conducted. Secondly, to investigate whether there were any statistically significant differences between female and male students, a t-test for continuous variables and chi-square test for categorical variables were performed. Thirdly, univariable logistic regression models were conducted to test the potential factors that are associated with sleep disturbance. Finally, multivariable logistic regression models were used to explore the independent associations of lifetime and past-year NMPOU with sleep disturbance, and the covariates that were associated (p value < 0.05) with sleep disturbance in univariable analyses were entered simultaneously as control variables.

Statistical significance was set at the $p < 0.05$ using two-sided tests.

3. Results

3.1. Population Characteristics by Sex

Table 1 presents the basic demographic information of this study. Of the 148,687 students, 48.0% (71,442) were boys and 52.0% (77,245) were girls. The age range was 12–18 years and the mean age of the students was 15.0 (SD: ±1.8). Overall, 1.8% and 0.7% of the students admitted that they were a "frequent user" of lifetime or past-year NMPOU, respectively. Among the total sample, 35.7% of the students rated their academic pressures as above average and 8.2% of the students had bullying experience. Approximately 5.3% of adolescents reported current smoking and 15.9% of the students currently drank alcohol. A total of 21.6% students reported having sleep disturbance. Statistically significant differences were observed in the sex distribution of age, grade, academic achievement, teacher–classmate and classmate relations, academic pressure, bullying experience, current smoking, current drinking, lifetime, and past-year NMPOU ($p < 0.05$).

Table 1. Sex difference of the sample characteristics (n = 148,687).

Variable	Total, No. (%)	Boys	Girls	p-Value [1]
Total	148,687	71,442 (48.0)	77,245 (52.0)	<0.001
Age				<0.001
12 to 13	34,890 (23.5)	16,844 (23.6)	18,046 (23.4)	
14 to 15	51,225 (34.5)	25,782 (36.1)	25,443 (32.9)	
16 to 18	62,572 (42.1)	28,816 (40.3)	33,756 (43.7)	

Table 1. Cont.

Variable	Total, No. (%)	Boys	Girls	p-Value [1]
Grade				
7th to 9th	77,936 (52.4)	39,717 (55.6)	38,219 (49.5)	<0.001
10th to 12th	70,751 (47.6)	31,725 (44.4)	39,026 (50.5)	
Academic achievement [596]				
Above average	52,839 (35.7)	24,364 (34.2)	28,475 (37.0)	<0.001
Average	49,782 (33.6)	21,172 (29.7)	28,610 (37.2)	
Below average	45,470 (30.7)	25,651 (36.0)	19,819 (25.8)	
Teacher classmate relations [515]				
Good	81,130 (54.8)	39,494 (55.5)	41,636 (54.1)	<0.001
Average	61,886 (41.8)	28,094 (39.5)	33,792 (43.9)	
Poor	5156 (3.5)	3564 (5.0)	1592 (2.1)	
Classmate relations [465]				
Good	108,178 (73.0)	52,656 (74.0)	55,522 (72.1)	<0.001
Average	37,389 (25.2)	16,873 (23.7)	20,516 (26.6)	
Poor	2655 (1.8)	1664 (2.3)	991 (1.3)	
Academic pressure [182]				
Below average	23,238 (15.6)	12,712 (17.8)	10,526 (13.6)	<0.001
Average	68,591 (49.2)	31,494 (44.1)	37,097 (48.1)	
Above average	56,676 (38.2)	27,147 (38.0)	29,529 (38.3)	
Bullying experience				
No	136,458 (91.8)	63,204 (88.5)	73,254 (94.8)	<0.001
Yes	12,229 (8.2)	8238 (11.5)	3991 (5.2)	
Current smoking				
No	140,855 (94.7)	64,708 (90.6)	76,147 (98.6)	<0.001
Yes	7832 (5.3)	6734 (9.4)	1098 (1.4)	
Current drinking				
No	125,120 (84.1)	56,357 (78.9)	68,763 (89.0)	<0.001
Yes	23,567 (15.9)	15,085 (21.1)	8482 (11.0)	
Lifetime NMPOU				<0.001
Abstainers	139,321 (93.7)	66,426 (93.0)	72,895 (94.4)	
Experimenters	6679 (4.5)	3529 (4.9)	3150 (4.1)	
Frequent users	2687 (1.8)	1487 (2.1)	1200 (1.6)	
Past-year NMPOU				<0.001
Abstainers	144,447 (97.1)	69,139 (96.8)	75,308 (97.5)	
Experimenters	3228 (2.2)	1738 (2.4)	1490 (1.9)	
Frequent users	1012 (0.7)	565 (0.8)	447 (0.6)	
Sleep disturbance				
No	116,522 (78.4)	56,694 (79.4)	59,828 (77.5)	<0.001
Yes	32,165 (21.6)	14,748 (20.6)	17,417 (22.5)	

NMPOU, non-medical prescription opioid use; Number of missing data were listed in superscript; [1] Chi-square tests were used to test the association between the above-mentioned categories and sex.

3.2. Prevalence of Sleep Disturbance by Sex

Among boys and girls, the prevalence of sleep disturbance was 20.6% and 22.5%, respectively (Table 1). Without adjusting for other variables, sleep disturbance was more prevalent among adolescents who were frequent lifetime NMPOU (36.2% among boys versus 41.8% among girls) and those with frequent past-year NMPOU (40.9% among boys versus 47.0% among girls). Among both boys and girls, lifetime and past-year NMPOU, age, grade, academic achievement, teacher–classmate, classmate relations, academic pressure, bullying experience, current smoking, and current drinking were associated with sleep disturbance (Table 2).

Table 2. Lifetime prevalence, crude odds ratios, and 95% CI of sleep disturbance among adolescents: stratified by sex.

Variable	Sleep Disturbance				
	Total n (%)	Boys n (%)	cOR (95%CI)	Girls n (%)	cOR (95%CI)
Lifetime NMPOU					
Abstainers	29,153 (20.9)	13,263 (20.0)	1	15,890 (21.8)	1
Experimenters	1972 (29.5)	946 (26.8)	1.49 (1.36–1.62)	1026 (32.6)	1.71 (1.57–1.87)
Frequent users	1040 (38.7)	539 (36.2)	2.25 (2.00–2.54)	501 (41.8)	2.65 (2.31–3.03)
Past-year NMPOU					
Abstainers	30,720 (21.3)	14,033 (20.3)	1	16,687 (22.2)	1
Experimenters	1004 (31.1)	484 (27.8)	1.50 (1.33–1.70)	520 (34.9)	1.90 (1.67–2.16)
Frequent users	441 (43.6)	231 (40.9)	2.74 (2.26–3.33)	210 (47.0)	2.99 (2.43–3.67)
Age					
12 to 13	3763 (10.8)	1723 (10.2)	1	2040 (11.3)	1
14 to 15	9838 (19.2)	4480 (17.4)	1.81 (1.67–1.95)	5358 (21.1)	2.11 (1.94–2.29)
16 to 18	18,564 (29.7)	8545 (29.7)	3.64 (3.35–3.95)	10,019 (29.7)	3.33 (3.07–3.61)
Grade					
7th to 9th	11,097 (14.2)	5328 (13.4)	1	5769 (15.1)	1
10th to 12th	21,068 (30.0)	9420 (30.0)	2.70 (2.54–2.88)	11,648 (30.0)	2.37 (2.21–2.53)
Academic achievement					
Above average	9762 (18.5)	4350 (17.9)	1	5412 (19.0)	1
Average	10,616 (21.3)	4194 (19.8)	1.15 (1.08–1.22)	6422 (22.4)	1.23 (1.17–1.29)
Below average	11,704 (25.7)	6177 (24.1)	1.48 (1.40–1.56)	5527 (27.9)	1.66 (1.57–1.74)
Teacher–classmate relations					
Good	13,605 (16.8)	6332 (16.0)	0.58 (0.55–0.61)	7273 (17.5)	0.55 (0.53–0.58)
Average	16,327 (26.4)	6956 (24.8)	1	9371 (27.7)	1
Poor	2145 (41.6)	1411 (39.6)	1.92 (1.75–2.10)	734 (46.1)	2.21 (1.95–2.50)
Classmate relations					
Good	20,772 (19.2)	9668 (18.4)	0.61 (0.58–0.64)	11,104 (20.0)	0.62 (0.59–0.65)
Average	10,288 (27.5)	4413 (26.2)	1	5875 (28.6)	1
Poor	1018 (38.3)	621 (37.3)	1.64 (1.45–1.86)	397 (40.1)	1.69 (1.44–1.98)
Academic pressure					
Below average	2918 (12.6)	1701 (13.4)	1	1217 (11.6)	1
Average	10,706 (15.6)	4569 (14.5)	0.62 (0.55–0.69)	6137 (16.5)	0.72 (0.62–0.83)
Above average	18,517 (32.7)	8472 (31.2)	1.35 (1.23–1.48)	10,045 (34.0)	1.89 (1.66–2.15)
Bullying experience					
No	27,600 (20.2)	11,858 (18.8)	1	15,742 (21.5)	1
Yes	4565 (37.3)	2890 (35.1)	2.38 (2.24–2.54)	1675 (42.0)	2.64 (2.44–2.85)
Current smoking					
No	29,223 (20.7)	12,328 (19.1)	1	16,895 (22.2)	1
Yes	2942 (37.6)	2420 (35.9)	2.39 (2.23–2.57)	522 (47.5)	3.43 (2.95–4.00)
Current drinking					
No	24,382 (19.5)	10,107 (17.9)	1	14,275 (20.8)	1
Yes	7783 (33.0)	4641 (30.8)	2.01 (1.90–2.12)	3142 (37.0)	2.26 (2.13–2.40)

NMPOU, non-medical prescription opioid use; cOR, crude odds ratio; 95% CI, 95% confidence interval.

3.3. Association Between Lifetime or Past-Year NMPOU and Sleep Disturbance

Table 3 and Figure 1 show the results of the final multivariable logistic regression models for sleep disturbance. After adjusting for age, grade, academic achievement, teacher–classmate and classmate relations, academic pressure, bullying experience, current smoking, and current drinking, lifetime and past-year NMPOU were significantly associated with sleep disturbance among both boys and girls. Among boys, frequent lifetime and past-year NMPOU was significantly associated with sleep disturbance, with aORs of 1.80 (95% CI, 1.57–2.05) and 2.07 (95%CI, 1.66–2.58), respectively. Among girls, frequent lifetime and past-year NMPOU were also positively associated with sleep disturbance, with aORs of 2.09 (95% CI, 1.80–2.44) and 2.16 (95%CI, 1.68–2.77), respectively. These results indicated that the associations between frequent lifetime and past-year NMPOU and sleep disturbance were higher among girls than boys. Moreover, the magnitudes of aORs for the significant associations between frequent lifetime or past-year NMPOU and sleep disturbance were greater than those between experimental use and sleep disturbance among both boys and girls.

Table 3. Adjusted odds ratios and 95%CI for measuring the association between opioids use and sleep disturbance stratified by sex.

Variable	Sleep Disturbance	
	Boys, aOR (95%CI) [1]	Girls, aOR (95%CI) [1]
Lifetime NMPOU		
Abstainers	1	1
Experimenters	1.25 (1.14–1.38)	1.44 (1.31–1.59)
Frequent users	1.80 (1.57–2.05)	2.09 (1.80–2.44)
Past-year NMPOU		
Abstainers	1	1
Experimenters	1.24 (1.09–1.42)	1.53 (1.33–1.76)
Frequent users	2.07 (1.66–2.58)	2.16 (1.68–2.77)

NMPOU, non-medical prescription opioid use; aOR, adjusted odds ratio; 95% CI, 95% confidence interval. [1] Adjusted for age (years), grade, academic achievement, teacher–classmate, classmate relations, academic pressure, bullying experience, cigarette smoking, current drinking.

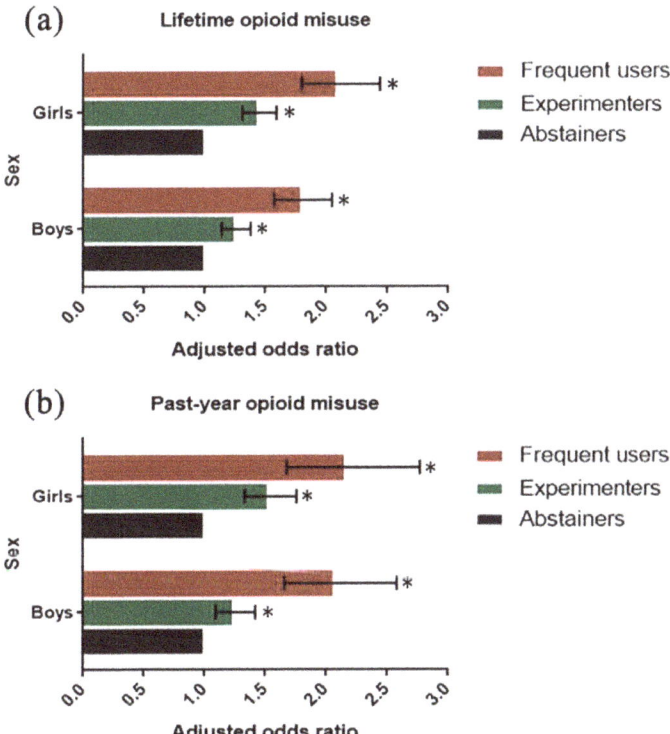

Figure 1. Adjusted OR and 95%CI for measuring the association of lifetime or past-year NMPOU with sleep disturbance stratified by sex.* $p < 0.05$.

4. Discussion

4.1. Main Findings

This is the large-scale study aimed to investigate the influence of lifetime or past year NMPOU on adolescents' sleep disturbance. The present results demonstrate that 21.6% of the sampled students reported having sleep disturbance. This prevalence is higher than that measured in a study conducted in Hefei of China, which indicated that 18.6% adolescents admitted having sleep disturbance [43]. To date, the role of sex for sleep disturbance among adolescents is not well characterized. Moreover, data from individual studies on the sex differences in sleep disturbance are not entirely consistent [44–46]. For example, Hartley et al. [44] found that girls reported more sleeping problems than did boys, while Russo et al. [45] reported the opposite results. Moreover, Morrison et al. [46] found that there were no significant differences between boys and girls regarding their number of sleep problems. With the large sample, our results demonstrate a higher prevalence of sleep disturbance among girls compared to boys.

Our results also illustrated that lifetime NMPOU was prevalent among Chinese adolescents, and the prevalence was higher for boys than girls. Furthermore, this study indicated that boys were found to have higher prevalence rates of experimental and frequent use of opioids in their lifetime or the past year. This finding is consistent with a previous study, which found that nonmedical use of opioids was more prevalent in boys than girls [47]. Some evidence also supported that males generally reported more substance use than females [48]. The observed sex differences in susceptibility to nonmedical opioids use may be useful to enhance the design of sex-sensitive surveillance, identification, prevention, and treatment decisions toward NMPOU [49].

The univariate analyses found that younger girls were more likely to have sleep disturbances. Previous studies also suggested that girls' sleep problems are usually manifested at an earlier age than boys [30,50]. Different social requirements for boys and girls and differences in the process of physiological changes linked to puberty might account for the difference [30,51]. In addition, we observed that adolescents who reported having bullying experience were at a higher risk of sleep disturbance. Similarly, Zhou et al. [8] found that adolescents who were victims of bullying had a twofold increased risk of having sleep disturbances. Unsurprisingly, compared to their corresponding groups, students who reported current smoking or drinking had a higher risk of having sleep disturbances. Higher grades (10th to 12th), poor relationships with teachers or classmates, and higher academic pressure were positively associated with higher risk for sleep disturbance. In light of the growth of sleep disturbance and the host of adverse consequences that are linked with it, it is critical to recognize the high-risk students who will be more prone to sleep disturbance. Specifically, sex, age, grades, bullying experience, current smoking or drinking, relationships with teachers or classmates, academic pressure and achievement were showed to be differentially associated with sleep disturbance among adolescents. Gaining a better understanding of the nuances of sleep disturbance trends will support more refined health promotion efforts. Therefore, we suggested that clinicians, schools, and families should pay more attention to these high-risk students mentioned above with the adverse characteristics to reduce the potential risk of sleep disturbance.

Our findings provide some evidence that compared with experimental opioid misuse, more frequent prescription opioid misuse was associated with a greater likelihood of reporting sleep disturbance after adjusting for covariates. We speculated that compared to experimental users of opioids, individuals who reported more frequent opioid misuse are more likely to progress to dependent users who experience more interpersonal conflict, which then can contribute to triggering negative effects on physical health, ultimately leading to sleep disturbance [52].

Notably, another novel discovery of the study was the effects of the separate analyses by sex, which suggested that the adjusted associations between lifetime or past-year NMPOU and sleep disturbance appeared slightly higher in girls than boys. A possible explanation is that females who reported opioids misuse were found to have greater levels of global psychiatric and emotional distress [53,54], and emotional trouble can lead to difficulty falling asleep in addition to further sleep disturbance [55].

4.2. Limitations

The limitations of the present study should be acknowledged when interpreting these findings. Firstly, it should be noted that a previous study found a bivariate relationship between the nonmedical use of prescription drugs and sleep among adolescents [56]. Furthermore, given the cross-sectional nature of the present study, our data cannot determine the exact timeline between lifetime or past-year NMPOU and sleep disturbance. Therefore, these issues should be further explored in a longitudinal study. Secondly, the data only included adolescents who were attending school, and on the day the survey was administered, adolescents who were not present at school or had dropped out of school were excluded. However, the anonymity of the questionnaires is assured and this method may have helped to collect accurate information from adolescents. Moreover, there could also be other potential confounders that were not included, such as mood disorders. Future surveys could collect the related information. Finally, our data only investigated the most widely used opioid drugs of Chinese adolescents. Hence, more prescription drugs need to be explored in future research.

Despite these limitations, the strength of the findings is that a large-scale sample of Chinese students was investigated, which ensures sufficient statistical power to measure the possible associations between lifetime or past-year NMPOU and sleep disturbance after adjusting for control variables. Besides, to our knowledge, the effect of sex on the association of lifetime or past-year NMPOU with sleep disturbance has not specifically been reported before. This is the first study that aimed to determine a sex-differential association among Chinese adolescents.

4.3. Implications

In China, NMPOU and sleep disturbance are both ongoing and rapidly evolving public health concerns. The findings clearly suggest that girls have a greater prevalence of sleep disturbance compared to boys and boys have a higher prevalence of experimental and frequent use of opioids in their lifetime and the past-year than girls. Furthermore, the study finds that although both boys and girls who reported lifetime or past-year NMPOU are at an increased risk of sleep disturbance, the association between frequency of opioid misuse and sleep disturbance is slightly stronger in girls. These results expand the areas of the literature, providing more specific information regarding the association between NMPOU and sleep disturbance. Also, the findings of this study highlight clinically relevant sex differences and may be helpful in guiding the design of sex-sensitive screening and treatment interventions for sleep disturbance [54]. Specific prevention and intervention programs are suggested: (1) to educate adolescents about avoiding the use of opioids as a way to deal with stress [57]; (2) to improve the awareness of the negative outcomes of NMPOU and sleep disturbance by educational campaigns; (3) to build a nation-wide active monitoring system to supervise NMPOU, sleep disturbance, and other health risk behavior (e.g., smoking, drinking alcohol, and bulling victimization, etc.) among Chinese adolescents.

5. Conclusions

To conclude, this report identified sex differences in the prevalence of lifetime or past-year NMPOU. Moreover, exposure to more frequent lifetime or past-year NMPOU is associated with a greater risk of sleep disturbance, especially among girls. Future intervention or prevention strategies should take into account the sex difference on the effects of sleep disturbance among adolescent nonmedical-opioid users in China.

Author Contributions: Design, C.L. and L.G., Formal analysis, D.X.; Investigation, M.Z., S.Z., and W.L.; Data Cleaning, L.G. and D.X.; Writing—original draft, D.X.; Writing—review and editing, C.L. and W.-H.Z.; supervision, C.L. and W.-H.Z.

Funding: This research was funded by the National Natural Science Foundation of China, grant number 81673252.

Acknowledgments: The authors are grateful for the local health professionals, the Department of Education, and the participating schools for their assistance and support. The authors also sincerely thank all the participants in our study.

Conflicts of Interest: The authors declare no conflict of interest.

References

1. Umlauf, M.G.; Bolland, A.C.; Bolland, K.A.; Tomek, S.; Bolland, J.M. The effects of age, gender, hopelessness, and exposure to violence on sleep disorder symptoms and daytime sleepiness among adolescents in impoverished neighborhoods. *J. Youth Adolesc.* **2015**, *44*, 518–542. [CrossRef]
2. Daly, B.P.; Jameson, J.P.; Patterson, F.; Mccurdy, M.; Kirk, A.; Michael, K.D. Sleep duration, mental health, and substance use among rural adolescents: Developmental correlates. *J. Rural Ment. Health* **2015**, *39*, 108–122. [CrossRef]
3. Colrain, I.M.; Baker, F.C. Changes in sleep as a function of adolescent development. *Neuropsychol. Rev.* **2011**, *21*, 5–21. [CrossRef]
4. Bailly, D.; Bailly-Lambin, I.; Querleu, D.; Beuscart, R.; Collinet, C. Sleep in adolescents and its disorders. A survey in schools. *L'Encephale* **2004**, *30*, 352–359. [CrossRef]
5. Garcia-Jimenez, M.A.; Salcedo-Aguilar, F.; Rodriguez-Almonacid, F.M.; Redondo-Martinez, M.P.; Monterde-Aznar, M.L.; Marcos-Navarro, A.I.; Torrijos-Martinez, M.P. The prevalence of sleep disorders among adolescents in Cuenca, Spain. *Rev. Neurol.* **2004**, *39*, 18–24. [PubMed]
6. Tang, D.; Li, P.; Guo, L.; Xu, Y.; Gao, X.; Deng, J.; Huang, J.; Huang, G.; Wu, H.; Yue, Y. The prevalences of and association between nonmedical prescription opioid use and poor sleep among Chinese high school students. *Sci. Rep.* **2016**, *6*. [CrossRef]
7. Guo, L.; Deng, J.; He, Y.; Deng, X.; Huang, J.; Huang, G.; Gao, X.; Lu, C. Prevalence and correlates of sleep disturbance and depressive symptoms among Chinese adolescents: A cross-sectional survey study. *BMJ Open* **2014**, *4*. [CrossRef] [PubMed]
8. Zhou, Y.; Guo, L.; Lu, C.; Deng, J.; He, Y.; Huang, J.; Huang, G.; Deng, X.; Gao, X. Bullying as a risk for poor sleep quality among high school students in China. *PLoS ONE* **2015**, *10*. [CrossRef]
9. Singh, G.K. Impact of neighborhood social conditions and household socioeconomic status on behavioral problems among US Children. *Matern. Child Health J.* **2012**, *16*, 158–169. [CrossRef] [PubMed]
10. Roberts, R.E.; Duong, H.T. The prospective association between sleep deprivation and depression among adolescents. *Sleep* **2014**, *37*, 239–244. [CrossRef]
11. Lunsford-Avery, J.R.; Krystal, A.D.; Kollins, S.H. Sleep disturbances in adolescents with ADHD: A systematic review and framework for future research. *Clin. Psychol. Rev.* **2016**, *50*, 159–174. [CrossRef]
12. Dewald, J.F.; Meijer, A.M.; Oort, F.J.; Kerkhof, G.A.; Bögels, S.M. The influence of sleep quality, sleep duration and sleepiness on school performance in children and adolescents: A meta-analytic review. *Sleep Med. Rev.* **2010**, *14*, 179–189. [CrossRef] [PubMed]
13. Goldstein, T.R.; Bridge, J.A.; Brent, D.A. Sleep disturbance preceding completed suicide in adolescents. *J. Consult. Clin. Psychol.* **2008**, *76*, 84–91. [CrossRef] [PubMed]
14. Lin, L.A.; Walton, M.A.; Bonar, E.E.; Blow, F.C. Trajectories of nonmedical use of prescription opioids among adolescents in primary care. *Addict. Res.* **2015**, *24*, 514–520. [CrossRef]
15. Hall, A.J.; Logan, J.E.; Toblin, R.L.; Kaplan, J.A.; Kraner, J.C.; Bixler, D.; Crosby, A.E.; Paulozzi, L.J. Patterns of abuse among unintentional pharmaceutical overdose fatalities. *J. Am. Med. Assoc.* **2008**, *300*, 2613–2620. [CrossRef] [PubMed]
16. Abuse, S.; Mental Health Services Administration. *Key Substance Use and Mental Health Indicators in the United States: Results from the 2016 National Survey on Drug Use and Health*; HHS Publication No. SMA 17-5044, NSDUH Series H-52; Center for Behavioral Health Statistics and Quality, Substance Abuse and Mental Health Services Administration: Rockville, MD, USA, 2017.
17. Hedden, S.L. *Behavioral Health Trends in the United States: Results from the 2014 National Survey on Drug Use and Health*; Substance Abuse and Mental Health Services Administration, Department of Heath & Human Services: Rockville, MD, USA, 2015.

18. Guo, L.; Xu, Y.; Deng, J.; Gao, X.; Huang, G.; Huang, J.; Deng, X.; Zhang, W.H.; Lu, C. Associations between childhood maltreatment and non-medical use of prescription drugs among Chinese adolescents. *Addiction* **2017**, *112*, 1600–1609. [CrossRef] [PubMed]
19. Guo, L.; Luo, M.; Wang, W.; Xiao, D.; Xi, C.; Wang, T.; Zhao, M.; Zhang, W.-H.; Lu, C. Association between nonmedical use of opioids or sedatives and suicidal behavior among Chinese adolescents: An analysis of sex differences. *Aust. New Zealand J. Psychiatry* **2019**, *53*, 559–569. [CrossRef]
20. Buttram, M.E.; Kurtz, S.P.; Surratt, H.L.; Levi-Minzi, M.A. Health and social problems associated with prescription opioid misuse among a diverse sample of substance-using MSM. *Subst. Use Misuse* **2014**, *49*, 277–284. [CrossRef] [PubMed]
21. Mateu-Gelabert, P.; Guarino, H.; Jessell, L.; Teper, A. Injection and sexual HIV/HCV risk behaviors associated with nonmedical use of prescription opioids among young adults in New York City. *J. Subst. Abus. Treat.* **2015**, *48*, 13–20. [CrossRef]
22. Edlund, M.J.; Forman-Hoffman, V.L.; Winder, C.R.; Heller, D.C.; Kroutil, L.A.; Lipari, R.N.; Colpe, L.J. Opioid abuse and depression in adolescents: Results from the National Survey on Drug Use and Health. *Drug Alcohol Depend.* **2015**, *152*, 131–138. [CrossRef]
23. Guo, L.; Xu, Y.; Deng, J.; Huang, J.; Huang, G.; Gao, X.; Wu, H.; Pan, S.; Zhang, W.H.; Lu, C. Association between nonmedical use of prescription drugs and suicidal behavior among adolescents. *JAMA Pediatrics* **2016**, *170*, 971–978. [CrossRef]
24. Kay, D.C.; Pickworth, W.B.; Neider, G.L. Morphine-like insomnia from heroin in nondependent human addicts. *Br. J. Clin. Pharmacol.* **2012**, *11*, 159–169. [CrossRef] [PubMed]
25. Pickworth, W.B.; Neidert, G.L.; Kay, D.C. Morphinelike arousal by methadone during sleep. *Clin. Pharmacol. Ther.* **1981**, *30*, 796–804. [CrossRef] [PubMed]
26. Ukponmwan, O. *Sleep-Waking States and the Endogenous Opioid System*; Erasmus University Rotterdam: Rotterdam, The Netherlands, 1986.
27. Walker, J.M.; Farney, R.J.; Rhondeau, S.M.; Boyle, K.M.; Valentine, K.; Cloward, T.V.; Shilling, K.C. Chronic opioid use is a risk factor for the development of central sleep apnea and ataxic breathing. *J. Clin. Sleep Med.* **2007**, *3*, 455–461. [PubMed]
28. Vaughn, M.G.; Nelson, E.J.; Salas-Wright, C.P.; Qian, Z.; Schootman, M. Racial and ethnic trends and correlates of non-medical use of prescription opioids among adolescents in the United States 2004–2013. *J. Psychiatr. Res.* **2016**, *73*, 17–24. [CrossRef] [PubMed]
29. Khooshabi, K.; Ameneh-Forouzan, S.; Ghassabian, A.; Assari, S. Is there a gender difference in associates of adolescents' lifetime illicit drug use in Tehran, Iran? *Arch. Med. Sci.* **2010**, *6*, 399–406. [CrossRef] [PubMed]
30. Ipsiroglu, O.S.; Fatemi, A.; Werner, I.; Paditz, E.; Schwarz, B. Self-reported organic and nonorganic sleep problems in schoolchildren aged 11 to 15 years in Vienna. *J. Adolesc. Health* **2002**, *31*, 436–442. [CrossRef]
31. Cross, C.P.; Cyrenne, D.L.; Brown, G.R. Sex differences in sensation-seeking: A meta-analysis. *Sci. Rep.* **2013**, *3*. [CrossRef]
32. Ahmadi, J.; Hasani, M. Prevalence of substance use among Iranian high school students. *Addict. Behav.* **2003**, *28*, 375–379. [CrossRef]
33. Galizio, M.; Stein, F.S. Sensation seeking and drug choice. *Int. J. Addict.* **1983**, *18*, 1039–1048. [CrossRef]
34. Krishnan, V.; Collop, N.A. Gender differences in sleep disorders. *Curr. Opin. Pulm. Med.* **2006**, *12*, 383–389. [CrossRef] [PubMed]
35. Wang, H.; Deng, J.; Zhou, X.; Lu, C.; Huang, J.; Huang, G.; Gao, X.; He, Y. The nonmedical use of prescription medicines among high school students: A cross-sectional study in southern China. *Drug Alcohol Depend.* **2014**, *141*, 9–15. [CrossRef] [PubMed]
36. Li, P.; Huang, Y.; Guo, L.; Wang, W.; Xi, C.; Lei, Y.; Luo, M.; Pan, S.; Deng, X.; Zhang, W.H.; et al. Sexual attraction and the nonmedical use of opioids and sedative drugs among Chinese adolescents. *Drug Alcohol Depend.* **2018**, *183*, 169–175. [CrossRef] [PubMed]
37. Tsai, P.S.; Wang, S.Y.; Wang, M.Y.; Su, C.T.; Yang, T.T.; Huang, C.J.; Fang, S.C. Psychometric evaluation of the Chinese version of the Pittsburgh Sleep Quality Index (CPSQI) in primary insomnia and control subjects. *Qual. Life Res.* **2005**, *14*, 1943–1952. [CrossRef] [PubMed]
38. Yang, J.; Guo, Y.; Du, X.; Jiang, Y.; Wang, W.; Xiao, D.; Wang, T.; Lu, C.; Guo, L. Association between problematic Internet use and sleep disturbance among adolescents: The role of the child's sex. *Int. J. Environ. Res. Public Health* **2018**, *15*, 2682. [CrossRef] [PubMed]

39. Olweus, D. The Olweus bully/victim questionnaire. *Br. J. Educ. Psychol.* **1996**. [CrossRef]
40. Wu, J.; He, Y.; Lu, C.; Deng, X.; Gao, X.; Guo, L.; Wu, H.; Chan, F.; Zhou, Y. Bullying behaviors among Chinese school-aged youth: A prevalence and correlates study in Guangdong province. *Psychiatry Res.* **2015**, *225*, 716–722. [CrossRef]
41. Kandra, K.L.; Anna, M.C.; Leah, R.; Goldstein, A.O. Support among middle school and high school students for smoke-free policies, North Carolina, 2009. *Prev. Chronic Dis.* **2013**, *10*, 675–681. [CrossRef]
42. Huang, R.; Ho, S.Y.; Wang, M.P.; Lo, W.S.; Lam, T.H. Sociodemographic risk factors of alcohol drinking in Hong Kong adolescents. *J. Epidemiol. Community Health* **2015**, *70*, 374–379. [CrossRef]
43. Xu, Z.; Su, H.; Zou, Y.; Chen, J.; Wu, J.; Chang, W. Sleep quality of Chinese adolescents: Distribution and its associated factors. *J. Paediatr. Child Health* **2012**, *48*, 138–145. [CrossRef]
44. Hartley, S.L.; Sikora, D.M. Sex differences in autism spectrum disorder: An examination of developmental functioning, autistic symptoms, and coexisting behavior problems in toddlers. *J. Autism Dev. Disord.* **2009**, *39*. [CrossRef] [PubMed]
45. Russo, P.M.; Caponera, E.; Barbaranelli, C. Personality, sleep habits and sleep problems in a representative sample of Italian eighth grade students. *Personal. Individ. Differ.* **2014**, *60*, S65–S66. [CrossRef]
46. Morrison, D.N.; Mcgee, R.; Stanton, W.R. Sleep problems in adolescence. *J. Am. Acad. Child Adolesc. Psychiatry* **1992**, *31*, 94–99. [CrossRef]
47. Wang, J.; Deng, J.X.; Lan, G.; Yuan, H.; Xue, G.; Huang, J.H.; Huang, G.L.; Lu, C.Y. Non-medical use of psychoactive drugs in relation to suicide tendencies among Chinese adolescents. *Addict. Behav.* **2015**, *51*, 31–37.
48. Cotto, J.H.; Davis, E.; Dowling, G.J.; Elcano, J.C.; Staton, A.B.; Weiss, S.R. Gender effects on drug use, abuse, and dependence: A special analysis of results from the National Survey on Drug Use and Health. *Gend. Med.* **2010**, *7*, 402–413. [CrossRef]
49. Back, S.E.; Payne, R.L.; Simpson, A.N.; Brady, K.T. Gender and prescription opioids: Findings from the National Survey on Drug Use and Health. *Addict. Behav.* **2010**, *35*, 1001–1007. [CrossRef] [PubMed]
50. Lazaratou, H.; Dikeos, D.G.; Anagnostopoulos, D.C.; Sbokou, O.; Soldatos, C.R. Sleep problems in adolescence. A study of senior high school students in Greece. *Eur. Child Adolesc. Psychiatry* **2005**, *14*, 237–243. [CrossRef] [PubMed]
51. Murata, K.; Araki, S. Menarche and sleep among Japanese schoolgirls: An epidemiological approach to onset of menarche. *Tohoku J. Exp. Med.* **1993**, *171*, 21–27. [CrossRef]
52. Ashrafioun, L.; Bishop, T.M.; Conner, K.R.; Pigeon, W.R. Frequency of prescription opioid misuse and suicidal ideation, planning, and attempts. *J. Psychiatr. Res.* **2017**, *92*, 1–7. [CrossRef]
53. Luthar, S.S.; Gushing, G.; Rounsaville, B.J. Gender differences among opioid abusers: Pathways to disorder and profiles of psychopathology. *Drug Alcohol Depend.* **1996**, *43*, 179–189. [CrossRef]
54. Back, S.E.; Lawson, K.M.; Singleton, L.M.; Brady, K.T. Characteristics and correlates of men and women with prescription opioid dependence. *Addict. Behav.* **2011**, *36*, 829–834. [CrossRef] [PubMed]
55. Vandekerckhove, M.; Weiss, R.; Schotte, C.; Exadaktylos, V.; Haex, B.; Verbraecken, J.; Cluydts, R. The role of presleep negative emotion in sleep physiology. *Psychophysiology* **2011**, *48*, 1738–1744. [CrossRef] [PubMed]
56. Ayres, C.G.; Pontes, N.M.; Pontes, M.C.F. Understanding the nonmedical use of prescription medications in the U.S. high school adolescents. *J. Sch. Nurs.* **2017**, *33*, 269–276. [CrossRef] [PubMed]
57. Jamison, R.N.; Butler, S.F.; Budman, S.H.; Edwards, R.R.; Wasan, A.D. Gender differences in risk factors for aberrant prescription opioid use. *J. Pain* **2010**, *11*, 312–320. [CrossRef] [PubMed]

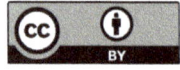 © 2019 by the authors. Licensee MDPI, Basel, Switzerland. This article is an open access article distributed under the terms and conditions of the Creative Commons Attribution (CC BY) license (http://creativecommons.org/licenses/by/4.0/).

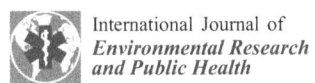

Article

Computerized Clinical Decision Support System for Prompting Brief Alcohol Interventions with Treatment Seeking Smokers: A Sex-Based Secondary Analysis of a Cluster Randomized Trial

Nadia Minian [1,2,3], Anna Ivanova [1], Sabrina Voci [1], Scott Veldhuizen [1], Laurie Zawertailo [1,4], Dolly Baliunas [1,5], Aliya Noormohamed [1], Norman Giesbrecht [5,6] and Peter Selby [1,2,3,5,7,*]

1. Nicotine Dependence Service, Centre for Addiction and Mental Health, 175 College St, Toronto, ON M5T 1P7, Canada; nadia.minian2@camh.ca (N.M.); anna.ivanova@camh.ca (A.I.); sabrina.voci@camh.ca (S.V.); scott.veldhuizen@camh.ca (S.V.); laurie.zawertailo@camh.ca (L.Z.); dolly.baliunas@camh.ca (D.B.); aliya.noormohamed@camh.ca (A.N.)
2. Department of Family and Community Medicine, University of Toronto, 500 University Ave, Toronto, ON M5G 1V7, Canada
3. Campbell Family Mental Health Research Institute, Centre for Addiction and Mental Health, 60 White Squirrel Way, Toronto, ON M6J 1H4, Canada
4. Department of Pharmacology and Toxicology, University of Toronto, 1 King's College Cir, Toronto, ON M5S 1A8, Canada
5. Dalla Lana School of Public Health, University of Toronto, 155 College, Toronto, ON M5T 3M7, Canada; norman.giesbrecht@camh.ca
6. Institute for Mental Health Policy Research, Centre for Addiction and Mental Health, 33 Russell St, Toronto, ON M5S 2S1, Canada
7. Department of Psychiatry, University of Toronto, 250 College Street, Toronto, ON M5T 1R8, Canada
* Correspondence: peter.selby@camh.ca

Received: 23 December 2019; Accepted: 4 February 2020; Published: 6 February 2020

Abstract: Although brief alcohol intervention can reduce alcohol use for both men and women, health care providers (HCPs) are less likely to discuss alcohol use or deliver brief intervention to women compared to men. This secondary analysis examined whether previously reported outcomes from a cluster randomized trial of a clinical decision support system (CDSS)—prompting delivery of a brief alcohol intervention (an educational alcohol resource) for patients drinking above cancer guidelines—were moderated by patients' sex. Patients ($n = 5702$) enrolled in a smoking cessation program at primary care sites across Ontario, Canada, were randomized to either the intervention (CDSS) or control arm (no CDSS). Logistic generalized estimating equations models were fit for the primary and secondary outcome (HCP offer of resource and patient acceptance of resource, respectively). Previously reported results showed no difference between treatment arms in HCP offers of an educational alcohol resource to eligible patients, but there was increased acceptance of the alcohol resource among patients in the intervention arm. The results of this study showed that these CDSS intervention effects were not moderated by sex, and this can help inform the development of a scalable strategy to overcome gender disparities in alcohol intervention seen in other studies.

Keywords: alcohol; tobacco; smoking cessation; clinical decision support systems; brief intervention; sex differences

1. Introduction

Alcohol use is a leading cause of death and disability worldwide [1]. In Canada, 3.3 million persons drink alcohol at levels that put them at risk of immediate harm, such as injury, and 4.7 million drink at levels that put them at risk of developing chronic conditions such as cancer and liver disease [2,3]. Co-use of other substances with alcohol can further increase the risk of harm [4–7]. For example, co-use of tobacco with alcohol leads to a multiplicative increase in the risk of aero-digestive and other cancers [8–11].

There is substantial evidence that brief intervention in primary health care settings can reduce hazardous or harmful alcohol consumption in patients compared to minimal or no intervention [12]. However, fewer than one in four Canadians report discussing alcohol use with a health care provider (HCP) in the previous two years [13]. Despite recommendations to screen all adults in primary care for risky alcohol use [14,15], there is evidence that discussions about alcohol use and delivery of brief alcohol interventions vary by patient sociodemographic characteristics [16,17]. While brief intervention is effective for both men and women [12], HCPs are less likely to discuss alcohol use [17–20] or provide a brief alcohol intervention to women compared to men [16,21–24]. This might be due to the research showing that HCP decisions to provide a brief intervention are associated with the social acceptability of alcohol [25,26], and findings pointing out that drinking is seen as an appropriate masculine behavior [27] but which defies feminine stereotypes [28].

Although men generally consume more alcohol than women [2,29], women have higher levels of blood alcohol after drinking an equivalent amount of alcohol and are more vulnerable to many of the negative consequences of alcohol use [29,30]. In addition, there is evidence that harm due to the use of alcohol is increasing among women in Canada. The rate of alcohol-related deaths has increased among women in Canada by 26% since 2001, compared to an approximately 5% increase among men [31]. In Ontario, emergency room visits due to alcohol use increased 87% for women between 2003 and 2016, compared to an increase of 53% for men during the same period [32]. Thus, the need for intervention with women that consume risky levels of alcohol is critical.

Computer-based clinical decision support systems (CDSSs) are one promising method of promoting HCP adherence to recommended best practices [33,34]. A CDSS uses information technology to provide clinicians with patient-specific assessments or recommendations in a timely manner to assist with clinical decision-making, for example by providing real-time alerts and reminders [35]. There is evidence from research conducted internationally that CDSSs improve various provider behaviours including prescribing practices (e.g., adjustment of drug dose or duration) [36,37], performance of preventive services (e.g., vaccinations) [37–39], and ordering tests [37,40]. However, evidence for the positive impact of CDSSs on practice have been inconsistent [41] and sometimes small to modest in magnitude [37]. Studies with predominantly male, veteran samples in the United States have found that the results of an electronic clinical reminder on HCP delivery of a brief alcohol intervention are mixed, with either positive [42] or no effect [43].

We previously reported findings from the COMBAT study [44], a pragmatic cluster randomized trial conducted in 2016 to 2017 in Ontario, Canada, to test the effectiveness of a CDSS that prompted HCPs in primary care to deliver a brief alcohol intervention—providing an educational alcohol resource—with patients flagged for drinking alcohol above cancer guidelines [45]. The CDSS was integrated into a web-based assessment HCPs completed with patients enrolling in the Smoking Treatment for Ontario Patients (STOP) program, a smoking cessation program implemented in primary care clinics across Ontario that provides behavioural support and up to 26 weeks of nicotine replacement therapy to eligible patients at no cost. In the original sample, a total of 15,150 patients (99.6% of patients) were screened; 5715 patients were identified as drinking above the Canadian Cancer Society (CCS) guidelines; 2578 were offered an appropriate alcohol resource; and 483 accepted the resource. The CDSS prompt had no statistically significant effect on HCP offering of an educational alcohol resource but significantly increased patient acceptance of the resource, when offered, from 16% to 21% [44].

Health information technology has been raised as a potential means to promote health equity by encouraging more equitable treatment [46–48], and there is some evidence demonstrating its capability to reduce disparities in care [49,50]. As such, a CDSS prompt might be one tool with the potential to reduce disparities based on sex or gender in the assessment and management of alcohol use by HCPs. Previous efforts to implement a CDSS have had an inconsistent impact on sex and gender disparities. Integration of a CDSS into the electronic health record of an internal medicine practice did not result in equitable practice, as female patients were less likely to be screened for alcohol use compared to men, although they were not less likely to receive a brief intervention if they screened positive [51]. Another study found that implementation of a performance measure and clinical decision support tool enhanced sex disparities, such that implementation of the performance measure led to a greater increase in rates of brief intervention for men [24]. However, both of these studies had limitations due to the use of single cut-off score to identify risky alcohol use, rather than applying a lower cut-off score for women as recommended [52]. As such, it remains unclear whether the impact of CDSS implementation on HCP delivery of brief intervention for risky alcohol use is similar for men and women and whether a CDSS reduces disparities in brief intervention between men and women. Thus, the purpose of this secondary analysis was to examine whether the effect of a CDSS on HCP offering of an alcohol resource to patients or patient acceptance of the alcohol resource differed based on patient sex.

2. Materials and Methods

2.1. Study Design and Sample

This was a sex-based, secondary analysis of the COMBAT study [44]. The patients in the trial were cigarette smokers who had enrolled in clinics across Ontario to obtain help with quitting smoking, who were also drinking above CCS guidelines [53]. Further trial eligibility criteria included enrolling in English and enrolling in person with their HCP completing the enrollment using the online portal designed for the program. As this secondary analysis was interested in the effects of patient sex on the main outcomes, the sample was further restricted to those who specified their sex as either male or female at enrollment, resulting in an analytic sample size of 5,702. Treatment arm randomization in the COMBAT study was performed at the site level to account for similarities among patient outcomes at the same clinic, as patients would have all been seen by the same HCP. Randomization was stratified by clinic type (family health team, community health center, nurse practitioner-led clinic) and predicted enrollment size at each clinic (i.e., small, large). Clinics were allocated on a 1:1 treatment versus control ratio to create balance between the two study arms. Further details about the cluster randomization can be found in previously published papers [44,53]. The COMBAT study was retrospectively registered at ClinicalTrials.gov, number NCT03108144, on 11 April 2017.

2.2. Study Variables

2.2.1. Treatment Arms

Eligible patients enrolling at clinics in the treatment arm were screened for risky drinking based on CCS guidelines. If patients were found to be drinking at a level that exceeded the CCS safe drinking cut off (defined as having consumed in the previous week at least seven alcoholic beverages for women and at least 14 alcoholic beverages for men and/or any patient consuming 5 or more alcoholic beverages on a single occasion), the HCP conducting the enrollment received a computer generated prompt to provide a brief alcohol intervention and hand out an appropriate resource to address risky drinking behavior during that enrollment visit. The recommended brief intervention and resources differed depending on the severity of the patient's risky drinking. More information about scoring of the CCS safe drinking cut off as well as descriptions of the brief interventions and resources offered by the HCPs in the study can be found in COMBAT's protocol manuscript [53] and in the manuscript describing the design of the alcohol resources [54]. The HCPs of patients who did not exceed the CCS safe drinking cut off did not receive any prompting by the CDSS.

Patients enrolling at clinics allocated to the control arm were asked the same alcohol consumption screening questions but were not flagged for HCPs if they drank above the CCS safe guidelines. The HCPs were still able to provide a brief intervention and offer a resource to address risky drinking behavior, but the CDSS did not prompt them to do so and did not provide any guidance regarding which type of resource the HCP should offer.

2.2.2. Patients' Sex

Patient sex was collected at baseline. As per STOP's registration questionnaire, patients were asked to self-identify as male, female, or other. Only 15 patients (0.3%) in the COMBAT sample selected "other". As this group lacked sufficient variability in outcomes and site level clustering variables for regression model convergence or detection of any differential effect, the analyses were limited to patients who self-identified as either male or female at enrollment.

2.2.3. Outcomes

This analysis had two outcomes of interest, both recorded by the HCPs in the online enrollment portal: (1) the offer of an appropriate alcohol resource by the HCP and (2) the acceptance of the offered alcohol resource by the patient. The primary outcome, offer of an appropriate alcohol resource, was coded dichotomously, yes or no, for each eligible patient enrollment. An outcome of yes was defined as the HCP offering an alcohol reduction resource for patients who drank above the CCS guidelines but scored below 20 points on the AUDIT-10 [55], or an offer of an alcohol abstinence resource to patients who drank above CCS guidelines and also had an AUDIT-10 score of 20 points or more. An outcome of no appropriate offer made was defined as the HCP stating they will not offer an alcohol resource, or an offer of an inappropriate resource (i.e., an offer of a reduction resource to patients requiring an abstinence resource or vice versa).

The secondary outcome, acceptance of the alcohol resource by the patient, was also coded dichotomously, yes or no, for each eligible patient enrollment. An outcome of yes was defined as the HCP offering any alcohol education resource, and the patient not declining it. An outcome of no was defined as the patient declining the offered resource. Due to the functionality of the CDSS, an incorrect resource could only be offered to patients in the control arm, and the type of resource was recorded only after it was accepted. This outcome reflects the acceptance of any resource, regardless of appropriateness.

2.3. Statistical Analyses

Descriptive statistics were used to describe males and females within each of the treatment arms on baseline characteristics including age, educational attainment, household income, employment status, smoking status, Heaviness of Smoking Index score [56], alcohol consumption, AUDIT-C [57] and AUDIT-10 scores, past year and lifetime attempts to quit smoking, recent marijuana and opioid use, and other health comorbidities. Descriptive statistics were also used to calculate crude primary and secondary outcomes within male and female subgroups of each treatment arm. To examine intervention and patients' sex effects, three logistic generalized estimating equations (GEE) models were then fit for each outcome with clinical site as a cluster variable (with an exchangeable correlation matrix), robust standard errors, and the site stratification variables (i.e., site size and type) included as covariates. The first model tested the intervention effect and included treatment arm, clinic size, and clinic type which replicated the model presented in a previous manuscript reporting the study's main findings [44]. Patient sex was added to a second model, to test for an overall sex difference. A treatment arm × sex interaction term was added to a third model, to test whether the intervention effect varied by sex. To better understand the range of likely true differences, we then calculated adjusted absolute differences and relative risks, along with 95% confidence intervals, for the differences among the treatment arm-specific sex effects.

With the exception of the addition of patient sex, the models were identical to those used in the original COMBAT analysis [44], as the goal of this work was to build on the previous analysis. As with the original COMBAT analysis, we adopted an intention to treat approach with clinics and patients analyzed in the originally assigned treatment arm. All analyses were conducted using Stata 14 [58].

2.4. Ethical Considerations

All patients gave their informed consent to participate in this research. The study was conducted in accordance with the Declaration of Helsinki and the COMBAT study protocol was reviewed and approved by the Research Ethics Board at the Centre for Addiction and Mental Health on 17 July 2015 (protocol number 035-2015).

3. Results

Baseline characteristics of our analytic sample by sex and treatment arm are presented in Table 1. There were some minor differences between males and females on several baseline characteristics. Specifically, the males in both treatment arms were slightly older, had lower rates of high school completion, were heavier smokers, had more lifetime quit attempts, and had greater rates of past 30 day marijuana use. Male patients in our sample also consumed more alcoholic beverages than females; however, this difference was due to the differential screen-in criteria for males versus females in the study. Overall, alcohol consumption and other Table 1 sex differences were similar between the intervention and control arms.

Table 1. Baseline patient characteristics for the main analytic sample ($n = 5702$).

Variables	Control		Intervention	
	Male	Female	Male	Female
	($n = 1547$)	($n = 1246$)	($n = 1597$)	($n = 1312$)
Age in years (mean, SD)	49.1 (13.5)	46.9 (13.8)	48.5 (13.6)	46.8 (13.4)
Graduated high school	1033 (67)	977 (78)	1071 (68)	997 (76)
Household income above $40,000	532 (34)	373 (30)	495 (31)	372 (28)
Currently employed	827 (53)	660 (53)	829 (52)	693 (53)
Daily smoking status	1430 (92)	1177 (94)	1506 (94)	1238 (94)
Heaviness of smoking index > 3	417 (29)	229 (19)	441 (29)	273 (22)
Number of alcoholic drinks in past week (mean, SD)	12.9 (14.3)	7.6 (9.4)	12.5 (14.7)	8.2 (10.6)
Above AUDIT-C cut off	1270 (82)	1018 (82)	1290 (81)	1080 (82)
Above AUDIT-10 cut off	67 (4)	33 (3)	97 (6)	43 (3)
Past year attempts to quit smoking	797 (52)	631 (51)	808 (51)	685 (52)
Lifetime attempts to quit smoking ≥ 11	261 (17)	180 (14)	293 (18)	185 (14)
Marijuana use in past 30 days	546 (35)	303 (24)	599 (38)	367 (28)
Opioid use in past 30 days	244 (16)	175 (14)	244 (15)	189 (14)
Number of comorbid conditions endorsed [1] (mean, SD)	2.3 (2.0)	2.4 (2.0)	2.5 (2.1)	2.4 (2.0)

Note: Values are numbers (percentages) unless stated otherwise. SD = standard deviation. [1] Possible comorbid conditions (lifetime history of diagnosis) included: high blood pressure, high cholesterol, heart disease, stroke, diabetes, chronic bronchitis/emphysema/chronic obstructive pulmonary disease, rheumatoid arthritis, chronic pain, cancer, depression, anxiety, schizophrenia, bipolar disorder, substance use disorder, alcohol use disorder, or problem gambling.

Figure 1a,b show the crude rates of primary and secondary outcomes in each of the patients' sex by treatment subgroups. In the control arm, 45% of males (702 patients) and 44% of females (548 patients) were offered an appropriate resource and 14% of males (100 patients) accepted the resource versus 18% of females (101 patients); in the intervention arm, 48% of males (760 patients) and 43% of females (560 patients) were offered an appropriate resource and 21% of males (157 patients) and 21% of females (120 patients) accepted it. Of the 201 accepted resources in the control arm, 45 (22%) were inappropriate, as defined by the study; 19% for females (19 of 101 patients) and 26% for males (26 of 100 patients), $F(1,49) = 1.55, p = 0.22$.

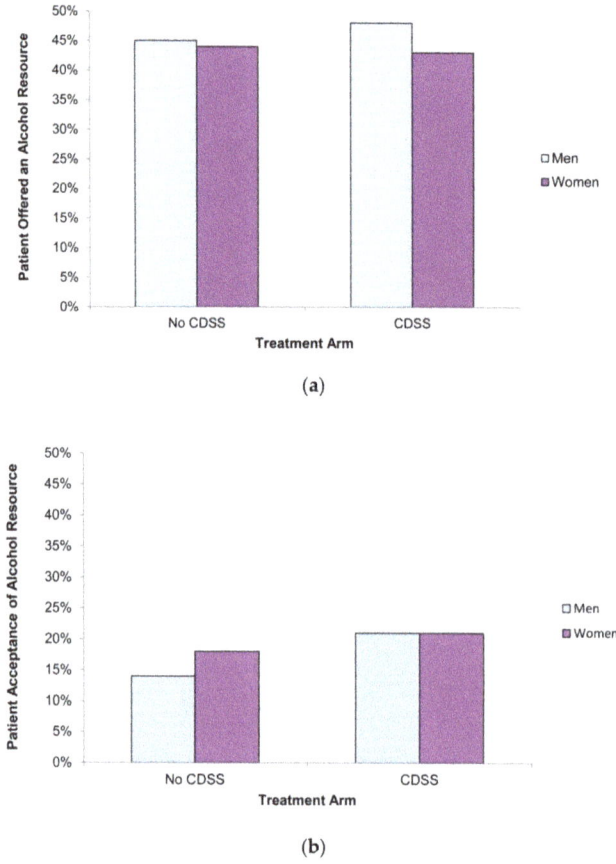

Figure 1. Proportion of men and women exceeding safe drinking guidelines (**a**) that were offered an appropriate educational alcohol resource by their health care provider in each treatment arm; (**b**) that accepted the offer of an educational alcohol resource by their health care provider in each treatment arm. CDSS = clinical decision support system.

Results from the GEE analysis are presented in Table 2. The original model (presented in a previously published manuscript [44]) did not find implementation of the CDSS to be a significant predictor of patients exceeding safe drinking guidelines being offered an appropriate educational alcohol resource [44]. In the present analysis, patients' sex was also non-significant as a covariate, and there was no evidence of a differential effect by sex.

Table 2. Adjusted odds ratios and 95% confidence intervals for offer and acceptance of an educational alcohol resource.

	CDSS as predictor of being OFFERED an appropriate alcohol resource n = 5702					
	Original model		With sex as covariate		With interaction term	
	OR (95% CI)	p-value	OR (95% CI)	p-value	OR (95% CI)	p-value
CDSS	1.20 (0.88–1.64)	0.25	1.20 (0.88–1.64)	0.25	1.24 (0.90–1.72)	0.19
Female patient	-	-	0.92 (0.82–1.03)	0.13	0.95 (0.82–1.11)	0.51
CDSS × Sex interaction term	-	-	-	-	0.93 (0.74–1.16)	0.53
	CDSS as a predictor of ACCEPTANCE of offered alcohol resource n = 2615					
	Original model		With sex as covariate		With interaction term	
	OR (95% CI)	p-value	OR (95% CI)	p-value	OR (95% CI)	p-value
CDSS	1.49 (1.01–2.18)	0.04	1.48 (1.01–2.16)	0.046	1.70 (1.12–2.57)	0.01
Female patient	-	-	1.12 (0.93–1.37)	0.24	1.33 (0.96–1.86)	0.09
CDSS × Sex interaction term	-	-	-	-	0.74 (0.50–1.09)	0.13

Note: Site stratification variables (i.e., clinic size and clinic type) were included as covariates.

The original model assessing the effect of the treatment arm on patient acceptance of the alcohol resource found that patients in the CDSS arm had significantly greater odds of accepting the alcohol resource when it was offered, compared to those in the control arm. The main effect of sex, when added, was not significant and neither was the sex × intervention interaction. There was therefore no evidence that the intervention effect with respect to resource acceptance differed by sex. Post-estimation calculations yielded an adjusted absolute difference in sex-specific intervention effects $(Mint - Mcontrol) - (Fint - Fcontrol)$ of 3.7% (95% CI = −1.9% to 9.3%) and a relative risk ratio $\frac{(Mint/Mcontrol)}{(Fint/Fcontrol)}$ of 1.27 (95% CI = 0.86 to 1.68). These confidence intervals indicate that any sex difference in the intervention effect is unlikely to be large, and suggest that the analysis was adequately powered to detect such a difference.

4. Discussion

The present study was a sex-based secondary analysis of the COMBAT study, a cluster randomized control trial which examined if the addition of a CDSS prompt influenced HCPs' provision of a brief alcohol intervention to patients in a smoking cessation program who drank above recommended alcohol consumption guidelines, compared to HCPs who did not receive a CDSS prompt. The results of the COMBAT trial showed that the CDSS did not increase the likelihood of HCPs offering an educational alcohol resource; however, it did increase the likelihood of patients' accepting the resource [44]. In this study, we found that these intervention effects were not moderated by sex.

The CDSS might have led to an increase in acceptance of alcohol resources among both men and women by influencing the way HCPs communicate with their patients. The CDSS provided guidance and concrete steps on what to do which might have made the resource more appealing to both male and female patients.

Less than half of eligible patients in the study were offered an alcohol resource, regardless of their sex or treatment arm, and less than a quarter of those offered an intervention actually accepted it, regardless of their sex. Prior research has shown similar or lower rates of alcohol intervention in primary care settings [42,59–61]. Thus, in this context—with this study showing that the CDSS led to an increase in the acceptance of alcohol resources and did not contribute to the sex inequities other interventions have shown [24]—the CDSS might be considered a success, as it led to more eligible patients receiving the alcohol resource.

Almost one quarter of resources accepted in the control arm conflicted with the study's guidelines for what type of resource was appropriate (abstinence or reduction), but this was similar for males and females. The HCP may have deemed the resource appropriate for their patient based on other characteristics known about the patient that would influence the HCP's judgment. For example, an HCP may choose to provide an alcohol reduction resource to a patient exceeding the AUDIT-10 cut off if they had intimate knowledge of the patient's case and felt it unnecessary to offer an alcohol abstinence resource during that appointment.

Perhaps one reason we did not find a differential impact of the CDSS prompt on offering of the resource for males and females was due to the fact that we framed our study around cancer prevention, instead of alcohol abuse. Many researchers have pointed out that HCPs do not provide a brief alcohol intervention to their patients, especially female patients, due to fear of stigmatizing them [26,62–64]. Alcohol stigma attached to women is related to societal views of alcohol use being more masculine and women who drink not being able to be a good caretaker as expected [65]. Thus, framing the advice as a cancer prevention strategy might have felt less stigmatizing for the HCPs. Findings from other cancer prevention strategies, such as cancer screening or diet and physical activity advice, have found no sex- or gender-based disparities in HCPs recommendations [66,67].

These findings need to be understood in the general context where the intervention is taking place: a country where drinking among women has been increasing [2,68]; multi-million marketing campaigns encourage and normalize the use of alcohol, especially among women [69]; where alcohol has become increasingly accessible [70]; and where few Ontarians are aware of the association between alcohol drinking and cancer risks [45]. This is problematic given that researchers have found stronger alcohol control policies are associated with lower levels of alcohol consumption [71,72]. While a CDSS was not a good solution to prompt HCPs to deliver a brief alcohol intervention, without changing the social climate around alcohol and without policy interventions which have been shown to reduce alcohol consumption worldwide (such as tax increases [73–78], restricting setting use [72,78–80], and placing upper limits on the density of outlets [78,79,81]), it might continue to be hard to increase the proportion of males and females who receive an alcohol intervention beyond that achieved using the current CDSS.

The current study has several limitations. Although our analysis shows that large sex differences in the effectiveness of the CDSS are unlikely to be present, some caution is appropriate. Patients in the COMBAT study were asked to self-identify as male, female, or other; by not including specific questions about sex at birth and additional gender response options, this study is limited in its interpretability. Further, it is also possible that sex differences in intervention effects might be masked by sex differences in the severity of alcohol-related problems. This is a possibility we were able to address only partially via the testing of a possible effect for the AUDIT-C that was done during selection of the covariates for the original model published previously [44]. We did not ask participants to report if they were pregnant. While we presumed there were only a small number of pregnant women in our sample, it warrants examination in future studies, as this could have had an impact on our primary and secondary outcomes. For example, HCPs may have been motivated to offer an alcohol resource to pregnant patients due to the increased perception of risk, and pregnant women might have been more motivated to accept an alcohol intervention for similar reasons.

While a CDSS has the potential for reducing or removing disparities, it is important to note that in our sample, there was no apparent disparity in offering the alcohol resource in the control arm (without CDSS). Thus, it will be valuable to replicate this study in a setting where there is a gender disparity. Also important to note is that the CDSS was implemented in clinics that have a robust infrastructure for smoking cessation. All clinics had implemented the STOP program, which offers various supports such as a community of practice, an active listserv, several webinars a year on topics related to smoking cessation (including alcohol use), and ongoing operational support. These supports might make it hard to generalize these findings to other clinics that don't have these supports.

Further research is needed to identify pragmatic implementation approaches that increase the delivery of brief alcohol interventions in primary care clinics. As other researchers have suggested, these might include the addition of a champion who can encourage HCPs to conduct a brief intervention to all patients who are drinking above guidelines and to problem solve barriers [74,82] as well as having ongoing training in alcohol screening and brief intervention. This might be particularly important in clinics with high staff turnover [82–85]. Both the champion and the training should emphasize the importance of making sure that sex and gender are taken into consideration when delivering brief alcohol intervention (e.g., addressing stigma and fear associated with reporting alcohol use during pregnancy and motherhood) [86–89]. Given that research has shown that the methods of program implementation can have a differential effect on males and females, it is critical to integrate a sex and gender lens to the conceptualization and evaluation of these approaches [90]. This will in turn ensure that more equitable health outcomes are achieved. In addition, future research should be conducted to understand the specific mechanisms through which the CDSS helped increase the proportion of patients' acceptance of the alcohol resource, including an examination of whether there are different mechanisms for men and women.

5. Conclusions

We previously reported that implementation of a CDSS in primary care clinics across Ontario did not increase the offer of an alcohol resource to patients drinking above cancer guidelines but did increase acceptance of the resource. Given that implementation science as a field has been criticized for neglecting sex and gender considerations from its analysis [90] and widespread evidence of gender disparities in HCP delivery of brief interventions, it was important to examine whether sex moderated our results. The findings of this study suggest that CDSS effects were not moderated by patient sex. Regardless of patient sex, the CDSS prompt did not increase delivery of a brief alcohol intervention but did lead to increased acceptance of the resource. In increasing patient acceptance, the CDSS successfully increased the number of both male and female patients that ultimately received the alcohol resource that was appropriate. These findings can help inform future program and policy development needed to increase rates of brief alcohol intervention without creating, maintaining, or worsening any gender disparities in alcohol screening and intervention.

Author Contributions: Conceptualization of this secondary analysis, N.M., A.I., S.V. (Sabrina Voci), and P.S.; Formal analysis, A.I. and S.V. (Scott Veldhuizen); Authors of this manuscript that were part of funding acquisition, N.M., L.Z., D.B., N.G. and P.S.; Investigation, N.M., A.I., and D.B.; Project administration, N.M.; Supervision, N.M. and Peter Selby; Writing—original draft, N.M., A.I. and S.V. (Sabrina Voci); Writing—review and editing, N.M., A.I., S.V. (Sabrina Voci), S.V. (Scott Veldhuizen), L.Z., D.B., A.N., N.G., and P.S. All authors have read and agreed to the published version of the manuscript.

Funding: This research was funded by the Canadian Cancer Society, grant number 703404.

Acknowledgments: We would like to thank the staff and patients that participated in this trial. Peter Selby would like to acknowledge salary support for his clinician-scientist position from the Centre for Addiction and Mental Health and the Department of Family and Community Medicine at the University of Toronto.

Conflicts of Interest: The authors have no conflict of interest to declare. However, Peter Selby has the following general disclosures to report: grants and/or salary and/or research support from the Centre for Addiction and Mental Health, Health Canada, Ontario Ministry of Health and Long-term care (MOHLTC), Canadian Institutes of Health Research (CIHR), Canadian Centre on Substance Use and Addiction, Public Health Agency of Canada (PHAC), Ontario Lung Association, Medical Psychiatry Alliance, Extensions for Community Healthcare Outcomes, Canadian Cancer Society Research Institute (CCSRI), Cancer Care Ontario, Ontario Institute for Cancer Research, Ontario Brain Institute, McLaughlin Centre, Academic Health Sciences Centre, Workplace Safety and Insurance Board, National Institutes of Health (NIH), and the Association of Faculties of Medicine of Canada. Peter Selby also reports receiving funding and/or honoraria from the following commercial organizations: Pfizer Inc./Canada, Shoppers Drug Mart, Bhasin Consulting Fund Inc., Patient-Centered Outcomes Research Institute, ABBVie, and Bristol-Myers Squibb. Further, Peter Selby reports receiving consulting fees from Pfizer Inc./Canada, Evidera Inc., Johnson & Johnson Group of Companies, Medcan Clinic, Inflexxion Inc., V-CC Systems Inc., MedPlan Communications, Kataka Medical Communications, Miller Medical Communications, Nvision Insight Group, and Sun Life Financial. Through an open tender process Johnson & Johnson, Novartis, and Pfizer Inc. are vendors of record for providing smoking cessation pharmacotherapy, free or discounted, for research studies in which Peter Selby is the principal investigator or co-investigator. The funders had no role in the design of the study; in the collection, analyses, or interpretation of data; in the writing of the manuscript, or in the decision to publish the results.

References

1. Yasin, Y.J.; Banoub, J.A.M. GBD 2016 Alcohol Collaborators. Alcohol use and burden for 195 countries and territories, 1990–2016: A systematic analysis for the Global Burden of Disease Study 2016. *Lancet* **2018**, *392*, 1015–1035.
2. Statistics Canada. Canadian Tobacco, Alcohol and Drugs Survey (CTADS): Summary of Results for 2017. Available online: https://www.canada.ca/en/health-canada/services/canadian-tobacco-alcohol-drugs-survey/2017-summary.html (accessed on 9 December 2019).
3. Young, S.W.; Candido, E.; Klein-Geltink, J.; Giesbrecht, N. Preventing alcohol-related cancer: What if everyone drank within the guidelines? *Can. J. Public Health* **2018**, *109*, 70–78. [CrossRef]
4. Pennings, E.J.; Leccese, A.P.; Wolff, F.A.D. Effects of concurrent use of alcohol and cocaine. *Addiction* **2002**, *97*, 773–783. [CrossRef] [PubMed]
5. Chihuri, S.; Li, G.; Chen, Q. Interaction of marijuana and alcohol on fatal motor vehicle crash risk: A case–control study. *Inj. Epidemiol.* **2017**, *4*, 8. [CrossRef] [PubMed]
6. Yurasek, A.M.; Aston, E.R.; Metrik, J. Co-use of alcohol and cannabis: A review. *Curr. Addict. Rep.* **2017**, *4*, 184–193. [CrossRef]
7. Pennay, A.; Lubman, D.I.; Miller, P. Combining energy drinks and alcohol: A recipe for trouble? *Aust. Fam. Physician* **2011**, *40*, 104.
8. Franceschi, S.; Talamini, R.; Barra, S.; Barón, A.E.; Negri, E.; Bidoli, E.; Serraino, D.; La Vecchia, C. Smoking and drinking in relation to cancers of the oral cavity, pharynx, larynx, and esophagus in northern Italy. *Cancer Res.* **1990**, *50*, 6502–6507.
9. Pelucchi, C.; Gallus, S.; Garavello, W.; Bosetti, C.; La, C.V. Cancer risk associated with alcohol and tobacco use: Focus on upper aero-digestive tract and liver. *Alcohol Res. Health* **2006**, *29*, 193–198.
10. Dawson, D.A. Drinking as a risk factor for sustained smoking. *Drug Alcohol Depend.* **2000**, *59*, 235–249. [CrossRef]
11. Falk, D.E.; Yi, H.-Y.; Hiller-Sturmhöfel, S. An epidemiologic analysis of co-occurring alcohol and tobacco use and disorders: Findings from the National Epidemiologic Survey on Alcohol and Related Conditions. *Alcohol Res. Health* **2006**, *29*, 162.
12. Kaner, E.F.; Beyer, F.R.; Muirhead, C.; Campbell, F.; Pienaar, E.D.; Bertholet, N.; Daeppen, J.B.; Saunders, J.B.; Burnand, B. Effectiveness of brief alcohol interventions in primary care populations. *Cochrane Database Syst. Rev.* **2018**. [CrossRef] [PubMed]
13. Canadian Institute of Health Information (CIHI). *How Canada Compares: Results From The Commonwealth Fund's 2016 International Health Policy Survey of Adults in 11 Countries—Accessible Report 2017*; Canadian Institute of Health Information: Ottawa, ON, Canada, 2017.
14. Curry, S.J.; Krist, A.H.; Owens, D.K.; Barry, M.J.; Caughey, A.B.; Davidson, K.W.; Doubeni, C.A.; Epling, J.W.; Kemper, A.R.; Kubik, M. Screening and behavioral counseling interventions to reduce unhealthy alcohol use in adolescents and adults: US Preventive Services Task Force recommendation statement. *JAMA* **2018**, *320*, 1899–1909. [PubMed]
15. RNAO. *Engaging Clients Who Use Substances*; Registered Nurses' Association of Ontario: Toronto, ON, Canada, 2015.
16. Kaner, E.; Heather, N.; Brodie, J.; Lock, C.A.; McAvoy, B.R. Patient and practitioner characteristics predict brief alcohol intervention in primary care. *Br. J. Gen. Pract.* **2001**, *51*, 822–827. [PubMed]
17. McKnight-Eily, L.R.; Liu, Y.; Brewer, R.D.; Kanny, D.; Lu, H.; Denny, C.H.; Balluz, L.; Collins, J. Vital signs: Communication between health professionals and their patients about alcohol use—44 states and the District of Columbia, 2011. *Mmwr. Morb. Mortal. Wkly. Rep.* **2014**, *63*, 16. [PubMed]
18. Bertakis, K.D.; Azari, R. Determinants of physician discussion regarding tobacco and alcohol abuse. *J. Health Commun.* **2007**, *12*, 513–525. [CrossRef] [PubMed]

19. Volk, R.J.; Steinbauer, J.R.; Cantor, S.B. Patient factors influencing variation in the use of preventive interventions for alcohol abuse by primary care physicians. *J. Stud. Alcohol* **1996**, *57*, 203–209. [CrossRef]
20. Denny, C.H.; Serdula, M.K.; Holtzman, D.; Nelson, D.E. Physician advice about smoking and drinking: Are US adults being informed? *Am. J. Prev. Med.* **2003**, *24*, 71–74. [CrossRef]
21. Angus, C.; Brown, J.; Beard, E.; Gillespie, D.; Buykx, P.; Kaner, E.F.; Michie, S.; Meier, P. Socioeconomic inequalities in the delivery of brief interventions for smoking and excessive drinking: Findings from a cross-sectional household survey in England. *BMJ Open* **2019**, *9*, e023448. [CrossRef]
22. Bachrach, R.L.; Blosnich, J.R.; Williams, E.C. Alcohol screening and brief intervention in a representative sample of veterans receiving primary care services. *J. Subst. Abus. Treat.* **2018**, *95*, 18–25. [CrossRef]
23. Lock, C.A.; Kaner, E.F. Implementation of brief alcohol interventions by nurses in primary care: Do non-clinical factors influence practice? *Fam. Pract.* **2004**, *21*, 270–275. [CrossRef]
24. Williams, E.C.; Lapham, G.T.; Rubinsky, A.D.; Chavez, L.J.; Berger, D.; Bradley, K.A. Influence of a targeted performance measure for brief intervention on gender differences in receipt of brief intervention among patients with unhealthy alcohol use in the Veterans Health Administration. *J. Subst. Abus. Treat.* **2017**, *81*, 11–16. [CrossRef] [PubMed]
25. Rapley, T.; May, C.; Kaner, E.F. Still a difficult business? Negotiating alcohol-related problems in general practice consultations. *Soc. Sci. Med.* **2006**, *63*, 2418–2428. [CrossRef] [PubMed]
26. Tam, C.W.M.; Zwar, N.; Markham, R. Australian general practitioner perceptions of the detection and screening of at-risk drinking, and the role of the AUDIT-C: A qualitative study. *Bmc Fam. Pract.* **2013**, *14*, 121. [CrossRef] [PubMed]
27. Capraro, R.L. Why college men drink: Alcohol, adventure, and the paradox of masculinity. *J. Am. Coll. Health* **2000**, *48*, 307–315. [CrossRef] [PubMed]
28. Ricciardelli, L.A.; Connor, J.P.; Williams, R.J.; Young, R.M. Gender stereotypes and drinking cognitions as indicators of moderate and high risk drinking among young women and men. *Drug Alcohol Depend.* **2001**, *61*, 129–136. [CrossRef]
29. Erol, A.; Karpyak, V.M. Sex and gender-related differences in alcohol use and its consequences: Contemporary knowledge and future research considerations. *Drug Alcohol Depend.* **2015**, *156*, 1–13. [CrossRef]
30. National Institute on Alcohol Abuse and Alcoholism. Are Women More Vulnerable to Alcohol's Effects? Available online: https://pubs.niaaa.nih.gov/publications/aa46.htm#:~{}:targetText=In%20general%2C%20women%20have%20less,the%20blood%20faster%20than%20men (accessed on 29 January 2020).
31. Canadian Institute for Health Information. Alcohol Harm on the Rise for Canadian Women. Available online: https://www.cihi.ca/en/alcohol-harm-on-the-rise-for-canadian-women (accessed on 9 December 2019).
32. Myran, D.T.; Hsu, A.T.; Smith, G.; Tanuseputro, P. Rates of emergency department visits attributable to alcohol use in Ontario from 2003 to 2016: A retrospective population-level study. *CMAJ* **2019**, *191*, E804–E810. [CrossRef]
33. Lobach, D.F.; Hammond, W.E. Computerized decision support based on a clinical practice guideline improves compliance with care standards. *Am. J. Med.* **1997**, *102*, 89–98. [CrossRef]
34. Coma, E.; Medina, M.; Méndez, L.; Hermosilla, E.; Iglesias, M.; Olmos, C.; Calero, S. Effectiveness of electronic point-of-care reminders versus monthly feedback to improve adherence to 10 clinical recommendations in primary care: A cluster randomized clinical trial. *Bmc Med. Inform. Decis. Mak.* **2019**, *19*, 245. [CrossRef]
35. Kawamoto, K.; Houlihan, C.A.; Balas, E.A.; Lobach, D.F. Improving clinical practice using clinical decision support systems: A systematic review of trials to identify features critical to success. *BMJ* **2005**, *330*, 765. [CrossRef]
36. Pearson, S.-A.; Moxey, A.; Robertson, J.; Hains, I.; Williamson, M.; Reeve, J.; Newby, D. Do computerised clinical decision support systems for prescribing change practice? A systematic review of the literature (1990–2007). *Bmc Health Serv. Res.* **2009**, *9*, 154. [CrossRef] [PubMed]
37. Shojania, K.G.; Jennings, A.; Mayhew, A.; Ramsay, C.R.; Eccles, M.P.; Grimshaw, J. The effects of on-screen, point of care computer reminders on processes and outcomes of care. *Cochrane Database Syst. Rev.* **2009**, *3*, CD001096. [CrossRef] [PubMed]
38. Bright, T.J.; Wong, A.; Dhurjati, R.; Bristow, E.; Bastian, L.; Coeytaux, R.R.; Samsa, G.; Hasselblad, V.; Williams, J.W.; Musty, M.D. Effect of clinical decision-support systems: A systematic review. *Ann. Intern. Med.* **2012**, *157*, 29–43. [CrossRef] [PubMed]

39. Dexter, P.R.; Perkins, S.; Overhage, J.M.; Maharry, K.; Kohler, R.B.; McDonald, C.J. A computerized reminder system to increase the use of preventive care for hospitalized patients. *N. Engl. J. Med.* **2001**, *345*, 965–970. [CrossRef] [PubMed]
40. Kastner, M.; Straus, S.E. Clinical decision support tools for osteoporosis disease management: A systematic review of randomized controlled trials. *J. Gen. Intern. Med.* **2008**, *23*, 2095–2105. [CrossRef]
41. Groenhof, T.K.J.; Asselbergs, F.W.; Groenwold, R.H.; Grobbee, D.E.; Visseren, F.L.; Bots, M.L. The effect of computerized decision support systems on cardiovascular risk factors: A systematic review and meta-analysis. *BMC Med. Inform. Decis. Mak.* **2019**, *19*, 108. [CrossRef]
42. Lapham, G.T.; Achtmeyer, C.E.; Williams, E.C.; Hawkins, E.J.; Kivlahan, D.R.; Bradley, K.A. Increased documented brief alcohol interventions with a performance measure and electronic decision support. *Med. Care* **2012**, *50*, 179–187. [CrossRef]
43. Williams, E.C.; Achtmeyer, C.E.; Kivlahan, D.R.; Greenberg, D.; Merrill, J.O.; Wickizer, T.M.; Koepsell, T.D.; Heagerty, P.J.; Bradley, K.A. Evaluation of an electronic clinical reminder to facilitate brief alcohol-counseling interventions in primary care. *J. Stud. Alcohol Drugs* **2010**, *71*, 720–725. [CrossRef]
44. Minian, N.; Baliunas, D.; Noormohamed, A.; Zawertailo, L.; Giesbrecht, N.; Hendershot, C.S.; Le Foll, B.; Rehm, J.; Samokhvalov, A.V.; Selby, P.L. The effect of a clinical decision support system on prompting an intervention for risky alcohol use in a primary care smoking cessation program: A cluster randomized trial. *Implement. Sci.* **2019**, *14*, 85. [CrossRef]
45. Canadian Cancer Society. The Truth About Alcohol. Available online: http://www.cancer.ca/en/about-us/news/on/2016/february/story4/?region=on (accessed on 23 December 2019).
46. Pérez-Stable, E.J.; Jean-Francois, B.; Aklin, C.F. Leveraging Advances in Technology to Promote Health Equity. *Med. Care* **2019**, *57*, S101–S103. [CrossRef]
47. US Department of Health and Human Services. *National Healthcare Disparities Report 2011*; Agency for Healthcare Research and Quality: Rockville, MD, USA, 2012.
48. Graham, G.N.; Spengler, R.F. Collaborating to end health disparities in our lifetime. *Am. J. Public Health* **2009**, *99*, 1930–1932. [CrossRef] [PubMed]
49. Lee, J. The impact of health information technology on disparity of process of care. *Int. J. Equity Health* **2015**, *14*, 34. [CrossRef] [PubMed]
50. Lau, B.D.; Haider, A.H.; Streiff, M.B.; Lehmann, C.U.; Kraus, P.S.; Hobson, D.B.; Kraenzlin, F.S.; Zeidan, A.M.; Pronovost, P.J.; Haut, E.R. Eliminating healthcare disparities via mandatory clinical decision support: The venous thromboembolism (VTE) example. *Med. Care* **2015**, *53*, 18. [CrossRef] [PubMed]
51. Bachhuber, M.A.; O'Grady, M.A.; Chung, H.; Neighbors, C.J.; DeLuca, J.; D'Aloia, E.M.; Diaz, A.; Cunningham, C.O. Delivery of screening and brief intervention for unhealthy alcohol use in an urban academic Federally Qualified Health Center. *Addict. Sci. Clin. Pract.* **2017**, *12*, 33. [CrossRef] [PubMed]
52. Bradley, K.A.; Boyd-Wickizer, J.; Powell, S.H.; Burman, M.L. Alcohol screening questionnaires in women: A critical review. *JAMA* **1998**, *280*, 166–171. [CrossRef] [PubMed]
53. Minian, N.; Baliunas, D.; Zawertailo, L.; Noormohamed, A.; Giesbrecht, N.; Hendershot, C.S.; Le Foll, B.; Rehm, J.; Samokhvalov, A.; Selby, P.L. Combining alcohol interventions with tobacco addictions treatment in primary care—The COMBAT study: A pragmatic cluster randomized trial. *Implement. Sci.* **2017**, *12*, 65. [CrossRef]
54. Minian, N.; Noormohamed, A.; Zawertailo, L.; Baliunas, D.; Giesbrecht, N.; Le Foll, B.; Rehm, J.; Samokhvalov, A.; Selby, P.L. A method for co-creation of an evidence-based patient workbook to address alcohol use when quitting smoking in primary care: A case study. *Res. Involv. Engagem.* **2018**, *4*, 4. [CrossRef]
55. Gomez, A.; Conde, A.; Santana, J.; Jorrin, A. Diagnostic usefulness of brief versions of Alcohol Use Disorders Identification Test (AUDIT) for detecting hazardous drinkers in primary care settings. *J. Stud. Alcohol* **2005**, *66*, 305–308. [CrossRef]
56. Heatherton, T.F.; Kozlowski, L.T.; Frecker, R.C.; Rickert, W.; Robinson, J. Measuring the heaviness of smoking: Using self-reported time to the first cigarette of the day and number of cigarettes smoked per day. *Br. J. Addict.* **1989**, *84*, 791–800. [CrossRef]
57. Bush, K.; Kivlahan, D.R.; McDonell, M.B.; Fihn, S.D.; Bradley, K.A. The AUDIT alcohol consumption questions (AUDIT-C): An effective brief screening test for problem drinking. *Arch. Intern. Med.* **1998**, *158*, 1789–1795. [CrossRef]
58. StataCorp. *Stata Statistical Software: Release 14*; StataCorp LP: College Station, TX, USA, 2015.

59. Gomel, M.K.; Wutzke, S.E.; Hardcastle, D.M.; Lapsley, H.; Reznik, R.B. Cost-effectiveness of strategies to market and train primary health care physicians in brief intervention techniques for hazardous alcohol use. *Soc. Sci. Med.* **1998**, *47*, 203–211. [CrossRef]
60. Kaner, E.F.; Heather, N.; Mcavoy, B.R.; Lock, C.A.; Gilvarry, E. Intervention for excessive alcohol consumption in primary health care: Attitudes and practices of English general practitioners. *Alcohol Alcohol.* **1999**, *34*, 559–566. [CrossRef] [PubMed]
61. Seale, J.P.; Shellenberger, S.; Tillery, W.K.; Boltri, J.; Barton, B.; McCauley, M.; Vogel, R. Implementing alcohol screening and intervention in a family medicine residency clinic. *Subst. Abus.* **2006**, *26*, 23–31. [CrossRef] [PubMed]
62. Weisner, C.; Schmidt, L. Gender disparities in treatment for alcohol problems. *JAMA* **1992**, *268*, 1872–1876. [CrossRef]
63. Thom, B.; Téllez, C. A difficult business: Detecting and managing alcohol problems in general practice. *Br. J. Addict.* **1986**, *81*, 405–418. [CrossRef]
64. Nygaard, P.; Aasland, O.G. Barriers to implementing screening and brief interventions in general practice: Findings from a qualitative study in Norway. *Alcohol Alcohol.* **2011**, *46*, 52–60. [CrossRef]
65. Gomberg, E. Alcoholic women in treatment: The question of stigma and age. *Alcohol Alcohol.* **1988**, *23*, 507.
66. Brawarsky, P.; Brooks, D.; Mucci, L.; Wood, P. Effect of physician recommendation and patient adherence on rates of colorectal cancer testing. *Cancer Detect. Prev.* **2004**, *28*, 260–268. [CrossRef]
67. Sinclair, J.; Lawson, B.; Burge, F. Which patients receive on diet and exercise?: Do certain characteristics affect whether they receive such advice? *Can. Fam. Physician* **2008**, *54*, 404–412.
68. Bulloch, A.G.; Williams, J.V.; Lavorato, D.H.; Patten, S.B. Trends in binge drinking in Canada from 1996 to 2013: A repeated cross-sectional analysis. *CMAJ Open* **2016**, *4*, E599. [CrossRef]
69. Johnston, A.D. *Drink: The Intimate Relationship Between Women and Alcohol*; Harper Collins: New York, NY, USA, 2013.
70. Stockwell, T.; Wettlaufer, A.; Vallance, K.; Chow, C.; Giesbrecht, N.; April, N.; Asbridge, M.; Callaghan, R.; Cukier, S.; Davis-MacNevin, P.; et al. *Strategies to Reduce Alcohol-Related Harms and Costs in Canada: A Review of Provincial and Territorial Policies*; Canadian Institute for Substance Use Research, University of Victoria: Victoria, BC, Canada, 2019.
71. Brand, D.A.; Saisana, M.; Rynn, L.A.; Pennoni, F.; Lowenfels, A.B. Comparative analysis of alcohol control policies in 30 countries. *PLos Med.* **2007**, *4*, e151. [CrossRef] [PubMed]
72. Madureira-Lima, J.; Galea, S. Alcohol control policies and alcohol consumption: An international comparison of 167 countries. *J. Epidemiol. Community Health* **2018**, *72*, 54–60. [CrossRef] [PubMed]
73. Patra, J.; Giesbrecht, N.; Rehm, J.; Bekmuradov, D.; Popova, S. Are alcohol prices and taxes an evidence-based approach to reducing alcohol-related harm and promoting public health and safety? A literature review. *Contemp. Drug Probl.* **2012**, *39*, 7–48. [CrossRef]
74. Cook, P.J. *Paying the Tab: The Costs and Benefits of Alcohol Control*; Princeton University Press: Princeton, NJ, USA, 2007.
75. Elder, R.W.; Lawrence, B.; Ferguson, A.; Naimi, T.S.; Brewer, R.D.; Chattopadhyay, S.K.; Toomey, T.L.; Fielding, J.E.; Services, T.F.o.C.P. The effectiveness of tax policy interventions for reducing excessive alcohol consumption and related harms. *Am. J. Prev. Med.* **2010**, *38*, 217–229. [CrossRef]
76. Naimi, T.S.; Brewer, R.D.; Miller, J.W.; Okoro, C.; Mehrotra, C. What do binge drinkers drink?: Implications for alcohol control policy. *Am. J. Prev. Med.* **2007**, *33*, 188–193. [CrossRef]
77. Sornpaisarn, B.; Shield, K.D.; Rehm, J. Alcohol taxation policy in Thailand: Implications for other low-to middle-income countries. *Addiction* **2012**, *107*, 1372–1384. [CrossRef]
78. Anderson, P.; Chisholm, D.; Fuhr, D.C. Effectiveness and cost-effectiveness of policies and programmes to reduce the harm caused by alcohol. *Lancet* **2009**, *373*, 2234–2246. [CrossRef]
79. Giesbrecht, N.; Wettlaufer, A.; April, N.; Asbridge, M.; Cukier, S.; Mann, R.; McAllister, J.; Murie, A.; Pauley, C.; Plamondon, L.; et al. *Strategies to Reduce Alcohol-Related Harms and Costs in Canada: A Comparison of Provincial Policies*; Centre for Addiction and Mental Health: Toronto, ON, Canada, 2013.
80. Agardh, E.; Högberg, P.; Miller, T.; Norström, T.; Österberg, E.; Ramstedt, M.; Rossow, I.; Stockwell, T. *Alcohol Monopoly and Public Health: Potential Effects of Privatization of the Swedish Alcohol Retail Monopoly*; Statens Folkhälsoinstitut: Östersund, Sweden, 2008.

81. Chikritzhs, T.; Catalano, P.; Pascal, R.; Henrickson, N. *Predicting Alcohol-Related Harms from Licensed Outlet Density: A Feasibility Study*; National Drug Law Enforcement Research Fund: Hobart, Austrilia, 2007.
82. Vendetti, J.; Gmyrek, A.; Damon, D.; Singh, M.; McRee, B.; Del Boca, F. Screening, brief intervention and referral to treatment (SBIRT): Implementation barriers, facilitators and model migration. *Addiction* **2017**, *112*, 23–33. [CrossRef]
83. Hargraves, D.; White, C.; Frederick, R.; Cinibulk, M.; Peters, M.; Young, A.; Elder, N. Implementing SBIRT (Screening, Brief Intervention and Referral to Treatment) in primary care: Lessons learned from a multi-practice evaluation portfolio. *Public Health Rev.* **2017**, *38*, 31. [CrossRef]
84. Mertens, J.R.; Chi, F.W.; Weisner, C.M.; Satre, D.D.; Ross, T.B.; Allen, S.; Pating, D.; Campbell, C.I.; Lu, Y.W.; Sterling, S.A. Physician versus non-physician delivery of alcohol screening, brief intervention and referral to treatment in adult primary care: The ADVISe cluster randomized controlled implementation trial. *Addict. Sci. Clin. Pract.* **2015**, *10*, 26. [CrossRef]
85. Muench, J.; Jarvis, K.; Vandersloot, D.; Hayes, M.; Nash, W.; Hardman, J.; Grover, P.; Winkle, J. Perceptions of clinical team members toward implementation of SBIRT processes. *Alcohol. Treat. Q.* **2015**, *33*, 143–160. [CrossRef]
86. Greaves, L.; Poole, N. Victimized or validated? Responses to substance-using pregnant women. *Can. Woman Stud.* **2004**, *24*, 87–92.
87. Jacobs, L. 'Bad' mothers have alcohol use disorder: Moral panic or brief intervention? *Gend. Behav.* **2014**, *12*, 5971–5979.
88. Nathoo, T. *Doorways to Conversation: Brief Intervention on Substance Use With Girls and Women*; Centre of Excellence for Women's Health: Vancouver, Austrilia, 2018.
89. Wagner, E.; Babaei, M. *Provincial Guideline for the Clinical Management of High-Risk Drinking and Alcohol Use Disorder*; British Columbia Centre on Substance Use: Vancouver, BC, Canada, 2019.
90. Tannenbaum, C.; Greaves, L.; Graham, I.D. Why sex and gender matter in implementation research. *Bmc Med. Res. Methodol.* **2016**, *16*, 145. [CrossRef] [PubMed]

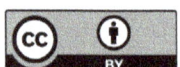

© 2020 by the authors. Licensee MDPI, Basel, Switzerland. This article is an open access article distributed under the terms and conditions of the Creative Commons Attribution (CC BY) license (http://creativecommons.org/licenses/by/4.0/).

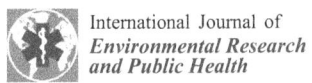

Article

Multi-Service Programs for Pregnant and Parenting Women with Substance Use Concerns: Women's Perspectives on Why They Seek Help and Their Significant Changes

Carol Hubberstey [1,*], Deborah Rutman [1], Rose A. Schmidt [2], Marilyn Van Bibber [1] and Nancy Poole [2]

1. Principal, Nota Bene Consulting Group, Victoria, BC V8R 3M4, Canada
2. Centre of Excellence for Women's Health, Vancouver, BC V6H 3N1, Canada
* Correspondence: carolmarie@shaw.ca

Received: 21 July 2019; Accepted: 6 September 2019; Published: 8 September 2019

Abstract: Within Canada, several specialized multi-service prevention programs work with highly vulnerable pregnant and early parenting women with substance use issues. Experiences of trauma, mental health, poverty, and other factors associated with the social determinants of health complete the picture. Program evaluations have demonstrated their value, but less has been said as to women's reasons for choosing to seek help from these programs, what they were hoping to gain, or what difference they believe has occurred as a result. The Co-creating Evidence project is a multi-year (2017–2020) national evaluation of holistic programs serving women at high risk of having an infant with prenatal alcohol or substance exposure. The evaluation uses a mixed methods design involving quarterly program output and "snapshot" client data, as well as in-person, semi-structured interviews and questionnaires with clients, program staff, and program partners. This article presents findings from interviews with women regarding why they sought help, how they used the services, and what they perceived to be the most significant change in their lives as a result. Obtaining help with substance use was the top theme for what women hoped to get from their participation in their program; however, women's reasons were often intertwined. Additional motivations included wanting information, support or assistance with: child welfare; pregnancy; housing; getting connected to health care or prenatal care; and opportunities for peer support. With respect to the most significant life change, themes included: reduced substance use; improved housing; stronger mother–child connection; and improved wellness and social connections. Findings demonstrated that vulnerable, marginalized pregnant and parenting women who are using substances will seek help when health and social care services are configured in such a way as to take into consideration and address their unique roles, responsibilities, and realities.

Keywords: gender; alcohol; substance use; FASD prevention; program evaluation; multi-service program delivery; client perspectives; pregnancy

---

1. Introduction

Prenatal consumption of alcohol and drugs continues to be a major health, social, and public policy issue in Canada [1,2]. Indeed, surveys have found that upward of 11% of women report consuming alcohol and between 1% and 5% reported using street drugs during pregnancy; both rates are considered to be underestimates given the inherent risks and stigma that go hand in hand with revealing prenatal consumption of alcohol and other substances. As well, a large percentage of the women who use substances prenatally are polysubstance users [3], with one report stating that the rate of (prenatal) poly substance "is as high as 50% in some studies" [4].

Women's reasons for prenatal substance use are both complex and gendered. Research suggests that women's prenatal substance use is often driven by a host of social determinants of health factors such as deep poverty, a history of physical or sexual abuse and neglect or other forms of trauma, intimate partner violence, mental health concerns, precarious living conditions including homelessness, child welfare involvement including maternal–child separation, and physical health problems [5–8]. Moreover, women who are struggling with substance use are typically isolated, are more likely to be living with a partner with problematic substance use, experience lower levels of social support, and have fewer resources at their disposal relative to their male counterparts [1,7,9]. These factors contribute to women's reluctance to reveal the full extent of their substance use [3].

Systemic barriers compound the situation as standard systems of care often don't meet the needs of women with prenatal or postnatal substance use issues, especially not women trying to raise children. Indeed, substance use and child protection services tend to operate in discrete silos with their own distinct goals, policies, expectations, and legislative responsibilities that in the past have resulted in high rates of child apprehensions from families wherein parental alcohol and drug use is a factor [10–14].

As a result, when seeking help for their substance use, vulnerable, marginalized women commonly experience numerous barriers including: stigmatization, lack of mental health supports, negative attitudes of health care providers, and adversarial approach of child welfare authorities [1,9,10,15]. Not surprisingly, fear of child welfare authorities is another factor in women's avoidance of services, as is inadequate transportation and/or lack of child care [16]. These factors together make the decision to seek addiction treatment and support services by vulnerable, pregnant, and early parenting and substance using women all the more challenging. For service providers this also makes it all the more important that the programs they offer meet women's needs [7,17–19].

Despite these hurdles, for many vulnerable women, pregnancy is a time of increased motivation to contemplate significant life changes, particularly prompted by women's desire to keep their newborn in their care [20]. Indeed, the research literature suggests that women will respond to prevention services that are aimed at improving their health, including efforts to decrease or stop substance use or to increase their safer use of substances [19–21]. There also is strong evidence that outcomes for mothers and infants improve when accessible, women-centered substance use services or treatment are offered in conjunction with prenatal care [2,9,19,22]; moreover, care that is also tailored to the specific and evolving needs of women, their children, and the mother–child dyad is viewed as the most effective [12]. Programs that integrate practical and social supports with prenatal and postnatal health services, such as culture, transportation, child care, and meals, and that address the fear of child apprehensions may have an advantage in terms of engaging women who otherwise have few reasons to trust the formal health care system [23]. Moreover, programs that use non-judgmental, relationship-based, trauma-informed, and harm reduction approaches and that acknowledge women's unique realities when it comes to the mother–child relationship have been found to be most effective in reaching vulnerable pregnant and parenting women with substance use issues [8,15,19,24,25].

Research indicates that many women who use substances during pregnancy are polysubstance-using [3,4]; further, once they engage with supportive services, they tend to be selective with respect to which substances they continue to use throughout pregnancy and which they reduce or stop using altogether [3]. In addition, women are inclined to underreport their substance use until they have built a relationship with their service provider that helps them to feel safe enough to disclose the full extent of their use [13]. Hence, community-based programs that have been leaders in the field of fetal alcohol spectrum disorder (FASD) prevention in Canada focus on problematic substance use more broadly, within the context of a social determinants of health context and women's lived experiences as a way of engaging very vulnerable women without further stigmatizing them for their choices [22]. In keeping with this practice approach, in this study, "problematic substance use" is defined as the use of substances, including alcohol, that result in negative consequences in a person's daily life, including adverse health consequences [26], as well as "social, financial, psychological, physical, or legal problems as a result of the drug use" [27].

Despite the evidence that exists with respect to promising approaches, further study would help to enhance our understanding of their implementation in community settings, including a better understanding of what motivates clients to seek services and supports as well as their perspectives on what changed the most in their lives as a result of their involvement in the service(s). To address this, a multi-site evaluation of "wrap-around" FASD prevention programs serving women at risk was envisaged.

Co-Creating Evidence Evaluation Study

In keeping with the internationally recognized four-part FASD prevention model [28], women at highest risk of having an infant with prenatal alcohol exposure are those who who have substance use, mental health, and/or trauma-related issues and/or related social or financial concerns; "Level 3" FASD prevention programs offer holistic, multi-service programming to these women in ways that are specialized, culturally safe, and accessible. The Co-creating Evidence project, a multi-site three-year evaluation of eight different holistic wrap-around programs serving highly vulnerable women at high risk of having an infant with prenatal substance exposure and/or affected by FASD is the first of its kind in Canada. Funded by the Public Health Agency of Canada, the study runs from 2017 to 2020 and brings together many of Canada's multi-service prevention programs with the aim of: sharing knowledge of their practices; demonstrating the effectiveness of prevention programming serving women with substance use and complex issues; and identifying characteristics that make these programs successful. The eight program sites volunteered to be part of the study.

Summary descriptions of the programs taking part in the study are provided in Box 1. The seventh program specifically serves pregnant or early parenting women who have substance use issues and/or other complex challenges. The eighth program serves women who are at risk by virtue of being young, i.e., 16 to 24 years of age; while problematic substance use may be an issue, it is not the program's primary focus. Nevertheless, given the region's very limited availability of substance use services, it is an issue that comes up with regularity. While the programs taking part in the co-creating evidence study are doing FASD prevention work, because they approach women's issues holistically and employ a social determinants of health lens, the programs typically do not depict themselves as FASD prevention programs. At the same time, staff at all programs have training in FASD and trauma-informed practice (as well as other types of training) and also are members of a national FASD prevention research network. All of the programs have a mandate to support healthy birth outcomes, including helping to reduce the likelihood of FASD.

Box 1. Capsule descriptions of co-creating evidence study's program sites.

HerWay Home (Victoria BC) offers drop-in and outreach support, on-site wellness and prenatal/post-natal groups as well as other health/medical services for women and their children, through a combination of program staff and in-kind support from the Island Health Authority. Women can participate in HWH until their child is approximately three years old.

Sheway (Vancouver BC) is a partnership between Vancouver Coastal Health Authority, Ministry for Children and Family Development, Vancouver Native Health Society and the YWCA of Vancouver. A range of on-site health and social services is offered on the first floor; an on-site health clinic is on the second floor; and child care and housing operated by the YWCA is on the third floor. Voluntary child welfare services are provided on-site through a partnership agreement with the provincial Ministry. The length of time that women can participate in Sheway is flexible and not set by the child's age.

Maxxine Wright (Surrey BC) offers health and social supports through co-location with Atira Women's Resource Society, which operates transition housing and second stage housing on-site. Atira offers most of the social programming, with participation from Fraser Health. Health/medical care is provided by Fraser Health. Child welfare and income assistance services are provided on-site through a partnership agreement with relevant provincial Ministries. Women can participate in MW until their child enters school.

Healthy, Empowered, and Resilient (Edmonton AB) is located within the Boyle Street Community Services, which provides an array of social, mental health, family, and cultural services in Edmonton's downtown core. H.E.R. provides outreach to highly street-involved clients; through its staffing and partnership with Boyle McCauley Health Centre, H.E.R. clients have access to prenatal care and post-natal support. Women can participate in H.E.R. until six months post-partum.

Raising Hope (Regina SK) is a residential program located in an 18-unit apartment building (purchased by a non-profit housing society for the program's exclusive use). A range of health/medical, social/cultural supports and programming including child care is offered on-site; residents are required to take part in daily programming. Women and their children can stay for 18 months.

The Mothering Project (Winnipeg MB) is a program of Mt Carmel Clinic and is co-located with the clinic. Through its staffing and partnerships, the MP offers a broad range of drop-in, outreach, and on-site supports and health/medical services along with a dedicated space for cultural ceremony. A licensed day care is co-located with MP with spaces set aside for program clients. Women can participate in the MP until their child reaches the age of five.

Breaking the Cycle (Toronto ON) is one of the first FASD prevention programs in Canada. The program provides children's developmental assessment and mental health services with wrap-around services for women. Each woman is connected to a counsellor and each child is connected to a Child Development Worker. Women can participate in BTC until their child is six years old.

Baby Basics (New Glasgow NS) is a weekly drop-in parenting program operated by Kids First Family Resource Program, for women under age 25 and their children age 0–6. Although not specifically directed at women who are using substances, there are very few such options available to women in the region. BB offers a safe place for women to access support and talk about a range of issues. Women can participate in BB until their infant is one year old.

A previous article [29] described the study overall, with an emphasis on presenting: an overall theory of change for the programs; the services, activities and common components offered by the eight programs; women's situations at intake; and interim qualitative findings regarding what clients like best about their program. This article shares additional interim findings from the study, based on data gathered between April and December 2018. In this article we focus on:

- What women hoped to get from engaging in their program;
- How women used their program's services/activities; and
- The most significant changes that women experienced as a result of their program.

2. Materials and Methods

2.1. Study Design

The co-creating evidence study is employing a mixed-methods design, guided by principles of collaboration and partnership. The study is guided by collaborative and participatory principles [30], including the principles of "fostering meaningful relationships" (with program staff and stakeholders), "developing a shared understanding of the program," "promoting appropriate participatory processes," and "promoting evaluative thinking" [31,32]. In June 2017, the project team convened an introductory face-to-face meeting with program leaders to create a theory of change and the theoretical/philosophical foundations, approaches, activities, and anticipated outcomes of the programs collectively. Since that time, bi-monthly web-based teleconferences have been held to discuss key issues related to data collection and analysis, and to solicit the program managers' feedback regarding interim project findings, draft reports, and knowledge translation. These meetings also provided the program leaders with opportunities to exchange information about their practices, shared issues, common understandings, programming shifts, and contextual issues of significance such as the ongoing opioid crisis. In addition, a National Advisory Committee was established at the beginning of the study, comprised of people with expertise in policy, programming, research and evaluation related to FASD. The Advisory Committee meets about 2–3 times a year.

2.2. Data Collection Processes and Instruments

Data are gathered through two separate processes:

1. The project team is undertaking two visits with each site, to conduct face-to-face, semi-structured, qualitative interviews, focus groups and questionnaires with staff, clients, and program partners.
2. The program manager/coordinator at each site is compiling and remitting quantitative output data and client-based data from April 2018 to September 2019, for a total of 18 months.

This article focuses on the qualitative interviews conducted with clients/participants during the first site visits between April and July 2018 and questionnaire data collected as part of the interview process. It is supplemented with interview data with staff and program managers/leaders.

2.3. On-site Data Collection by Project Team

The project team conducted individual qualitative interviews with clients, using an interview guide that was created for this project. Interview questions include: how the woman first learned about the program; what she hoped to get out of her involvement with the program; her life situation just prior to becoming involved with the program; her satisfaction with the program (e.g., what she liked most about the program, didn't like, and would change); and what was most important to her about the program. As well, the interview contained open-ended questions pertaining to the client's use of the program's various services and activities. Clients were also asked about perceived impacts of the program. A modified version of the most significant change (MSC) technique was employed [33], informants are asked to share what was "the most significant change that happened" as a result of the program. The MSC technique was modified in this study in that the analysis of clients' stories did not involve formal review by external stakeholders or hierarchical selection and quantification of the stories.. The interviews were conducted in a private office, using a guided conversation approach that enabled interviewees to speak freely about which was most important to them.

After the interview, women were invited to complete the client questionnaire, which most often was administered verbally by the project team member, but which the participant could complete on her own if she preferred. The client questionnaire utilized a five-point Likert-type scale and focused both on participants' experiences with their program (e.g., sense of physical safety and emotional safety; being respected; being a partner in planning and having a voice in decision-making; feeling that staff are sensitive when asking about difficult experiences, and so forth), and their perspectives on program impacts and how helpful the program had been in relation to outcomes in various facets of their life (e.g., in relation to accessing safe housing, accessing prenatal/postnatal care, and having a healthy birth, keeping or regaining their child(ren) in their care, and quitting or reducing their substance use). The questionnaire was created specifically for this study; at the same time, it included standardized questionnaire items that have been used in evaluations of trauma-informed and/or harm reduction focused programs [34].

All participants were provided with an honorarium ($25) for completing the interview and questionnaire. Program staff were available afterwards should clients have questions, comments, or concerns regarding the interview. Prior to launching the formal data collection, the project team pilot tested the interview guides and interview process with four sites. The purpose was to garner feedback from clients and staff regarding the process and the questions including how clients felt about answering potentially difficult questions about their lives.

2.4. Participants and Sampling Approach

Eligibility criteria for client participation in the interview and questionnaire were as follows: (a) the woman had to be accessing services from the program in the month of data collection; (b) women were 16 years or older; and, (c) women were English-speaking. Recruitment was handled by program staff who, approximately one month prior to the site visit, posted notices in program space regarding the interviews and made announcements during group and/or drop-in programming, inviting clients to come to the program for an interview or otherwise express their desire to do the interview off-site. Both forms of recruitment reinforced that the interviews were confidential and anonymous. For clients, a voluntary sampling approach was employed as program coordinators and the research team thought it was important for all clients who wanted to take part in an interview and who were available during the team's site visit to be able to do so. At the same time, program staff did not formally track the number of clients whom they told about the site visit and interview opportunity, nor did they keep track of the number of clients who expressed disinterest in doing an interview; thus, it was not possible to know how many, if any, clients refused to participate in the in-person data collection process. A nominated sampling approach was used to create the sample of service partners; program staff at all sites provided the researchers with contact information for each program's closest service partners.

A total of 125 program participants/clients (of whom 123 completed the client questionnaire) took part in an in-person interview between April and July 2018. The number of interviews with clients varied across sites, from $n = 32$ at one of the largest sites to $n = 8$ at two sites; there were three sites at which more than 20 clients were interviewed and five sites at which 8–11 women were interviewed. Differences in terms of the number of interviews conducted per site reflect the size and scale of the programs and was roughly proportional to the number of clients per site. As well, events outside of the program, including crises in the community and/or in clients' lives also impacted response to the invitation to take part in the study.

All of the program participants identified their gender as female, and more than half were older than 30 years old (see Table 1). Every participant who completed the client questionnaire completed the demographic questions. Most often women self-identified their cultural background as Indigenous, followed by European/White. The length of time women had participated in the programs varied from less than one month to more than three years. Some of this variation is due to the policies of the individual program; for example, no participants from HER had participated in the program for more than one year as the discharge from the program occurs at six months post-partum.

2.5. Data Analysis

A frequency analysis of the client questionnaire was conducted in SPSS 26 (SPSS Inc., Chicago, IL, USA) to describe the participants. Missing data for each question ranged from $n = 0$ to $n = 45$, and percentages reported in the results did not include the women who did not answer each question in the denominator.

Table 1. Characteristics of client questionnaire participants.

Program Site	Herway Home	Sheway	Maxx Wright	HER	Raising Hope	Mothering Project	Breaking the Cycle	Baby Basics	Total
	n	n	n	n	n	n	n	n	N (%)
Number of participants									
	8	35	20	9	10	25	8	8	123
Age									
16–24	1	4	3	5	3	3	1	6	26 (21%)
25–30	2	5	6	3	5	5	3	2	31 (25%)
30+	5	26	11	1	2	17	4	0	66 (54%)
Cultural background (top 3)									
Indigenous	2	19	8	7	8	20	0	1	65 (53%)
European/White	3	9	4	1	2	2	5	7	33 (27%)
Mixed Race	3	6	5	0	0	3	1	0	18 (15%)
Length of time participating in program									
<1 month	0	0	1	1	0	0	0	1	3 (2%)
1–6 months	3	3	3	4	5	5	3	1	27 (22%)
7–12 months	1	5	2	4	3	2	2	1	20 (16%)
1–3 years	3	12	4	0	1	7	3	3	33 (27%)
>3 years	1	15	10	0	1	11	0	2	40 (33%)

As the interviews with clients, staff and service partners involved open-ended questions, qualitative data analysis techniques were used, and qualitative data analysis software (NVivo12) (QRS International, Melbourne, Australia) was utilized to facilitate the analyses. In keeping with these techniques, written transcripts from all interviews were read multiple times by the researchers to begin the process of identifying themes and analytic ideas. Initially, each researcher coded the transcripts separately and identified preliminary themes inductively. The three researchers involved in carrying out the interviews highlighted naturally occurring patterns in the data, including words, phrases, or ideas most commonly voiced by participants, which formed the basis of the thematic analysis [35,36]. As means to strengthen the study's rigor, the project team engaged in numerous discussions wherein they presented and reviewed one another's emerging reflections, insights, and ideas about the data. Any differences in the researchers' interpretations were resolved through discussion, review of the supportive textual evidence for each theme, knowledge of and comparisons with findings from the literature and previous relevant research, and consensus decision-making. Themes were ranked in strength based on a combination of the frequency with which they emerged and the intensity with which the speakers voiced the theme as evidenced by repetition of the theme/idea within the same utterance and/or the speaker's emphasis or tone of voice when speaking, which was recorded by the researchers in their interview transcripts.

2.6. Ethics Approval

The evaluation study received ethics approval from the University of British Columbia Office of Research Ethics (H17-02168), Fraser Health Authority, Vancouver Coastal Health Authority, Island Health Authority, and York University. Study participants provided informed consent to participate in the interviews. All study participants were competent to provide their own informed consent and all were over age 18.

3. Results

3.1. Overview of the Programs' Services

Drawing on interviews with staff and program leaders/managers and written program descriptions, Table 2 shows that, through a combination of their own staff or staff from partner organizations providing services on site, all co-creating evidence programs offer a mix of accessible health and social services and supports aimed at meeting clients' holistic health, social, cultural, and practical needs. The programs' core philosophical pillars include being relationship-based, trauma-informed, women-centered, culturally-informed, and employing non-stigmatizing harm reduction approaches. Many services were offered in group format, though nearly all programs offered one-to-one services as well. Programs connected to a health authority were more likely to offer health services on site (e.g., public health nurse, physician, nurse practitioner, or midwife).

Table 2. Services/activities offered by programs via staff or service partners or via referrals.

Service/Activity	Number of Programs Offering Service/Activity on Site via Program Staff or Service Partners	Number of Programs Linking Clients to Service/Activity via Referral to Service Partners	Total Number of Programs Offering or Facilitating Access to Service
Basic needs support	8	0	8
Child assessment and early intervention	5	2	7
Child care on site	7	0	7
Child health	6	2	8
Child welfare support	7	0	7
Cultural programming	5	1	6
Drop in; peer connection	8	0	8
Food; nutrition	8	0	8
Health; medical services	6	2	8
Housing	4	4	8
Life skills	6	1	7
Mental health; trauma	8	0	8
Outreach	6	0	6
Parenting programs	7	1	8
Prenatal and postnatal care	7	1	8
Substance use counselling	7	1	8

3.2. What Women Hoped to Get from Participating in Their Program

Clients were asked what they had hoped to get by participating in their program. The themes were often interconnected, as clients generally provided several reasons for program involvement. The top themes to emerge were (in order of frequency):

- Wanted support in relation to problematic substance use and/or trauma
- Wanted support with child welfare and/or mother–child connection
- Wanted support and information related to pregnancy
- Wanted help in getting housing
- Wanted help in getting connected to health care or prenatal care
- Wanted healthy peer connections or peer support
- Brief discussion of the key themes follows.

3.2.1. Wanted Support in Relation to Problematic Substance Use and/or Trauma

The most frequently emerging theme—voiced by nearly half of the clients interviewed—was that women were seeking help in addressing their substance use. However, for many women, this was intertwined with wanting help in dealing with effects of trauma because of experiences of violence or abuse and with wanting help with housing and with child welfare issues. (Child protection/child welfare terms are used interchangeably. Provinces/territories within Canada hold the legislated mandate to protect children and if need be to remove them from their parent(s). Generally speaking child protection social workers investigate and will remove children if deemed necessary, whereas child welfare social workers are tasked with working with the family to mitigate the risk factors. Nevertheless, any involvement of child protection/child welfare authorities means that the parent(s) is/are under scrutiny, that risk factors or concerns are present and that the parent(s) could lose their child if they are unable to satisfy the expectations of child welfare/child protection staff.)

> I wanted to get sober. I wanted my children back, my family back. . . . . I was using drugs and alcohol. I was going through a rough time—breaking up with my partner who was abusive mentally and emotionally.

> [I wanted] better housing, support to keep me away from drugs and alcohol, and help with nutrition. [I wanted] to keep my baby.

> [I wanted] connections with other mothers and knowing that there were groups I could do that would help me with being a mother with trauma and addiction.

3.2.2. Wanted Support with Child Welfare and/or Mother–Child Connection

Hand in hand with women's desire for support in relation to their substance use was their desire for support in relation to keeping or regaining their child(ren) in their care and/or in having a strong mother–child connection. Clients often sought participation in specific program activities (e.g., substance use/recovery groups or parenting groups) and/or sought connection with program staff who would be able to speak to their motivation and capacity to care for their child(ren); most often, the programs were already known to clients for their support and advocacy in relation to child welfare.

> I wanted a different way of bonding with my child, a different community.

> I wanted connections with other mothers and knowing that there were groups I could do that would help me with being a mother with trauma and addiction.

> I wanted sobriety and to learn to parent my kids; I had lost custody.

> I wanted to get support and bring my child home and parent in a healthy lifestyle for her and for me.

While wanting to demonstrate that they were capable of parenting may have been the initial impetus for attending their program, as women made gains, some realized that they wanted more, whether that was a better quality of life or a more stable foundation for building a life for their children.

> To start with, I only wanted to get my children back. Now I want a better quality of life for me and my kids.

> I also wanted to connect with a therapist. I wanted to have a stable foundation to work with. I knew [child protection] would be involved, so I wanted to create a healthy foundation for that involvement.

3.2.3. Wanted Support and Information Related to Pregnancy

Another strong theme and reason for engagement with their program was a desire for guidance and information in relation to their pregnancy as well as help with other issues such as finding safe and stable housing, child welfare, and substance use. Many women spoke of wanting this pregnancy to be different from their previous one(s).

> I was pregnant and had addictions and I wanted to have support through my pregnancy.

> Initially, I didn't know where or how I'd go with the pregnancy. I needed guidance and support. When I first found out I was pregnant, I cried for 48 hours straight. I also wanted information. I didn't know where to go and what my next step would be.

> Support to keep moving forward. I wanted to make changes in my life.

3.2.4. Wanted Help in Getting Housing

As noted previously, at intake over half of clients (ranging up to 85% at some program sites) had precarious and/or inadequate housing. Clients voiced their desire for program assistance in helping them access safe and stable housing, as they also recognized the inextricable connection between housing and child welfare authorities' safety concerns.

> Support, because I have [child protection] involvement. I wanted support and stable housing and getting addictions out of the way. I want to go home with my baby.

> I was in a really shitty situation. I was living with a friend; she was using drugs. I ended up in a shelter. I needed resources to help me with my pregnancy and with raising my baby, and I wanted help getting into different housing.

3.2.5. Wanted Help in Getting Connected to Health Care or Prenatal Care

Approximately 20% of the clients interviewed stated that they were looking for health or prenatal care. Some women sought a health/prenatal care provider because they had recently moved to the community—often to flee an abusive ex-partner or to shed ties with people who used substances—while others may have been in the community for a while but sought a prenatal care provider in order to focus on having a healthy pregnancy. As well, some women emphasized that they wanted to connect with a health or perinatal care provider who would not judge or stigmatize them for their substance use.

> My family doctor set me up with a maternity doctor who specialized in working with women with addictions. She suggested that I network with someone. I was afraid that the nurses at the hospital would see my medical history, see that I was on suboxone, and be judgmental and call child welfare.

> I was looking for prenatal care. I was looking for programs and people to help support me to have a healthy pregnancy.

3.2.6. Wanted Healthy Peer Connections or Peer Support

Finally, wrapped up in the notion of finding support was a desire by clients for healthy peer connections, partly born of a desire to be amongst women with similar backgrounds and with whom they could safely share their story.

> I was looking for support and advocacy for my situation. I was needing a group for women like me who have been through years of trauma and abuse. I did not want to be the only woman in the room with that kind of lived experience.

> [I wanted] to open up more; learn how to speak to others when they needed help; to share my story with others who were struggling; to help guide others on a positive path.

Some women wanted the sense of community that could come from being in a prenatal group and to have answers to their questions.

> The sense of community here. Support group. I didn't know other pregnant women.

3.3. Clients' Experiences of Utilizing Their Program's Services/Activities

As part of the qualitative interviews, clients were asked to describe ways in which they used the various activities or services offered by programs. A sample of their comments, presented in Table 3, provides a more complete picture of the services listed in Table 2 and sheds light on women's perspectives on the value of a "one-stop" approach to health care, poverty, child protection issues, parenting, social connections, substance use, and culture.

Table 3. Examples of ways that clients utilized their program's services.

Service/Activity	Examples of Ways That Clients Utilized the Service/Activity
Basic needs support	Lots of practical support such as a bag of clothes for the baby and items for myself such as a sports bra when I gave birth recently. I got help with income security.
Child assessment and early intervention	A speech language pathologist was linked to my son—the referral from [the program] sped up the process. We were referred to the hospital and introduced to a dentist for the children. The staff made sure the children were up to date for their immunizations and referred them to an Infant Development worker.
Child care on site	My baby is in daycare sometimes. I want to get a regular spot in the daycare. They have the daycare here. You can take "self-care" breaks and have the kids go into daycare.
Child health	My son had vaccinations with the Public Health Nurse and saw the dental hygienist. He is getting dental surgery soon as a result. I brought my older daughter to see the doctor; my baby is in care still.
Child welfare support	When my partner assaulted me in November, child welfare was automatically involved. I was concerned they would take my kids away. I met with child protection services with [program] as my support. [The program] advocated for me to get my kids back early and to have visits, and then extended visits with my kids—and then my kids came back to me.
Cultural programming	I went to the Round Dance organized by [program's partner organization]. I do drumming and Talking Circle here.
Drop in; peer connection	A lot of the women who come here I've known since childhood. Now we're moms together. All my friends are here; they're getting sober and are moms. The other women are role models—they help us develop skills and increase confidence. I have connections with other women coming to [the program].
Food; nutrition	Lunch program; weekly bag of nutrition; fresh bread; prenatal and postnatal minerals and supplements plus education and workshops on healthy nutrition. Every week I get a four-liter jug of milk, eggs and cheese. That weekly food bag really helps.
Health; medical	I see the Public Health Nurse at the [program] regularly. She is the one who wanted me on Methadone—she said would it be better for the baby than T3s. We discuss sexual health information in group.
Housing	I got help with housing through another agency but [the program] helped me to switch the lease to be in my name, which means that I have to be more responsible. My support worker got me into a nice place for women. People are getting their kids back and staying off drugs.
Life skills	We had someone come and talk about the food guide. The nurse from [program's partner organization] provided nutrition education. We learned how to make baby food and we did fire prevention education.
Mental health; trauma	I spoke with the trauma counsellor about some of the things I have seen in the last year. I've been living a very high-risk life—drugs, violence, lots of money. I'm working with the trauma worker now. I'm doing that to get my son back.
Outreach	My Outreach Worker is my mainstay. My Outreach Worker will go to court with me as an advocate.
Parenting programs	I took a couple of parenting groups. That helps me with how I play with my daughter. I learned about her development and how to talk with my teenage son. I've done lots of programs, like wellness, circle of security, and rediscovering parenting. They are all very useful because as my kids age, new problems arise and I retake the group to see how the information applies to my current situation. I like that the groups repeat regularly.
Prenatal; postnatal care	I'm seeing the doctor here, getting Methadone, and going to prenatal classes. They give me rides to [program's partner organization] for prenatal care. We learn about breastfeeding, traditional teachings, abuse and violence there.
Substance use counselling	I had stopped cocaine and alcohol in 2017. [The program] helps me deal with and address the urges. Fear of [child protection] also motivates me. I have a one-to-one counsellor I was seeing weekly until recently. Now we meet biweekly. I'm going to be starting Group (struggling with addictions group) tomorrow. I talk with the counsellor all the time about my use and where I live. It is hard to stop using when you are selling drugs all the time.

3.4. Most Significant Change(s) That Women Experienced (as a Result of Their Program)

As a key component of the qualitative interview, clients were asked what had been the most significant change(s) that had taken place for them and their family since they started participating in their program. As was the case with other open-ended interview questions, women's responses often contained multiple themes, and the themes were clearly intertwined. The top themes were (reported in order of frequency):

- Quit or reduced substance use;
- Strengthened mother–child connection;
- Kept/regained custody/care of child(ren);
- Improved wellness/mental health;
- Increased support;
- Safer, improved housing.

3.4.1. Quit or Reduced Substance Use

The most frequently emerging theme of the "most significant change," voiced by approximately 40% of the clients interviewed ($n = 51$), was that they had quit or reduced their substance use. Many attributed their program with helping them to quit using substances.

> If I hadn't been at this program, it would have been harder to stay sober, and my baby would have gone to live with my mom.
>
> Because the staff care so much about their clients, I've gotten clean. I've been in and out of addiction for 18 years, but because of them, my using time has reduced—it's down to two days. They've reached out to me. They've made a huge difference to me.

In keeping with these findings, on the client questionnaire, 79% ($n = 93$, 4% missing;) agreed or strongly agreed that the program had helped them quit, reduce or engage in safer substance use, and 70% ($n = 83$, 3% missing) agreed or strongly agreed that the program had helped them access substance use services or supports. Approximately 20% of women indicated on the client questionnaire that these items were not applicable to them, as they had not sought help from their program for substance use concerns.

3.4.2. Strengthened Mother–Child Connection

The second theme, voiced by nearly the same number of clients ($n = 49$), pertained to the existence or strengthening of the connection between the woman and her child(ren). This important theme focused on the presence and preservation of the mother–child relationship rather than on whether women had retained or regained custody of their child(ren), and thus it was voiced both by women who did not have their child(ren) in their care as well as those who did. Similarly, most women ($n = 93$, 79%, 5% missing) agreed or strongly agreed on the questionnaire that the program had helped them improve their connection to their children. This theme also relates to the situation voiced by some women that, had they not had support from their program, they likely would not have continued with their pregnancy:

> My baby and I have a home. We know we're not alone—both because I can call the [program] staff and because of other women. Without [program], I probably wouldn't have had my baby.
>
> My stress level has gone down quite a bit. I know that no matter what, they'll be here. The program helps with everything: prenatal care, housing, [child protection] advocacy, baby stuff. Before coming into this program, I felt hopeless.

3.4.3. Kept/Regained Custody/Care of Child(ren)

In keeping with the previous point, the third strongest theme was that women had retained and/or regained their children in their care. As reflected in clients' comments, keeping their infant in their care and/or getting their child back from foster care nearly always occurred in tandem with other pivotal life events, such as reducing or ending their substance use, accessing stable housing, and breaking away from a high-risk "past lifestyle."

> Getting my daughter back from foster care and having my baby come home from the hospital with me. Getting my kids back is the biggest thing. That showed me I'm done with my past lifestyle.

> I've been clean and sober for 22 months. Getting clean changed my whole life. I got my son back, and I'm about to get the older two children back in September.

3.4.4. Improved Wellness/Mental Health

The fourth top theme, voiced by about a third of the clients interviewed ($n = 39$), had to do with women's experience of improved wellness and well-being. Along these lines, clients described feeling happier, less stressed, more self-confident, self-aware and emotionally equipped to deal with personal triggers, as well as being more socially engaged.

> Our household is more balanced. I know my triggers and deal with anger better. I am more balanced emotionally.

> Coming to [the program] is getting us out of our shells. My daughter and I, we really needed this. It's really made a difference in terms of our health, mental health and well-being

3.4.5. Increased Support

Strongly connected to all themes was clients' sense that they had increased supports—both from program staff and from other program participants—and a support network that they could count on. As well, for some women, a significant change was their newfound capacity to reach out to others for support when needed.

> I'm about to reach out for support. I couldn't do that before.

Paralleling these findings, on the client questionnaire, 93% ($n = 111$, 3% missing) agreed or strongly agreed with the statement "I feel supported and less isolated; I have social support."

3.4.6. Safer, Improved Housing

Approximately 25% of the clients interviewed reported that, for them, a/the significant change since becoming involved with their program was accessing safe and adequate housing. As noted previously, clients often spoke of housing in essentially the same breath as they talked about keeping/regaining their child(ren) and/or quitting or reducing their substance use, as the inter-connections between these outcomes were evident. In one client's words:

> Getting suitable housing and reuniting with my son. We were in the single room occupancy apartment when I had the baby. Then he went into a foster home. Then we got housing and the baby was returned to us.

3.4.7. Additional "Significant Changes"/Outcomes

Three additional "most significant change" themes are important to mention, given that they emerged in the comments of quite a few clients ($n = 20$ or roughly 16% of those interviewed). These were:

- Increased self-confidence/self-esteem;

- Reduced isolation and/or increased connection to peers;
- Increased self-compassion/self-determination.

As these clients stated:

They've helped me open up more. I feel more self-confident and happier. I've opened up a lot more.

I got back into my culture. I'm teaching my daughter how to smudge and do drumming.

I'm happy, have lots of friends. I've connected again with family, and I'm sober.

It helped me—the therapy and the groups—to reflect on myself, and I wanted to do that for myself. I have a better understanding of myself. They give us the tools to help ourselves.

3.5. Summary of Key Findings

By way of summary, Table 4 presents the top themes and their interconnection in relation to what women hoped to get from participating in their program and their most significant change.

Table 4. Top themes in relation to what women hoped to get from participating in their program and their most significant change.

What Women Hoped to Get from Participating in Their Program	Women's Most Significant Change
Support with problematic substance use and/or trauma ($n = 61$)	Quit, reduced or safer substance use ($n = 51$) Improved wellness/mental health ($n = 39$)
Support with child welfare and/or mother-child connection ($n = 58$)	Strengthened mother – child connection ($n = 49$) Women keep/regain children in their care ($n = 43$)
Support and information re: pregnancy ($n = 37$) Help in accessing health care or prenatal care ($n = 29$)	Increased support ($n = 34$)
Help in getting safe, stable housing ($n = 32$)	Safer, improved housing ($n = 29$)
Healthy peer connections or peer support ($n = 23$)	Reduced isolation/connection to identity, peers, culture ($n = 19$)

4. Discussion

The interim findings of the Co-creating Evidence multi-site evaluation make a valuable contribution to the literature by focusing on the perspectives of highly vulnerable, pregnant, and early parenting women with problematic substance use, and drawing an arc from their life circumstances prior to entering the program, to what it was they were hoping to gain by reaching out for help, and finally, to their views on the most significant changes in their lives as a result of their involvement with the program. In doing so, the preliminary findings support the already rich literature on the complexity of issues that this population of women face, including intimate partner violence, trauma/mental health, poverty, precarious housing, and child welfare involvement [1,5,6].

The study also contributes to a better understanding as to what prompts women to want to make a change in their life circumstances. In this vein, the study affirms the view that pregnancy can be a powerful catalyst for transformation for women who are marginalized from mainstream services by virtue of their circumstances and contributes to the literature that vulnerable pregnant and parenting women experiencing numerous personal and systemic barriers will seek help, ideally at a single point of access, when those services are non-judgmental and take into consideration and address their realities [2,19,37–39]. Additionally, from a gender perspective, women have also been found to respond to and benefit from programs that take into consideration their unique roles and responsibilities and that reduce obstacles to their participation, including those related to caring for children and family [18,19,40].

On that note, women's top priorities prior to joining their program and the areas of their lives in which they reported significant improvement were intertwined such that they rarely spoke of just one priority or benefit. In this regard, while obtaining support in relation to their problematic substance use was the most frequently cited theme, it was often entwined with issues of current or past trauma. Addressing these issues together was part of the programs' holistic, trauma-informed, and women-centered approach. Often closely associated with clients' desire for support in relation to their substance use was a yearning to retain and/or regain their children; a related goal was to create a better life for themselves and for their child(ren) including learning more about parenting and having opportunities for positive peer connections for themselves and their child(ren). This lends further weight to the tenet that when working with vulnerable women, the child is "undeniably part of the equation" [40]. At the same time, women who use substances pre and postnatally often experience parenting difficulties resulting in the further likelihood of child welfare involvement; hence, recommended best practices include not only being responsive to the mother–child dyad but also development of a collaborative working relationship between substance use services and child welfare agencies [12,23,41].

For almost one-quarter of clients, improved housing was reported as a, if not the, most significant change in their lives. As four of the co-creating evidence study programs offered housing to at least some clients either on-site (for example, through the program's own services or through co-location with a housing agency) and others achieved this through partnerships with local or provincial housing providers, clients were able to more readily access supported/social housing as a result of their association with their program. Safe and stable housing is fundamental to satisfying the safety concerns of child welfare authorities—i.e., enabling women to be able to go home with their infant after giving birth and/or to regain custody of older children—as well as to sustaining other positive life changes.

Poor health or mental health were key issues at intake and were areas in which clients experienced positive change as a result of their involvement with the programs. For women, this "significant change" was characterized as an overall sense of wellness and social connections; a frequent theme was their experience of improved mental well-being, increased support, and self-confidence/self-esteem, reduced isolation, and increased self-compassion and self-determination. In describing the pathways that mothering women take toward quitting their substance use, Marcellus similarly found that restoring their sense of self—described as gaining and sustaining recovery, becoming more socially connected and less isolated, improving personal well-being, and regaining credibility in multiple domains—was a key trajectory for women [42]. In this regard the findings to date of the co-creating evidence study are consistent with client perceptions of integrated treatment programs in Ontario, in that those participating in integrated programs reported positive psycho-social outcomes, including improved self-confidence and greater sense of self [2].

Finally, it has also been noted in the literature that women respond differently to substance use services than do men, showing a preference for services and programs that engender an atmosphere of hope, acceptance, and support [43]. Earlier qualitative findings from the Co-creating Evidence study [29] described that what clients liked best about their program was the caring, non-judgmental, supportive, helpful approach of staff. This along with the availability of multiple services in one place was among the top themes, indicating that it is possible for vulnerable pregnant and parenting women with complex challenges including problematic substance use to achieve positive outcomes when presented with the right mix of services and approaches that adequately address their health and social support needs as women and mothers.

Limitations

Despite the strong congruence between this study's findings and the existing literature, the study's limitations should be noted. With regard to the on-site client-related data collection (i.e., interviews and questionnaires with clients), we understand that the voluntary sampling approach could have resulted in biases, in that clients with more positive views about their program would have been disproportionately inclined to take part in the evaluation study. As well, without the denominator in terms of potential participation in the evaluation, we cannot assess bias nor the representativeness of the sample. Further, with a circumscribed number of days for each site visit and on-site data collection, clients had a narrow window of opportunity to take part. As such, we cannot know for certain that we achieved "saturation," nor was the concept of saturation the means by which we determined the number of interviews to conduct at each site. Nonetheless, we have no reason to believe that clients who held fewer positive perspectives were disinclined to participate in the study nor were they prevented from doing so. The confidential, conversational approach to interviewing also facilitated participants sharing their diverse experiences and perspectives. Given that there will be a second round of on-site data collection with clients, there will be an opportunity to explore the issue of sampling bias and determine whether saturation was achieved.

5. Conclusions

Women's prenatal alcohol use and other substance use frequently occur within the context of inadequate housing, intimate partner violence, trauma, poverty, and social isolation. These burdens combined with systemic barriers affect their ability and willingness to engage with formal health care services. Often, women reveal the full extent of their substance use, including alcohol, only when they feel safe, accepted, not stigmatized, and when their program/service is meeting their practical needs.

With its focus on clients' perspectives, this paper makes a valuable contribution to the literature regarding multi-service programs aimed at vulnerable pregnant and parenting women who use alcohol and other substances. The article highlights the multiple, interconnected reasons why women seek help from these programs, most notably the twin desires to address their substance use and to regain and/or keep their baby/children in their care. Rounding this out are women's desires for help with housing, prenatal/health care, and peer support, suggesting that pregnancy can be an important catalyst for making significant life changes.

This study affirms how capably women can provide such guidance to service providers as to their service needs. It also affirms the value of a holistic approach that addresses both problematic substance use and the social determinants of health in accessible, women-centered, and integrated programming.

To ensure that this population of vulnerable pregnant/parenting women receive such holistic services, funders too will need to consider how to integrate funding streams, to include health, social and cultural services, housing, income support, child welfare, and public safety resources to these multi-service programs.

Author Contributions: Conceptualization, C.H. and D.R.; methodology, D.R., C.H., R.A.S., N.P., and M.V.B.; funding acquisition, C.H., D.R., N.P., and M.V.B.; investigation, D.R., C.H., M.V.B., R.A.S.; formal analysis, C.H., D.R., R.A.S., M.V.B., and N.P.; project administration, C.H. and D.R.; visualization, D.R. and C.H.; writing—original draft preparation, C.H., D.R. and R.A.S.; writing—review and editing, C.H., D.R., M.V.B., R.A.S., and N.P.

Funding: This research was funded by the Public Health Agency of Canada, FASD National Strategic Projects Fund, Project #1617-HQ-000070.

Conflicts of Interest: The authors declare no conflict of interest.

References

1. Finnegan, L. *Substance Abuse in Canada: Licit and Illicit Drug Use During Pregnancy: Maternal, Neonatal and Early Childhood Consequences*; Canadian Centre on Substance Abuse: Ottawa, ON, Canada, 2013.
2. Tarasoff, L.; Milligan, K.; Le, T.; Usher, A.; Urbanoski, K. Integrated treatment programs for pregnant and parenting women with problematic substance use: Service descriptions and client perceptions of care. *J. Subst. Abus. Treat.* **2018**, *90*, 9–18. [CrossRef] [PubMed]
3. Latuskie, K.; Leibson, T.; Andrews, N.; Motz, M.; Pepler, D.; Ito, S. Substance use in pregnancy among vulnerable women seeking addiction and parenting Support. *Int. J. Ment. Health Addict.* **2018**, *17*, 137–150. [CrossRef]
4. Forray, A. Substance use during pregnancy [version 1; peer review: 2 approved]. *F1000 Res.* **2016**, *5*, 887. [CrossRef] [PubMed]

5. Boyd, S.; Marcellus, L. *With Child: Substance Use During Pregnancy: A Woman-Centred Approach*; Fernwood Publishing: Halifax, NS, Canada, 2007.
6. Espinet, S.; Jeong, J.; Motz, M.; Racine, N.; Major, D.; Pepler, D. Multimodal assessment of the mother-child relationship in a substance-exposed sample: Divergent associations with the Emotional Availability Scales. *Infant Ment. Health J.* **2013**, *34*, 496–507. [CrossRef]
7. Gelb, K.; Rutman, D. *Substance Using Women with FASD and FASD Prevention: A Literature Review on Promising Approaches in Substance Use Treatment and Care for Women with FASD*; School of Social Work, University of Victoria: Victoria, BC, Canada, 2011.
8. Pepler, D.; Motz, M.; Leslie, M.; Jenkins, J.; Espinet, S.; Reynolds, W. *A Focus on Relationships*; Mothercraft Press: Toronto, ON, Canada, 2014.
9. Sword, W.; Niccols, A.; Fan, A. "New Choices" for women with addictions: Perceptions of program participants. *BMC Public Health* **2004**, *4*, 10. [CrossRef]
10. Choi, S.; Ryan, J.P. Co-occurring programs for substance abusing mothers in child welfare: Matching services to improve family reunification. *Child. Youth Serv. Rev.* **2007**, *29*, 1395–1410. [CrossRef]
11. Huebner, R.; Young, N.; Hall, M.; Posze, L.; Willauer, T. Serving families with child maltreatment and substance use disorders: A decade of learning. *J. Soc. Work* **2017**, *20*, 288–305. [CrossRef]
12. Meixner, T.; Milligan, K.; Urbanoski, K.; McShane, K. Conceptualizing integrated service delivery for pregnant and parenting women with addictions: Defining key factors and processes. *Can. J. Addict.* **2016**, *7*, 57–65.
13. Marsh, J.; Smith, B. Integrated substance abuse and child welfare services for women: A progress Review. *Child. Youth Serv. Rev.* **2011**, *33*, 466–472. [CrossRef]
14. Grant, T.; Graham, C.; Ernst, C.; Peavy, M.; Novick Brown, N. Improving pregnancy outcomes among high-risk mothers who abuse alcohol and drugs: Factors associated with subsequent exposed births. *Child. Youth Serv. Rev.* **2014**, *46*, 11–18. [CrossRef]
15. Motz, M.; Leslie, M.; Pepler, D.; Moore, T.; Freeman, P. Breaking the Cycle: Measures of Progress 1995–2005. *J. FAS Int.* **2006**, *4*, e22.
16. Stone, R. Pregnant women and substance use: Fear, stigma and barriers to care. *Health Justice* **2015**, *3*, 2. [CrossRef]
17. Corse, S.; Smith, M. Reducing substance abuse during pregnancy: Discriminating among levels of response in a prenatal setting. *J. Subst. Abus. Treat.* **1998**, *15*, 457–467. [CrossRef]
18. Poole, N.; Isaac, B. *Apprehensions: Barriers to Treatment for Substance-Using Mothers*; British Columbia Centre of Excellence for Women's Health: Vancouver, BC, Canada, 2001; Available online: http://bccewh.bc.ca/wp-content/uploads/2012/05/2001_Apprehensions-Barriers-to-Treatment-for-Substance-Using-Mothers.pdf (accessed on 8 September 2019).
19. Nathoo, T.; Poole, N.; Bryans, M.; Dechief, L.; Hardeman, S.; Marcellus, L.; Poag, E.; Taylor, M. Voices from the community: Developing effective community programs to support pregnant and early parenting women who use alcohol and other substances. *First Peoples Child Fam. Rev.* **2013**, *8*, 93–107.
20. Rutman, D.; Callahan, M.; Lundquist, A.; Jackson, S.; Field, B. *Substance Use and Pregnancy: Conceiving Women in the Policy-making Process*; Status of Women Canada: Ottawa, ON, Canada, 2000.
21. Gopman, S. Prenatal and postpartum care of women with substance use disorders. *Obstet. Gynecol. Clin. N. Am.* **2014**, *41*, 213–228. [CrossRef] [PubMed]
22. Network Action Team on FASD Prevention from a Women's Health Determinants Perspective. Consensus on 10 Fundamental Components of FASD Prevention from a Women's Health Determinants Perspective. 2010. Available online: http://bccewh.bc.ca/2014/02/10-fundamental-components-of-fasd-prevention-from-a-womens-health-determinants-perspective/ (accessed on 8 September 2019).
23. Andrews, N.; Motz, M.; Pepler, D.; Jeong, J.; Khoury, J. Engaging mothers with substance use issues and their children in early intervention: Understanding use of service and outcomes. *Child Abus. Negl.* **2018**, *83*, 10–20. [CrossRef] [PubMed]
24. Rutman, D. Voices of women living with FASD: Perspectives on promising approaches in substance use treatment, programs and care. *First Peoples Child Fam. Rev.* **2013**, *8*, 107–121.
25. Nota Bene Consulting Group. *HerWay Home Final Evaluation Report*; Nota Bene Consulting Group: Victoria, BC, Canada, 2017.
26. Kelty Mental Health Resource Centre. Addiction and Substance Use. Available online: http://keltymentalhealth.ca/substance-use/addiction-substance-use-overview (accessed on 8 September 2019).

27. Atlantic Canada Council on Addiction. Problematic Substance Use That Impacts the Workplace. Available online: http://www.health.gov.nl.ca/health/publications/addiction_substance_abuse_workplace_toolkit.pdf (accessed on 8 September 2019).
28. Poole, N. *Fetal Alcohol Spectrum Disorder (FASD) Prevention: Canadian Perspectives*; Public Health Agency of Canada: Ottawa, ON, Canada, 2008.
29. Rutman, D.; Hubberstey, C. National evaluation of Canadian multi-service FASD prevention programs: Interim findings from the Co-Creating Evidence' study. *Int. J. Environ. Res. Public Health* **2019**, *16*, 1767. [CrossRef] [PubMed]
30. Berghold, J.; Thomas, S. Participatory research methods: A methodological approach in motion. *Qual. Soc. Res.* **2012**, *13*, 30.
31. Cousins, J.; Whitmore, E.; Shulha, L.K.; Al Hudib, H.L.; Gilbert, N. Principles to Guide Collaborative Approaches to Evaluation. Canadian Evaluation Society, 2015. Available online: https://evaluationcanada.ca/sites/default/files/20170131_caebrochure_en.pdf (accessed on 8 September 2019).
32. Shulha, L.; Whitmore, E.; Cousins, J.B.; Bilbert, N.; Al Hudib, H. Introducing evidence-based principles to guide collaborative approaches to evaluation: Results of an empirical process. *Am. J. Eval.* **2016**, *37*, 193–217. [CrossRef]
33. Davies, R.; Dart, J. *The 'Most Significant Change' (MSC) Technique: A Guide to Its Use*; CARE International: London, UK, 2005; Available online: https://www.mande.co.uk/wp-content/uploads/2005/MSCGuide.pdf (accessed on 8 September 2019).
34. Fallot, R.; Harris, M. *Creating Cultures of Trauma-Informed Care (CCTIC): A Self-Assessment and Planning Protocol*; Community Connections: Washington, DC, USA, 2009; Available online: https://www.theannainstitute.org/CCTICSELFASSPP.pdf (accessed on 8 September 2019).
35. Braun, V.; Clarke, V. Using thematic analysis in psychology. *Qual. Res. Psychol.* **2006**, *3*, 77–101. [CrossRef]
36. Thorne, S. Data analysis in qualitative research. *Evid. Based Nurs.* **2000**, *3*, 68–70. [CrossRef]
37. Revai, T.; Sheway team. Sharing the Journey: The Sheway Model of Care. 2015. Available online: http://sheway.vcn.bc.ca/files/2016/01/Sharing-the-Journey.pdf (accessed on 8 September 2019).
38. Niccols, A.; Milligan, K.; Sword, W.; Thabane, L.; Henderson, J.; Smith, A. Integrated programs for mothers with substance abuse issues: A systematic review of studies reporting on parenting outcomes. *Harm Reduct. J.* **2012**, *9*, 14. [CrossRef] [PubMed]
39. Sword, W.; Jack, S.; Niccols, A.; Milligan, K.; Henderson, J.; Thabane, L. Integrated programs for women with substance use issues and their children: A qualitative meta-synthesis of processes and outcomes. *Harm Reduct. J.* **2009**, *9*, 32. [CrossRef] [PubMed]
40. Schmidt, R.; Poole, N.; Greaves, L.; Hemsing, N. *New Terrain: Tools to Integrate Trauma and Gender Informed Responses into Substance Use Practice and Policy*; Centre of Excellence for Women's Health: Vancouver, BC, Canada, 2018. [CrossRef]
41. Women's Services Strategy Group. *Best Practices in Action: Guidelines and Criteria for Women's Substance Abuse Treatment Services*; (n.d.).; Jean Tweed Centre: Toronto, ON, Canada, 2006; Available online: http://jeantweed.com/wp-content/themes/JTC/pdfs/Best%20Practice-English.pdf (accessed on 8 September 2019).
42. Marcellus, L. A grounded theory of mothering in the early years for women recovering from substance use. *J. Fam. Nurs.* **2017**, *23*, 341–365. [CrossRef]
43. Substance Abuse and Mental Health Services Administration (SAMHSA). *Substance Abuse Treatment: Addressing the Specific Needs of Women*; Treatment Improvement Protocol (TIP) Series, No. 51; SAMHSA: Rockville, MD, USA, 2009. Available online: https://www.ncbi.nlm.nih.gov/books/NBK83252/ (accessed on 8 September 2019).

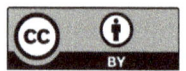

© 2019 by the authors. Licensee MDPI, Basel, Switzerland. This article is an open access article distributed under the terms and conditions of the Creative Commons Attribution (CC BY) license (http://creativecommons.org/licenses/by/4.0/).

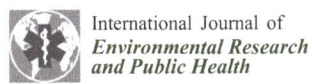

Review

Technology-Based Substance Use Interventions: Opportunities for Gender-Transformative Health Promotion

Julie Stinson [1,*], Lindsay Wolfson [1,2] and Nancy Poole [1]

1. Centre of Excellence for Women's Health, D404-4500 Oak St, Vancouver, BC V6H 3N1, Canada; lindsay.wolfson@gmail.com (L.W.); npoole@cw.bc.ca (N.P.)
2. Canada FASD Research Network, PO Box 11364, Vancouver, BC V5R 0A4, Canada
* Correspondence: juliestinson7@gmail.com

Received: 20 December 2019; Accepted: 4 February 2020; Published: 5 February 2020

Abstract: Drawing on data from a scoping review on sex, gender and substance use, this narrative review explores the use of gender-informed and technology-based approaches in substance use prevention and health promotion interventions. With an ever-changing landscape of new technological developments, an understanding of how technology-based interventions can address sex, gender, and intersecting equity considerations related to substance use is warranted. Current technology-based approaches to substance use prevention and health promotion are described and assessed for gender-specific and gender transformative outcomes, and limitations are discussed related to inclusivity, access, confidentiality, and a dearth of research on technological approaches that integrate gender-based analysis. A call for action designed to advance technology-based health promotion, prevention and brief interventions that address gender equity simultaneously with substance use is proposed.

Keywords: gender; technology; gender transformative; health promotion; substance use; SGBA+; substance use prevention

1. Introduction

Historically, substance use prevention and treatment interventions have employed directive, gender-blind and abstinence-oriented approaches [1–7]. However, research from the substance use field has demonstrated the importance of sex and gender considerations in substance use responses including prevention and treatment interventions [8–11]. The gendered factors, influences, and differences as to how individuals respond to substance use prevention and cessation cannot be ignored. For example, concerns surrounding weight gain have been found more often to be a reason for avoiding smoking cessation for women compared to men [12]. Other gender-mediated reasons for smoking cessation have demonstrated that men are more likely to quit as a result of tobacco policy, and that social unacceptability is more closely associated with quitting among women [13]. Such gender-informed influences are integral to understanding how to approach substance use health promotion, prevention and brief intervention efforts.

In understanding gender-responsive approaches, it is important to consider the range in which gender inclusions and considerations can impact gender equity outcomes. See Figure 1. Gender-blind programs ignore gender norms, roles and relations and may therefore reinforce gender-based discrimination, biases and stereotypes. Gender-specific programs acknowledge gender norms, consider women's and men's specific needs and act to accommodate these needs to some degree. Gender-transformative approaches focus on the dual goals of improving health, social or economic status as well as gender equity [14]. The benefits of gender-transformative approaches have been demonstrated globally, addressing gender norms, stereotypes or relations as a route to improved health outcomes when undertaking prevention and health promotion efforts [14–17]. Future programs and studies can be created or evaluated using sex and gender-based analysis plus (SGBA+) to determine their implementation (or lack of) of a gender-transformative approach or to analyze the effectiveness of programs for promoting inclusivity. This form of analysis provides an important perspective to evaluating programs and evidence for potential gaps in relation to sex, gender and intersectional equity [18].

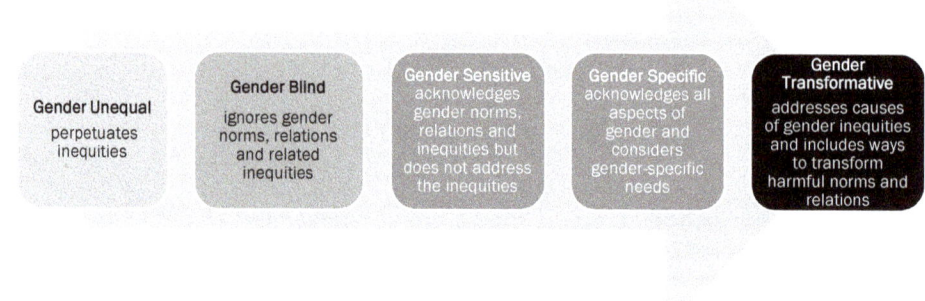

Figure 1. Gender Integration Continuum, reproduced adaptation with permission from Greaves, L., Pederson, A., Poole, N., Making it Better: Gender Transformative Health Promotion; published by Women's Press, 2014 [14] (p. 22).

Simultaneous to the growing commitment to SGBA+, there has been an increased interest in incorporating technology into substance use prevention and treatment. Technology has become more interwoven into day-to-day life and into the health care sector with the advancements of technology and Internet-based care (eHealth). In one regard, technology provides a significant opportunity for prevention and health promotion interventions to reach large audiences. Technology has more recently been used to connect with adolescents and young adults but also older generations and individuals of all genders, with a focus on health promoting and harm reducing decision making. However, gaps and cautions remain as to the reach and inclusivity of these technological approaches to date. Given the dearth of research beyond web-based tobacco and alcohol interventions [19], an understanding of the scope of technological approaches to prevention and health promotion for all substances is warranted. Further, it is timely to examine how sex and gender play into decision making surrounding substance use prevention efforts and how gender-informed harm reduction-oriented approaches might be further or more effectively achieved in technology-based interventions. This article will provide an examination of how technology-based substance use prevention approaches are integrating health promotion and harm reduction, and how sex, gender and intersecting factors of age, race, and socioeconomic status related to substance use are, or are not, being achieved in these efforts. It will further provide recommendations for the direction of future research on technology-based substance use prevention and health promotion approaches.

2. Methods

This narrative review is based on a subset of findings from a scoping review conducted on the integration of sex and gender in research on opioids, alcohol, tobacco and cannabis prevalence and patterns of use, health effects, and prevention, treatment and harm reduction interventions and outcomes. The four substances were chosen for having differential sex and gender impacts, and for their current critical concern in Canada.

The scoping review was based on two broad questions:

(1) How do sex- and gender-related factors impact: (a) patterns of use; (b) health effects of; and (c) prevention/treatment or harm reduction outcomes for opioid, alcohol, tobacco/nicotine and cannabis use?
(2) What harm reduction, health promotion/prevention and treatment interventions and programs are available that include sex, gender and gender-transformative elements and how effective are these in addressing opioid, alcohol, tobacco/ nicotine and cannabis use?

The scoping review methodology has been described in full in Hemsing et al. [20]. Over five thousand (5030) papers were included in the original review, which excluded research specific to pregnant women who use substances, but was inclusive of women, girls, men, boys, trans and gender diverse people of all other ages and demographics. The included papers were categorized by substance (alcohol, tobacco, opioid, and cannabis and multiple substances/substance use generally) as well as by research focus (i.e., prevalence, health effects and biological responses, and prevention and intervention type) in an Endnote library. This narrative review draws upon articles from the scoping review findings. The authors reviewed articles categorized in the prevention (64 articles), harm reduction (50 articles), and brief intervention (76 articles) fields for relevance and did additional key word searches in the full library using the terms: Tech(nology) (8 articles), Health Promotion (8 articles), Web(site) (15 articles), Internet (8 articles), App(s) (3 articles), Computer(s) (11 articles), Mobile (4 articles), Text Message (2 articles), (Tele)Phone (9 articles), Online (11 articles), Social Media (5 articles), Digital (3 articles), Fitbit (1) and Video(s) (3 articles). Due to the prevalence of articles that focused on technology-based brief interventions, an additional targeted search was done for the studies categorized as having a research focus on brief interventions, which identified 17 papers. 52 articles from the combined search were excluded for being duplicate values.

A total of 239 articles were analyzed for inclusion, 54 meet the criteria of examining sex and/or gender in technology-based substance use prevention approaches and outcomes, and 45 were included in this article. Of these articles, 11 were computer-based, 12 were phone-based, 19 were web-based and 3 examined multiple technological mediums. Since 'technology-based interventions' was not a specific category in the original scoping review, a narrative review approach was used for this article in order to examine all of the literature more broadly related to this topic.

3. Technology-Based Substance Use Prevention and Health Promotion Approaches

There were multiple ways in which substance use prevention and health promotion approaches incorporated gender and technology in the literature including brief web-based interventions (16 articles), targeted web-based messaging (three articles), social media, websites and virtual communities (eight articles), computer games (three articles), text messaging (three articles), mobile phone applications (apps) (seven articles) and telephone interventions (five articles). Of the 45 included articles, 11 reported on patterns and prevalence of use and 34 evaluated the efficacy of technology-based interventions. The interventions ranged from gender blind to gender transformative. Of the nine articles that described gender-transformative approaches, only five unique interventions were reported—all of which were conducted with only girls or women. Two of these interventions were brief web-based interventions, two were mobile phone apps, and one was a telephone-delivered intervention.

As a result of the dearth of gender-transformative interventions exemplified in the literature, the review findings have been categorized by technological approach in order to examine the literature more broadly and provide a critical analysis of how gender has been considered across all technology-based platforms (see Table S1 for details). The following section will examine gender inclusion by technological medium and how these platforms have incorporated variances of harm reduction, health promotion, prevention, and treatment.

4. Gender Considerations in Technology-Based Substance Use Interventions

4.1. Brief Web-Based Interventions

Brief web-based interventions represented web/computer-based programs often in module format that embodied an education and/or health promotion approach to substance use harm reduction. They were the most advanced in taking a gender-informed approach, though studies were often only conducted with single gender groups of girls or women. For example, one gender-transformative web-based brief intervention focused on girls (12–13 years old) and the relationship between mothers and daughters as a mechanism for health promotion and substance use prevention [21], promoted social skills (self-efficacy, communication) and decision making as ways of coping with stress, managing substance use, questioning peer norms, and understanding media influences [22]. This home-based module program was conducted on the internet or with a CD-ROM on gender-specific substance use prevention topics guided by family interaction theory, completed by mother–daughter dyads. Dyads were advised to complete one 45 min session/week [23]. Results showed stronger communication and closeness between the mother and daughter, stronger substance use refusal skills for girls, and improved parental monitoring and rule setting in regards to substance use [21,22,24]. Girls also showed improved conflict management, improved problem-solving skills, and reduced stress [21,24]. One of the most significant differences was the change in normative beliefs among the girls, and reduced substance use overall [24]. The results remained constant at one- and two-year follow ups, with decreased substance use and intention to use among girls who were involved in the program, as well as lower weekly alcohol consumption among mothers at two-year follow-up [24,25].

This program was tested with a variety of populations of mothers and daughters. When tested with girls aged 10 to 12 and their mothers who reside in public housing, similar positive results were seen, with mother–daughter communication and closeness, reduced stress, and stronger refusal skills reported by girls at 5 month follow up [21]. Similarly, with a population of Hispanic and African American girls aged 10 to 13 and their mothers, the intervention resulted in overall increased protective factors and reduced risk factors in connection to communication, knowledge and refusal skills. It also resulted in lowered girls' alcohol use and intention to use in the future for all substances [23]. When conducted with a population of Asian-American adolescent girls, results showed reduced depressed mood and reduced substance use/intention to use in the future [26]. Overall, this program, based in attachment and nurturing parental relationships as a means of promoting healthy behaviour, showed both change in behaviour and beliefs, as opposed to change in beliefs only. This web-based model also enables girls to engage with the program at their own pace and in their location of choice [22]. A similar gender-specific intervention, called RealTeen, that involved 13- and 14-year-old girls, rather than the mother–daughter dyad, also reported lower rates of substance use among girls, healthier normative beliefs, and stronger self-efficacy as they relate to substance use [27].

Other brief web-based interventions designed to reach and engage women often combined interventions on substance use with other gender-based health concerns such as sexual or relational violence [28,29]. For example, Gilmore et al. examined the impact of a combined brief web-based substance use intervention and sexual assault risk reduction intervention for college women [29,30]. The authors found that offering a dual intervention provided college-aged women with a comprehensive set of skills, resources and protective behavioural strategies to both reduce heavy episodic drinking and risk of sexual violence [29,30]. Another gender-transformative program, 'BSAFER' (Brief Intervention for Substance Use and Partner Abuse for Females in the Emergency Room), was designed for women who had accessed the emergency department for substance misuse and intimate partner violence. This brief web-based intervention was conducted on a tablet during an emergency department visit and included goal-setting questions and informational videos. The intervention resulted in decreased weekly substance use [28]. However, despite favourable results in reduced heavy drinking, the authors noted that the effectiveness of the program may be circumstantial to women with higher risk severity for sexual assault and intimate partner violence [28].

There were gender-sensitive interventions that reported gender differences in the uptake of brief web-based interventions. For example, in one study Hispanic men tended to respond more favourably to web-based brief interventions, compared to Hispanic women, who preferred in-person brief interventions [31]. Another study, focused on drinking self-assessment, found that the intervention appealed more to women, despite no significant differences in drinking outcomes between men and women (the intervention resulted in reduced consumption and reduced consequences from drinking for men and women) [32].

Many studies did not report on tailored gender-specific approaches, rather they reported on the gender differences in responsiveness to brief web-based interventions that were gender blind in design. However, the brief interventions described show positive results in reducing substance use and related health concerns for women and girls, when they intentionally address key gendered influences on substance use or protective factors known to be specifically helpful for girls/women.

Brief web-based interventions with personalized normative feedback have been able to address misperceptions about substance use norms by bringing in self-reflection, connecting an individual's harmful substance use to 'atypical' as opposed to 'normative' beliefs [33,34]. This method has resulted in reduced alcohol consumption, and changes in perceived norms, for both men and women, though with varying results when integrating gender-specific feedback [33,35]. Lewis et al. found that gender-specific normative feedback was effective for women who identified more strongly with their gender [35]. This finding demonstrates that perceived gender norms are a mediating factor for how much women drink, and that gender-specific programming works for women. These programs provide evidence that gender identity is a determining factor of the success of brief web-based interventions for substance use, which further evidences the need for gender-transformative programming. However, more work is warranted to demonstrate the efficacy of web-based normative feedback for men and gender-diverse individuals.

4.2. Virtual Communities, Social Media and Targeted Web-Based Messaging

Other computer-based interventions in the literature included the use of websites, virtual communities, and social media in substance use interventions. Websites dedicated to substance use prevention—most commonly smoking cessation—and/or health promotion were not as commonly researched or evaluated. Those included in the review appeared to be out of date for the target demographic's preferred technological delivery modality or they reinforced gender-stereotypes as opposed to being gender transformative [36]. Virtual communities and social media interventions were comparatively gender-informed [37,38].

Virtual communities primarily included chat forums as peer-support models (commonly located on prevention and harm reduction websites). Virtual communities and social networking chat fora have been correlated with increased alcohol use; a finding stronger among girls compared to boys [39] demonstrating that girls may be more susceptible to engage in harmful drinking via online pressures. This gender difference is especially present among adolescents at high risk who lack healthy coping strategies [39].

Social media approaches involved the creation of pages or purchased advertising space on social media platforms to relay prevention and health promotion messages, such as the health benefits incorporated with abstaining from smoking [38,40]. Targeted web-based messaging used similar approaches to social media campaigns but expanded beyond social media platforms to include all web-based platforms [41–43]. Both social media platforms and targeted web-based messaging have often been used as opportunities for marketers to promote alcohol use, which has resulted in increased substance use particularly among young people [39,44]. However, when used as a medium for prevention and health promotion messaging, these mediums have also been proven to increase smoking cessation and awareness of health effects of smoking and secondhand smoke, including its connections to breast cancer for both boys and girls [37,38,40–42]. Richardson et al. examined gender- and culture-specific web-based messages surrounding tobacco smoke and breast cancer. They found that Indigenous boys and girls involved the study were more likely to agree that secondhand smoke increased risks of breast cancer, compared to a control group that was presented a gender-neutral visual messages [41,42]. Participants also spent significantly more time viewing the messages and girls who received the gender- and culture-specific intervention were 52% more likely to request additional information about secondhand smoke and breast cancer, compared to those in the control group [41]. Though knowledge increased, messaging did not change smoking status, intention to try smoking, or intention to avoid second hand smoke [42].

4.3. Computer Game Programs

Computer game interventions used simulation to increase understanding of the effects of substance use, refusal skills, or changing patterns and behaviours [45,46]. Few computer game programs integrated gender considerations in design, delivery or specific audience to be reached. One game entitled Guardian Angel, though gender blind in design, was tested on male veterans to encourage practice of relapse prevention skills using simulation. Participants would make daily decisions to support the recovery of a simulated character, designed to address coping skills and high-risk environments. The findings demonstrated reductions in binge drinking and higher self-efficacy [45]. Another game, Game On: Know Alcohol (GO:KA), combined social marketing and education, alternating game and knowledge-based modules focused on a harm reduction approach. GO:KA demonstrated one of the more successful interventions, that effected behavioural change as opposed to an attitude change only [43]. However, while GO:KA did show attitude changes for boys and girls, behaviour changes and reductions in alcohol use/intended alcohol use were only evident for girls, and the intervention design was not gender informed [43]. Other studies have also shown education-based programs to be particularly effective in changing girls' substance use behaviours [43,47,48], but not boys. These gender differences in behavioural change could be connected to evidence suggesting that education-based programs need to be repeated in more long-term settings to be effective [43,47,48].

4.4. Mobile Health Applications (mHealth Apps)

Mobile health apps were more commonly described in the literature as traditional 'mHealth' approaches, where an application on a smartphone monitors certain activity and provides alerts based on behaviours. Much like step trackers or heart rate monitoring apps, the mobile apps focused on substance use behaviours, such as alcohol frequency or drinks consumed [49]. MHealth apps provide some of the leading examples of technological innovation, including in their ability to engage individuals in substance use prevention and health promotion [49]. However, the literature has described the functionality, technical issues, and security and privacy of the apps as key barriers and concerns to programmatic success [49,50]. In regards to gender-informed approaches in intervention design, programs have ranged from gender blind to gender transformative, with some reporting gendered differences to uptake and success.

The gender-transformative program See Me Smoke-Free addresses smoking, diet and physical activity among women who smoke. Findings showed significant increases in healthy eating and physical activity, as well as higher rates of smoking cessation [51]. However, for men, similar to other technology-based programming, mobile health apps did not appear to be as successful. For example, the Swedish app *Promillekoll* created to reduce heavy episodic drinking through awareness by allowing users to test blood alcohol content levels showed men increasing drinking frequency while using this app, which was not the case for women [19]. This may have been a result of the program design being gender blind or, by comparison, the increased use and interest by women in using technology for substance use interventions [52,53].

Apps in the form of wearable tech, such as with a Fitbit, can also provide health promotion and support for transitional recovery as people leave intensive inpatient treatment. Abrantes et al. tested a gender-transformative lifestyle activity program among women with depression involved in inpatient treatment for alcohol. In-person physical activity counseling during inpatient treatment, combined with a Fitbit to monitor a step-counting goal, resulted in 44% of women abstaining from alcohol during the 3 month program. The authors suggested testing the usefulness of this health promotion intervention with women as they transition from treatment to community [54].

4.5. Text Message

Text message programs [55–57] used short message service (SMS) to send harm reduction messages related to substance use to participants. While some text-based programs were person-assisted, where an in-person brief intervention was supplemented with two-way text message goal planning, others were more directed by technology, with participants receiving pre-programmed messages on personal control and behavioural change [55,56]. The text message programs primarily focused on brief alcohol interventions for socioeconomically disadvantaged men or for men and women on college and university campuses [56,57]. In the studies with men who were socioeconomically marginalized, the men in the intervention group tended to engage at high levels with the program and appeared to be more comfortable in regards to divulging sensitive personal information about their relationships and experiences with harmful drinking with this format compared to others [55,56]. In the mixed-gender campus study, setting drinking-limit goals via SMS were found to promote a decrease in drinking particularly for men in comparison to women [57]. Though the intervention for socioeconomically disadvantaged men describes some program adaptation to intersectional context in regards to topics and language, it lacked detailed solutions to inequities and harmful norms, falling more in line with a gender-sensitive approach. The campus-based intervention could be considered gender blind, lacking acknowledgement of any gender considerations in programming. This was a common occurrence in the literature, whereby gender was not considered in the intervention design or was not explained in the study findings beyond the gender disaggregation.

4.6. Telephone-Delivered Interventions

Telephone-delivered interventions that were gender informed were most commonly reported for women as alcohol [58,59] and tobacco [12,60] cessation interventions. Phone-delivered interventions, including quitlines, have shown some promising results in connection to women over the age of fifty, specifically for alcohol reduction; however, telephone-delivered interventions included in the review rarely used a sample other than women, and when they did the intervention was gender blind [58,59,61]. One qualitative study examining binge drinking, depression and Post Traumatic Stress Disorder (PTSD) among women veterans found the women showed high acceptability to using phone-based care for health monitoring, feedback, and counseling [58]. This may be because of the culture and stigma surrounding substance use and gender [61]. For example, Kim et al. describe the reluctancy of women of Korean ethnicity to pursue in-person smoking cessation treatment due to the stigma attached to women who smoke, and how telephone and online programs that can be accessed privately in their homes are preferred. In this study, the younger women preferred a videoconferencing intervention over a phone based model [61].

Phone-delivered interventions may be preferred among women of older generations due to their longer lifetime experience with this mode of technology, compared to newer forms such as mobile health apps. The longer length of the phone-delivered interventions may be too time consuming for younger women who have grown up with the internet and fast-paced technology all their lives [58]. Keeping with the pace of technology may also be a reason why phone-delivered interventions did not present as commonly used methods. However, considerations should be made to ensure that individuals who find phone-delivered interventions to be most effective can still be reached.

5. Future Directions for Gender Integration in Technology-Based Substance Use Interventions

5.1. Gender-Transformative Approaches

How gendered approaches have been integrated into substance use prevention and harm reduction efforts can be seen in the light of the gender response continuum—ranging from gender blind, to gender sensitive/specific, to gender transformative [14] whereby gender is ignored, accommodated to lesser or greater degree or transformed through attention to gender equity. Although progress has been made, particularly with girls in regards to gender-informed technology-based substance use programming [48], some programs have continued to reinforce negative gender stereotypes, such as focusing on heteronormative attractiveness as a reason for reducing consumption or positing sexual assault reduction as women's and girls' responsibility, as opposed to promoting health and critical thinking [27,36]. Although the effectiveness of programs in relation to the gendered outcomes achieved was explored in many of the studies, there continues to be a lack of programming that is tailored to address specific gendered influences on substance use, or that attempts to address some aspects of gender equity while also addressing substance use prevention or harm reduction (i.e., that is gender transformative). Due to its reach and low-cost in comparison to other substance use interventions, the online environment provides a key location for offering gender-transformative interventions.

5.2. Gender and Intersecting Equity Considerations

A lack of a gender-informed or transformative approach is paired with a lack of attention to other aspects of equity. These would be mitigated if SGBA+ had been applied in the design and delivery of programming. For example, although over 70% of young women look to the internet for health and substance use related prevention or cessation information, women of colour are less likely to seek out this information online [36,62]. Other findings suggest that, regardless of age, Caucasian men and women were more likely to use a smoking cessation website compared to men and women of colour, with the exception of a virtual community forum used by Hispanic young adult men and women [36].

The need for attention to interventions that move beyond the gender binary as well as consider sexual orientation and culture in the intervention design and implementation is also important as the prevalence of smoking among LGBTQ+ identified youth and young adults is significantly higher than among youth and young adults who identify as heterosexual [50]. The larger scoping review, from which the literature for this review was derived was inclusive of women, girls, men, boys, trans and gender diverse people of all ages and demographics, excluding pregnant women. However, there were no technology-based substance use interventions that were inclusive of or targeted to trans and gender diverse people, beyond one study that examined LGBTQ+ youth and young adults' perceptions of a culturally tailored mHealth app for smoking cessation. In this study by Baskerville et al., LGBTQ+ identified youth and young adults have expressed that substance use mobile health apps that are culturally-tailored and recognize their specific needs are highly valued when seeking out substance use prevention programming [50]. This has also been reflected in studies that have incorporated elements of Indigenous culture into interventions with Indigenous youth, which have seen that the boys and girls prefer this type of format, are more inclined to receive the messaging, and girls in particular are more inclined to want to learn more [41,42,47].

5.3. Gender, Inclusivity and Access

Technology-based interventions must consider gender, inclusivity and access to technology. Often individuals have differing and inequitable access to technology; however, participants in technology assisted programming are required to have their own access to a computer, the Internet, or a phone with data. In one study, although 80% of participants said they would be interested in participating in a mobile health treatment intervention, there was differing interest by gender—with women being more interested than men—and only 50% of interested participants indeed had access to data on their cellphones [52].

Age must also be considered. Age has shown to be a factor not only with technology use in general, but for how and what it is used for. For example, one study found that younger adults (aged 18–34) visited a smoking cessation website significantly less often than adults over 34 years old, viewed fewer pages, and were less likely to use the virtual community page [36]. Consistent with other research findings, young men in particular were less likely to use the website compared to young women [36]. This could be related to how younger generations, who have grown up on faster and more immediate technology-based resources, have considerably different knowledge and methods of using technology, use it at a different pace, and use considerably different platforms. These reflections of age, gender, and how they affect use should be taken into account when designing and implementing technology-based substance use prevention and health promotion initiatives.

5.4. Gender, Technological Interventions and Confidentiality

There is concern surrounding the collection of data by mobile technology. Studies have shown that both men and women have expressed concerns pertaining to how their private information will be used or communicated outside of face-to-face interactions [50,53,58]. These concerns are reflected in how individuals engage with technology-based programs. For example, female veterans have expressed reluctance to share their information, viewing the phone-delivered programming as 'too impersonal' [58] while younger men, appear to be more inclined to share their information [63]. Participants have expressed that having print and web-based versions of programs would help mitigate these concerns [50]. However, it has also been reported that both adolescent girls and boys are more comfortable with filling out web based surveys of alcohol and tobacco use, when compared to filling out printed surveys, reporting higher and possibly more accurate rates of use [63]. For example, girls have reported a younger age of drinking onset when filing out a web-based survey when compared to a printed version. This may reflect the differing concerns of confidentiality and privacy as they relate to age, gender, and access to technology.

5.5. Furthering the Efficacy of Gender and Technology-Based Interventions

A re-occurring challenge of many substance use prevention and health promotion programs was the challenge of not only shifting attitudes, but behaviours as well. Some studies have reported behavioural changes. For example, studies have shown that education-based programs, which are central to a health promotion approach, have resulted in significant changes in girls' behaviours towards substance use [47,48]. However, for boys and men, reported behavioural change was often less common than it was for girls and women [33,35,43]. A central issue to changing behaviours has been connected to the need for more longer term programs—an issue that some technology-based programs may find solutions to through the ability to provide wide-reaching interventions on relatively low cost platforms [43].

6. Limitations

The purpose of this review was to provide an examination of how technology-based substance use prevention approaches have integrated gender-informed health promotion and harm reduction, and how sex, gender and intersecting factors of age, race, and socioeconomic status related to substance use are, or are not, being achieved in these efforts. To identify the breadth of the literature on this topic, provide descriptive detail of the types of interventions that have been conducted, and to identify patterns and prevalence of use, a narrative review was conducted. Only four unique gender-transformative interventions were examined in the quantitative studies available, all of which included samples of only girls and/or women. Quantitative studies also varied in inclusion or measures of effect sizes, and thus there was an overall lack of data availability and consistency to conduct a meta-analysis that examined gender-comparative effects of gender-informed interventions. Future research in this field would benefit from more quantitative research that includes gender comparators, including trans and gender diverse individuals. This would also facilitate meta-analyses of the effects of gender-transformative interventions.

7. Conclusions

There has been a substantial amount of research conducted on the effects that sex and gender factors have on substance use and technological approaches to substance use prevention and health promotion. Compared to gender—and culturally-blind programming, the studies gathered and examined, demonstrated that gender—and culturally-tailored programming is more desired and effective at raising awareness and demonstrating measurable attitudinal and behavioural change related to substance use. And yet, few programs have incorporated sex and gender evidence into their program design, delivery and specific audiences to be reached, and fewer have analyzed the effectiveness of programs developed specifically through a SGBA+ lens. It is evident that there is still a considerable way to go to link the two and further incorporate sex, gender, and gender-transformative approaches in technology-based substance use prevention and health promotion efforts. Future research on this topic would benefit from additional quantitative analyses that incorporate gender comparisons to further identify effective gender-informed and transformative approaches.

The research has shown that compared to men, women tend to prefer technology-based substance use interventions, show higher substance use rates, and find these interventions more helpful. Generally, both men and women prefer technology-based interventions versus non technology-based interventions. Further, gender-specific and culturally-specific substance use programming is a preferential method for boys and girls. Programs that are educational and provide opportunities for self-reflection using personalized normative feedback and/or critical thinking are particularly successful. This research review demonstrates that health promotion-based technological approaches have some of the largest effects on women and girls—particularly in studies that focused on girls and reducing alcohol use and related harms. There is significant opportunity to partner with young men and women, and with technological platform designers, to increase the use, reach and effectiveness of health promotion, substance use prevention and brief interventions that take gender into account and advance gender equity.

With the advancements of technology-based health promotion and prevention efforts, there is a great opportunity to modify technological approaches to respond to the evidenced gaps, echoing the movement and progress of global eHealth and mHealth initiatives. These interventions have the opportunity to respond to shifts in technological engagement, reaching across generations with the goal and ability of streamlining the efficiency of substance use prevention and harm reduction, while keeping in mind how gender-transformative interventions can lead to successful health outcomes.

Supplementary Materials: The following are available online at http://www.mdpi.com/1660-4601/17/3/992/s1, Table S1: Included Studies.

Author Contributions: Conceptualization, J.S. and N.P.; Methodology, J.S.; Formal Analysis, J.S.; Data Curation, J.S. and L.W.; Writing—Original Draft Preparation, J.S.; Writing—Review and Editing, J.S., L.W., and N.P.; Visualization, J.S.; Supervision, N.P.; Funding Acquisition, N.P. All authors have read and agree to the published version of the manuscript.

Funding: This research was supported by the Canadian Institutes of Health Research (CIHR)—Institute of Gender and Health Team Grant #384548.

Conflicts of Interest: The authors declare no conflict of interest.

References

1. Longshore, D.; Ellickson, P.L.; McCaffrey, D.F.; St Clair, P.A. School-based drug prevention among at-risk adolescents: Effects of ALERT plus. *Health Educ. Behav.* **2007**, *34*, 651–668. [CrossRef] [PubMed]
2. Vigna-Taglianti, F.; Vadrucci, S.; Faggiano, F.; Burkhart, G.; Siliquini, R.; Galanti, M.R.; EU-Dap Study Group. Is universal prevention against youths' substance misuse really universal? Gender-specific effects

in the EU-Dap school-based prevention trial. *J. Epidemiol. Community Health* **2009**, *63*, 722–728. [CrossRef] [PubMed]
3. Putkonen, H.; Weizmann-Henelius, G.; Lindberg, N.; Rovamo, T.; Hakkanen-Nyholm, H. Gender differences in homicide offenders' criminal career, substance abuse and mental health care. A nationwide register-based study of Finnish homicide offenders 1995–2004. *Crim. Behav. Ment. Health* **2011**, *21*, 51–62. [CrossRef] [PubMed]
4. Degenhardt, L.; Gisev, N.; Trevena, J.; Larney, S.; Kimber, J.; Burns, L.; Shanahan, M.; Weatherburn, D. Engagement with the criminal justice system among opioid-dependent people: A retrospective cohort study. *Addiction* **2013**, *108*, 2152–2165. [CrossRef]
5. Valera, P.; Anderson, M.; Cook, S.H.; Wylie-Rosett, J.; Rucker, J.; Reid, A.E. The smoking behaviors and cancer-related disparities among urban middle aged and older men involved in the criminal justice system. *J. Cancer Educ.* **2015**, *30*, 86–93. [CrossRef]
6. Golder, S.; Logan, T.K. Violence, victimization, criminal justice involvement, and substance use among drug-involved men. *Violence Vict.* **2014**, *29*, 53–72. [CrossRef]
7. Hayatbakhsh, M.R.; Kinner, S.A.; Jamrozik, K.; Najman, J.M.; Mamun, A.A. Maternal partner criminality and cannabis use in young adulthood: Prospective study. *Aust. N. Z. J. Psychiatry* **2007**, *41*, 546–553. [CrossRef]
8. Minian, N.; Penner, J.; Voci, S.; Selby, P. Woman focused smoking cessation programming: A qualitative study. *BMC Womens Health* **2016**, *16*, 17. [CrossRef]
9. Greenfield, S.F.; Cummings, A.M.; Kuper, L.E.; Wigderson, S.B.; Koro-Ljungberg, M. A Qualitative Analysis of Women's Experiences in Single-Gender Versus Mixed-Gender Substance Abuse Group Therapy. *Subst. Use Misuse* **2013**, *48*, 750–760. [CrossRef]
10. D'Souza, D.C.; Cortes-Briones, J.A.; Ranganathan, M.; Thurnauer, H.; Creatura, G.; Surti, T.; Planeta, B.; Neumeister, A.; Pittman, B.; Normandin, M.D.; et al. Rapid Changes in Cannabinoid 1 Receptor Availability in Cannabis-Dependent Male Subjects After Abstinence From Cannabis. *Biol. Psychiatry Cogn. Neurosci. Neuroimaging* **2016**, *1*, 60–67. [CrossRef]
11. Reece, A.S.; Hulse, G.K. Elevation of the ACTH/cortisol ratio in female opioid dependent patients: A biomarker of aging and correlate of metabolic and immune activation. *Neuroendocrinol. Lett.* **2016**, *37*, 325–336. [PubMed]
12. Levine, M.D.; Bush, T.; Magnusson, B.; Cheng, Y.; Chen, X. Smoking-related weight concerns and obesity: Differences among normal weight, overweight, and obese smokers using a telephone tobacco quitline. *Nicotine Tob. Res.* **2013**, *15*, 1136–1140. [CrossRef] [PubMed]
13. Chow, C.K.; Corsi, D.J.; Gilmore, A.B.; Kruger, A.; Igumbor, E.; Chifamba, J.; Yang, W.; Wei, L.; Iqbal, R.; Mony, P.; et al. Tobacco control environment: Cross- sectional survey of policy implementation, social unacceptability, knowledge of tobacco health harms and relationship to quit ratio in 17 low-income, middle-income and high- income countries. *BMJ Open* **2017**, *7*. [CrossRef] [PubMed]
14. Greaves, L.; Pederson, A.; Poole, N. (Eds.) *Making It Better: Gender-Transformative Health Promotion*; Women's Press: Toronto, ON, Canada, 2014.
15. Barker, G.; Ricardo, C.; Nascimento, M. *Engaging Men and Boys in Changing Gender-Based Inequity in Health: Evidence from Programme Interventions*; World Health Organization: Geneva, Switzerland, 2007.
16. Hillenbrand, E.; Karim, N.; Mohanraj, P.; Wu, D. *Measuring Gender-Transformative Change: A Review of Literature and Promising Practices*; CARE USA. Atlanta, GA, USA, 2015.
17. Wilchins, R.; Gilmer, M. *Addressing Masculine Norms to Improve Life Outcomes for Young Black Men: Why We Still Can't Wait*; True Child: Washington, DC, USA, 2016.
18. Clow, B.; Pederson, A.; Haworth-Brockman, M.; Bernier, J. *Rising to the Challenge: Sex- and Gender-Based Analysis for Health Planning, Policy and Research in Canada*; Atlantic Centre of Excellence for Women's Health: Halifax, NS, Canada, 2009.
19. Gajecki, M.; Berman, A.H.; Sinadinovic, K.; Rosendahl, I.; Andersson, C. Mobile phone brief intervention applications for risky alcohol use among university students: A randomized controlled study. *Addict. Sci. Clin. Pract.* **2014**, *9*, 11. [CrossRef]
20. Hemsing, N.; Greaves, L. Gender norms, roles, and relations and cannabis-use patterns: A scoping review. *Int. J. Environ. Res. Public Health* **2020**, *17*, 3. [CrossRef]
21. Schwinn, T.M.; Schinke, S.; Fang, L.; Kandasamy, S. A web-based, health promotion program for adolescent girls and their mothers who. reside in public housing. *Addict. Behav.* **2014**, *39*, 757–760. [CrossRef]

22. Schinke, S.P.; Cole, K.C.; Fang, L. Gender-specific intervention to reduce underage drinking among early adolescent girls: A test of a computer-mediated, mother-daughter program. *J. Stud. Alcohol Drugs* **2009**, *70*, 70–77. [CrossRef]
23. Schinke, S.P.; Fang, L.; Cole, K.C.; Cohen-Cutler, S. Preventing Substance Use Among Black and Hispanic Adolescent Girls: Results From a Computer-Delivered, Mother-Daughter Intervention Approach. *Subst. Use Misuse* **2011**, *46*, 35–45. [CrossRef]
24. Schinke, S.P.; Fang, L.; Cole, K.C. Preventing substance use among adolescent girls: 1-year outcomes of a computerized, mother-daughter program. *Addict. Behav.* **2009**, *34*, 1060–1064. [CrossRef]
25. Schinke, S.P.; Fang, L.; Cole, K.C. Computer-delivered, parent-involvement intervention to prevent substance use among adolescent girls. *Prev. Med.* **2009**, *49*, 429–435. [CrossRef]
26. Fang, L.; Schinke, S.P.; Cole, K.C. Preventing substance use among early Asian-American adolescent girls: Initial evaluation of a web-based, mother-daughter program. *J. Adolesc. Health* **2010**, *47*, 529–532. [CrossRef]
27. Schwinn, T.M.; Schinke, S.P.; Di Noia, J. Preventing drug abuse among adolescent girls: Outcome data from an internet-based intervention. *Prev. Sci.* **2010**, *11*, 24–32. [CrossRef]
28. Choo, E.K.; Zlotnick, C.; Strong, D.R.; Squires, D.D.; Tape, C.; Mello, M.J. BSAFER: A Web-based intervention for drug use and intimate partner violence demonstrates feasibility and acceptability among women in the emergency department. *Subst. Abus.* **2016**, *37*, 441–449. [CrossRef]
29. Gilmore, A.K.; Lewis, M.A.; George, W.H. A randomized controlled trial targeting alcohol use and sexual assault risk among college women at high risk for victimization. *Behav. Res. Ther.* **2015**, *74*, 38–49. [CrossRef]
30. Gilmore, A.K.; Bountress, K.E. Reducing drinking to cope among heavy episodic drinking college women: Secondary outcomes of a web-based combined alcohol use and sexual assault risk reduction intervention. *Addict. Behav.* **2016**, *61*, 104–111. [CrossRef]
31. Gryczynski, J.; Carswell, S.B.; O'Grady, K.E.; Mitchell, S.G.; Schwartz, R.P. Gender and ethnic differences in primary care patients' response to computerized vs. in-person brief intervention for illicit drug misuse. *J. Subst. Abus. Treat.* **2018**, *84*, 50–56. [CrossRef]
32. Koski-Jannes, A.; Cunningham, J.A.; Tolonen, K.; Bothas, H. Internet-based self-assessment of drinking-3-month follow-up data. *Addict. Behav.* **2007**, *32*, 533–542. [CrossRef]
33. Lewis, M.A.; Neighbors, C.; Oster-Aaland, L.; Kirkeby, B.S.; Larimer, M.E. Indicated prevention for incoming freshmen: Personalized normative feedback and high-risk drinking. *Addict. Behav.* **2007**, *32*, 2495–2508. [CrossRef]
34. Thompson, K.; Burgess, J.; MacNevin, P.D. An Evaluation of e-CHECKUP TO GO in Canada: The Mediating Role of Changes in Social Norm Misperceptions. *Subst. Use Misuse* **2018**. [CrossRef]
35. Lewis, M.A.; Neighbors, C. Optimizing personalized normative feedback: The use of gender-specific referents. *J. Stud. Alcohol Drugs* **2007**, *68*, 228–237. [CrossRef]
36. Cantrell, J.; Ilakkuvan, V.; Graham, A.L.; Richardson, A.; Xiao, H.; Mermelstein, R.J.; Curry, S.J.; Sporer, A.K.; Vallone, D.M. Young Adult Utilization of a Smoking Cessation Website: An Observational Study Comparing Young and Older Adult Patterns of Use. *JMIR Res. Protoc.* **2016**, *5*, e142. [CrossRef]
37. Smith, A.D.; Smith, A.A. Gender perceptions of smoking and cessation via technology, incentives and virtual communities. *Int. J. Electron. Healthc.* **2011**, *6*, 1–33. [CrossRef] [PubMed]
38. Bottorff, J.L.; Struik, L.L.; Bissell, L.J.; Graham, R.; Stevens, J.; Richardson, C.G. A social media approach to inform youth about breast cancer and smoking: An exploratory descriptive study. *Coll. J. R. Coll. Nurs. Aust.* **2014**, *21*, 159–168. [CrossRef] [PubMed]
39. Larm, P.; Åslund, C.; Nilsson, K.W. The role of online social network chatting for alcohol use in adolescence: Testing three peer-related pathways in a Swedish population-based sample. *Comput. Hum. Behav.* **2017**, *71*, 284–290. [CrossRef]
40. Haines-Saah, R.J.; Kelly, M.T.; Oliffe, J.L.; Bottorff, J.L. Picture Me Smokefree: A qualitative study using social media and digital photography to engage young adults in tobacco reduction and cessation. *J. Med. Internet Res.* **2015**, *17*, e27. [CrossRef] [PubMed]
41. Richardson, C.G.; Struik, L.L.; Johnson, K.C.; Ratner, P.A.; Gotay, C.; Memetovic, J.; Okoli, C.T.; Bottorff, J.L. Initial impact of tailored web-based messages about cigarette smoke and breast cancer risk on boys' and girls' risk perceptions and information seeking: Randomized controlled trial. *JMIR Res. Protoc.* **2013**, *2*, e53. [CrossRef] [PubMed]

42. Schwartz, J.; Bottorff, J.L.; Ratner, P.A.; Gotay, C.; Johnson, K.C.; Memetovic, J.; Richardson, C.G. Effect of web-based messages on girls' knowledge and risk perceptions related to cigarette smoke and breast cancer: 6-month follow-up of a randomized controlled trial. *JMIR Res. Protoc.* **2014**, *3*, e53. [CrossRef] [PubMed]
43. Rundle-Thiele, S.; Russell-Bennett, R.; Leo, C.; Dietrich, T. Moderating teen drinking: Combining social marketing and education. *Health Educ.* **2013**, *113*, 392–406. [CrossRef]
44. Branley, D.B.; Covey, J. Is exposure to online content depicting risky behavior related to viewers' own risky behavior offline? *Comput. Hum. Behav.* **2017**, *75*, 283–287. [CrossRef]
45. Verduin, M.L.; LaRowe, S.D.; Myrick, H.; Cannon-Bowers, J.; Bowers, C. Computer simulation games as an adjunct for treatment in male veterans with alcohol use disorder. *J. Subst. Abus. Treat.* **2013**, *44*, 316–322. [CrossRef]
46. Wetter, D.W.; McClure, J.B.; Cofta-Woerpel, L.; Costello, T.J.; Reitzel, L.R.; Businelle, M.S.; Cinciripini, P.M. A Randomized Clinical Trial of a Palmtop Computer-Delivered Treatment for Smoking Relapse Prevention Among Women. *Psychol. Addict. Behav.* **2011**, *25*, 365–371. [CrossRef] [PubMed]
47. Bottorff, J.L.; Haines-Saah, R.; Oliffe, J.L.; Struik, L.L.; Bissell, L.J.L.; Richardson, C.P.; Gotay, C.; Johnson, K.C.; Hutchinson, P. Designing Tailored Messages about Smoking and Breast Cancer: A Focus Group Study with Youth. *Can. J. Nurs. Res. Arch.* **2014**, *46*, 66–86. [CrossRef] [PubMed]
48. Schwinn, T.M.; Hopkins, J.E.; Schinke, S.P. Developing a Web-Based Intervention to Prevent Drug Use Among Adolescent Girls. *Res. Soc. Work Pract.* **2016**, *26*, 8–13. [CrossRef] [PubMed]
49. Leonard, N.R.; Silverman, M.; Sherpa, D.P.; Naegle, M.A.; Kim, H.; Coffman, D.L.; Ferdschneider, M. Mobile Health Technology Using a Wearable Sensorband for Female College Students With Problem Drinking: An Acceptability and Feasibility Study. *JMIR Mhealth Uhealth* **2017**, *5*, e90. [CrossRef] [PubMed]
50. Baskerville, N.B.; Dash, D.; Wong, K.; Shuh, A.; Abramowicz, A. Perceptions Toward a Smoking Cessation App Targeting LGBTQ+ Youth and Young Adults: A Qualitative Framework Analysis of Focus Groups. *JMIR Public Health Surveill.* **2016**, *2*, e165. [CrossRef]
51. Gordon, J.S.; Armin, J.; M, D.H.; Giacobbi, P., Jr.; Cunningham, J.K.; Johnson, T.; Abbate, K.; Howe, C.L.; Roe, D.J. Development and evaluation of the See Me Smoke-Free multi-behavioral mHealth app for women smokers. *Transl. Behav. Med.* **2017**, *7*, 172–184. [CrossRef]
52. Antoine, D.; Heffernan, S.; Chaudhry, A.; King, V.; Strain, E.C. Age and gender considerations for technology-assisted delivery of therapy for substance use disorder treatment: A patient survey of access to electronic devices. *Addict. Disord. Treat.* **2016**, *15*, 149–156. [CrossRef]
53. Kim, D.J.; Choo, E.K.; Ranney, M.L. Impact of gender on patient preferences for technology-based behavioral interventions. *West. J. Emerg. Med.* **2014**, *15*, 593–599. [CrossRef]
54. Abrantes, A.M.; Blevins, C.E.; Battle, C.L.; Read, J.P.; Gordon, A.L.; Stein, M.D. Developing a Fitbit-supported lifestyle physical activity intervention for depressed alcohol dependent women. *J. Subst. Abus. Treat.* **2017**, *80*, 88–97. [CrossRef]
55. Crombie, I.K.; Irvine, L.; Falconer, D.W.; Williams, B.; Ricketts, I.W.; Jones, C.; Humphris, G.; Norrie, J.; Slane, P.; Rice, P. Alcohol and disadvantaged men: A feasibility trial of an intervention delivered by mobile phone. *Drug Alcohol Rev.* **2017**, *36*, 468–476. [CrossRef]
56. Irvine, L.; Melson, A.J.; Williams, B.; Sniehotta, F.F.; McKenzie, A.; Jones, C.; Crombie, I.K. Real Time Monitoring of Engagement with a Text Message Intervention to Reduce Binge Drinking Among Men Living in Socially Disadvantaged Areas of Scotland. *Int. J. Behav. Med.* **2017**, *24*, 713–721. [CrossRef] [PubMed]
57. Suffoletto, B.; Merrill, J.E.; Chung, T.; Kristan, J.; Vanek, M.; Clark, D.B. A text message program as a booster to in-person brief interventions for mandated college students to prevent weekend binge drinking. *J. Am. Coll. Health* **2016**, *64*, 481–489. [CrossRef] [PubMed]
58. Abraham, T.H.; Wright, P.; White, P.; Booth, B.M.; Cucciare, M.A. Feasibility and acceptability of shared decision-making to promote alcohol behavior change among women Veterans: Results from focus groups. *J. Addict. Dis.* **2017**, *36*, 252–263. [CrossRef] [PubMed]
59. McKay, J.R.; Van Horn, D.; Oslin, D.W.; Ivey, M.; Drapkin, M.L.; Coviello, D.M.; Yu, Q.; Lynch, K.G. Extended telephone-based continuing care for alcohol dependence: 24-month outcomes and subgroup analyses. *Addiction* **2011**, *106*, 1760–1769. [CrossRef] [PubMed]
60. Rasmussen, S.R. The cost effectiveness of telephone counselling to aid smoking cessation in Denmark: A modelling study. *Scand. J. Public Health* **2013**, *41*, 4–10. [CrossRef] [PubMed]

61. Kim, S.S.; Sitthisongkram, S.; Bernstein, K.; Fang, H.; Choi, W.S.; Ziedonis, D. A randomized controlled trial of a videoconferencing smoking cessation intervention for Korean American women: Preliminary findings. *Int. J. Womens Health* **2016**, *8*, 453–462. [CrossRef]
62. Laz, T.H.; Berenson, A.B. Racial and ethnic disparities in internet use for seeking health information among young women. *J. Health Commun.* **2013**, *18*, 250–260. [CrossRef]
63. Lygidakis, C.; Rigon, S.; Cambiaso, S.; Bottoli, E.; Cuozzo, F.; Bonetti, S.; Della Bella, C.; Marzo, C. A web-based versus paper questionnaire on alcohol and tobacco in adolescents. *Telemed. J. EHealth* **2010**, *16*, 925–930. [CrossRef]

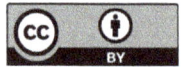

© 2020 by the authors. Licensee MDPI, Basel, Switzerland. This article is an open access article distributed under the terms and conditions of the Creative Commons Attribution (CC BY) license (http://creativecommons.org/licenses/by/4.0/).

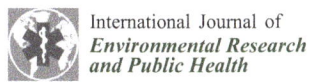

Review

Fathers' Views and Experiences of Creating a Smoke-Free Home: A Scoping Review

Rachel O'Donnell [1,*], Kathryn Angus [1], Peter McCulloch [1], Amanda Amos [2], Lorraine Greaves [3] and Sean Semple [1]

1. Institute for Social Marketing, Faculty of Health Sciences and Sport, University of Stirling, Stirling FK9 4LA, Scotland, UK
2. GRIT, Usher Institute, University of Edinburgh, Edinburgh EH8 9AG, Scotland, UK
3. Centre of Excellence for Women's Health, Vancouver, Canada & School of Population and Public Health, University of British Columbia, Vancouver, BC V6R 1Z3, Canada
* Correspondence: r.c.odonnell@stir.ac.uk; Tel.: +44-178-646-7460

Received: 21 November 2019; Accepted: 12 December 2019; Published: 17 December 2019

Abstract: Enabling parents to create a smoke-free home is one of the key ways that children's exposure to second-hand smoke (SHS) can be reduced. Smoke-free home interventions have largely targeted mothers who smoke, and there is little understanding of the barriers and facilitators that fathers experience in creating a smoke-free home. Systematic searches combining terms for fathers, homes, and SHS exposure were run in April 2019 in Web of Science's Citation Indices, PsycINFO, and PubMed for English-language studies published since 2008. The searches identified 980 records for screening, plus 66 records from other sources. Twelve studies reported in 13 papers were included in this scoping review. Eight of the studies were conducted in Asian countries (five in China, one in India, one in Japan, and one in Iran), three were conducted in Canada, and one in Turkey. Findings were extracted in verbatim text for thematic analysis. The review identified that attitudes and knowledge, cultural and social norms, gender power relations, and shifting perceptions and responsibilities related to fatherhood can impact on fathers' views of their role in relation to creating and maintaining a smoke-free home. There were too few published studies that had assessed smoke-free home interventions with fathers to draw conclusions regarding effective approaches. Research is clearly needed to inform our understanding of fathers' roles, successes and challenges in creating and maintaining a smoke-free home, so that father-inclusive rather than mother-led interventions can be developed to benefit entire households and improve gender equity as well as health.

Keywords: scoping review; barriers; facilitators; fathers; males; gender; smoking; smoke-free home; second-hand smoke

1. Introduction

Governments, health practitioners, and wider society all have a duty to protect non-smokers from the harms caused by second-hand smoke (SHS) exposure, which is estimated to cause nearly 900,000 deaths per annum and approximately 0.7% of global morbidity [1]. With substantial progress made in introducing smoke-free legislation in many countries in the past decade, most children's exposure to SHS now occurs in their own home [2], with 40% of children worldwide regularly exposed to SHS indoors [3]. Studies conducted in Japan [4], the USA [5], Australia [6], Germany [7], and Denmark [8] have documented social disparities in children's exposure to SHS at home, with children living in socio-economic disadvantage more likely to be exposed than children living in more affluent areas. In Scotland, 15% of children living in the most deprived areas are still exposed to SHS in their homes, compared to only 1% in the most affluent areas [9].

In the UK and elsewhere, smoke-free homes research has largely focused on the role of women and mothers in creating a smoke-free home [10], and the barriers and facilitators associated with women's (mother's) experiences of smoking behaviour change in these settings. There is a lack of available data estimating the proportion of fathers globally who smoke in the home, and little is known about their roles in creating and maintaining a smoke-free home, despite evidence that, with few exceptions, men are more likely to smoke than women [11]. These differences are particularly stark in East Asia and the Pacific region, where current figures suggest 49% of men smoke compared to less than 3% of women [12]. In households where relationships are vulnerable, gender power imbalances are strongly evident, with studies citing women's lack of agency in effecting change in male smoking behaviours in their relationships or household [10]. On this basis, there have been recent calls in China and Malaysia for smoke-free home interventions to be delivered at a household level, rather than specifically targeting mothers [13,14], highlighting the need for approaches that engage with all members of smoking households.

Developing smoke-free home interventions that work directly with fathers, rather than tasking mothers with reminding, persuading, or negotiating with fathers to take their smoking outside the home, could address gender-specific issues underlying fathers' smoking in the home as well as relieving mothers of this burden. It would also frame household smoking as a household responsibility, with family-wide impact. The call to include gender in tobacco control dates back 40 years to the 1980s–90s [15,16]. Gender-sensitive approaches have recently been used in Canada to develop father-friendly smoking cessation interventions [17,18] that are sensitive to gender-related factors that may influence the approach and outcomes [19]. Gender-transformative approaches go one stage further, applying gender theory in designing tobacco cessation/reduction initiatives with the dual aim of changing negative gender and social norms, and improving health and gender equity [20]. This goal explicitly aims to shift societal-level gender norms and stereotypes for both men and women in order to improve health, and in particular, to achieve equitable health opportunities for both men and women [21].

The aim of this scoping review was to synthesize findings on (1) the barriers and facilitators associated with changing fathers' smoking behaviour in the home, and (2) the development, delivery, and effectiveness of interventions aimed at changing fathers' smoking behaviour in the home.

2. Materials and Methods

A scoping review was carried out as they are increasingly used to examine the extent, range, and nature of existing research on a given topic or question. Scoping reviews are also used to identify gaps in the literature, and aid in the planning of future research [22,23], which also guided our choice of review method. In reporting this review, we have been guided by the PRISMA extension for scoping reviews (PRISMA-ScR) checklist [23]. A review protocol is available from the authors on request.

Studies were eligible for the scoping review if they met the following inclusion criteria:

- Populations: the study's sample comprised fathers, step-fathers, or male partners who smoked and lived in a home where a wife/partner and/or children also either lived or spent time there as their home, herein referred to as fathers.
- Interventions and Comparisons: the study could include none or any intervention and none or any comparison.
- Outcomes: the study investigated smoking behaviour in the home (evidenced by self-report and/or changes in objective measures of exposure to SHS (air quality, biological markers); and/or changes in SHS attitudes and/or knowledge; and/or any barriers and facilitators to changing smoking behaviour or creating a smoke-free home.
- Study types: the study collected qualitative and/or quantitative primary data, was written in English, and published since January 2008. This time frame was selected to limit the search to contemporary studies, and to acknowledge potential shifts in attitudes to smoking and smoke-free home environments associated with the increased focus on introducing comprehensive smoke-free

laws from 2005 since the entry into force of the WHO Framework Convention on Tobacco Control (WHO-FCTC) [24].
- Studies of expectant fathers or female partners were also excluded because pregnancy is a well-documented 'teachable moment' where women may be more motivated to stop smoking [25]. Although a smaller number of studies have examined the extent to which pregnancy is a motivator for expectant fathers who quit smoking, it has been suggested that fathers are willing to make changes to their smoking behaviour during this time [26–28] and that they may feel differently about their health habits during pregnancy because they are more focused on the family as a whole [29].
- Grey literature and other literature reviews were also excluded.

A systematic search for studies was run in the following databases on 2 April 2019: Web of Science Citation Indices (Science Citation Index Expanded, Social Sciences Citation Index and Arts and Humanities Citation Index), PsycINFO, and PubMed. The search strategy combined terms for fathers, smoking/second-hand smoke, and homes, and was limited to English language records published since 1 January 2008 (see Appendix A for a sample search strategy). Other sources of papers were recommendations from academic experts; the reference lists of two relevant literature review papers [19,30]; and a search of Web of Science Citation Indices for smoking-related papers authored by Dr. J.L. Bottorff or Prof. J.L. Oliffe (see also Appendix A). Search results were downloaded to reference management software and duplicates excluded. Records were single-screened for inclusion on titles initially [KA], then potentially-relevant records were double-screened for inclusion by abstract [PM, RO]. Finally, full-text papers were double-screened for inclusion [PM, RO]. This double-screening process incorporated checks on our interpretation of, and agreement on, the barriers and facilitators we identified in existing studies. Any disagreements for inclusion were resolved by a third reviewer [KA], with the final set of included studies checked by members of the wider review team (See Supplementary Materials for a list of papers excluded at the full text screening stage).

Data were extracted by a single reviewer [PM] initially into a simple table to collect each study's objective, sample, setting, country, study design, analysis method, intervention (if any), and the relevant findings. The latter were extracted in verbatim text from the papers' results and discussion sections for analysis. All extractions were checked for accuracy by a second reviewer [RO]. No quality assessments were made of individual studies included in this review, as scoping reviews do not aim to produce critically appraised and synthesized results, and are used to provide an overview or map of the evidence in a given topic area [31]. Study findings were read and re-read by two reviewers initially to (a) identify broad themes that were then categorized as barriers or facilitators to fathers creating a smoke-free home, and (b) identify efforts to test smoke-free home interventions with a sample or sub-sample of fathers in discussion with the wider review team.

3. Results

The systematic searches identified 980 records for screening by the reviewers plus 66 records from other sources (see Figure 1 for a depiction of the flow of information through the different phases of the review). A total of 12 studies reported in 13 papers were included in the review.

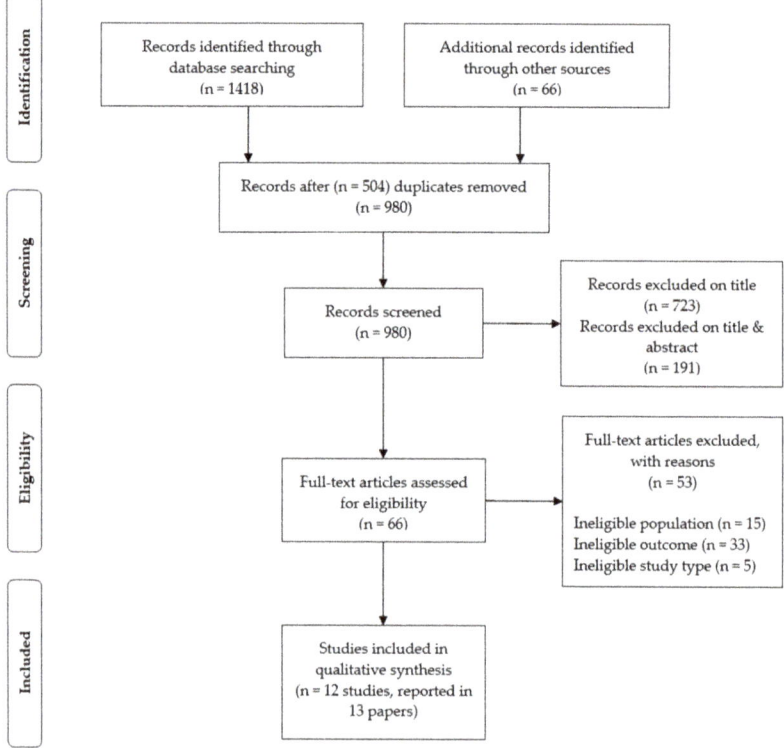

Figure 1. PRISMA flow diagram [32].

Most of the studies (*n* = 8) were conducted in Asian countries (five in China, one in India, one in Japan, and one in Iran), three were conducted in Canada (one study with Chinese-Canadian fathers (reported in two papers), and two with fathers of European, Asian, or Middle Eastern descent), and one in Turkey. Table 1 includes summaries of the seven articles that describe fathers' views on facilitators and barriers associated with creating/maintaining a smoke-free home. Table 2 includes summaries of the six articles that assessed efforts to test smoke-free home interventions with a sample or sub-sample of fathers. Note: The number of studies in Tables 1 and 2 are greater than 13 as one study [33] reported on barrier/facilitators and interventions.

Table 1. Studies that describe fathers' views on barriers and facilitators associated with creating/maintaining a smoke-free home.

Reference	Country	Purpose	Population	Study Design	Key Findings of Relevance to Fathers
Abdullah et al. 2012 [34]	China (Shanghai)	To explore attitudes to children's exposure to second-hand smoke in the home in order to inform more effective smoke-free home interventions and policies.	A convenience sample of 31 caregivers (12 fathers, 10 mothers, 9 grandparents) with children aged 5 and under.	Qualitative study: 4 focus groups and 10 in-depth interviews. Thematic analysis.	Facilitators: Most participants said they were willing to protect their child from SHS exposure. Barriers: There was a lack of knowledge about the health risks of SHS exposure. Many families did not openly discuss smoking restrictions at home, and had no rules in place. Other barriers to adopting a smoke-free home included the social acceptability of smoking, hosting social gatherings at home, authoritative attitudes of the father or father-in-law, and difficulties with visitors who smoked.
Berg et al. 2011 [35]	China (Shanghai)	To examine the reasons, processes and challenges associated with establishing smoke-free homes policies.	13 fathers who were current smokers and 17 mothers who were non-smokers living with at least one child.	Qualitative study; 30 face to face semi-structured interviews. Thematic analysis.	Facilitators: Mothers were credited with initiating discussion regarding creating a smoke-free home more often and were reported to have decision making authority. Barriers: Common responses to their request to establish a smoke-free home among fathers were agreement, ignoring it, temporarily acquiescing, insisting on smoking in the home anyway, and devaluing the benefits of creating smoke-free homes. Challenges to enforcement included weather, social situations, the smoker being home alone, ineffective harm reduction behaviours such as smoking near windows, and addiction.
Kwon et al. 2014 [36]	Canada	To explore the role of masculinity in new and expectant fathers' explanations of their continued smoking.	20 fathers (10 of European descent, and 10 of either Asian or Middle Eastern descent) from a previous study with a sample of 29 fathers.	Qualitative study; secondary analysis of interview data from a larger programme of research.	Facilitators: Most fathers reported reconciling with their partners to maintain a smoke-free home. In order to be responsible fathers and spousal partners, they accepted that their smoking routines needed to change. For some, new routines of parenting reduced their opportunities to smoke in the home. Domestic duties such as mowing the lawn and walking the dog provided them with opportunities to smoke outside. Fathers drew on masculine ideas such as protector and risk-taker, which influenced their smoking behaviour change efforts in the home.
Mao et al. 2015 [37], 2018 [38]	Canada (Ontario, Quebec, British Columbia)	To explore (1) the smoking-related experiences of immigrant Chinese fathers, and (2) the influence of denormalization in Canada on male Chinese immigrant smoking after migration.	22 fathers of Chinese origin who were currently smoking or had quit smoking in the past 5 years.	Qualitative study; semi-structured telephone interviews. Interpretive thematic analysis.	Facilitators: The message that exposure to SHS is harmful to pregnant women and young children was well understood. Fathers' changes in smoking were constructed as voluntary behaviour modifications, rather than forced practices. The Chinese fathers were willing to conform to Canadian smoking norms and extended the ban on indoor smoking in the public sphere into homes. Becoming a father strengthened efforts to maintain a smoke-free home, even during the cold Canadian winter months. Involvement in childcare also increased the Chinese fathers' determination to restrict their home smoking.
Nichter et al. 2015 [33] (see also Table 2)	India (Kerala)	To develop, refine and promote a community-based intervention to reduce SHS exposure among women and children at home.	Survey: 140 husband wife pairs, where the husband was a smoker Focus Groups/Intervention development: 3 focus groups of 8 wives, whose husbands smoked.	Quantitative survey measuring attitudes re: SHS exposure Qualitative; Focus groups discussing household gender relations and the ability of women to encourage a smoke-free home.	Barriers: Most women felt powerless to change their husband's behaviour, as (typically in this region of India) husbands do not listen to advice from their wives about their personal habits. Men and women underestimated the risks of SHS exposure to child health, but men more so—65% of women thought it could cause serious illness, compared to only 32% of men. 28% of women believed it could cause minor illness or was harmless, compared to 42% of men.

Table 1. *Cont.*

Reference	Country	Purpose	Population	Study Design	Key Findings of Relevance to Fathers
Oliffe et al. 2010 [39]	Canada (Vancouver)	To investigate smoking and masculinities by detailing the highly gendered nature of the everyday places where fathers smoke.	20 new fathers who cohabited with their female partner and smoked during the pregnancy and postpartum period.	Ethnographic study–fathers took part in a semi-structured interview in the first month postpartum, were given a camera and encouraged to take pictures of the places that they smoked in during their partner's pregnancy and afterwards. A second interview was then conducted to discuss photographs taken.	Facilitators: Most fathers understood the dangers of SHS exposure in the home. Fathers spoke of their preference to smoke at work rather than at home, as this gave them freedom to smoke without the surveillance from or risk to their child or partner. Some fathers linked the discussion of their outdoor smoking to notions of good fathering.
Saito et al. 2018 [40]	Japan	To test the potential mediating role of perceived smoking norms on the associations between education and indoor smoking among parents who smoke.	A convenience sample of 1645 parents (822 mothers, 823 fathers) from an online survey panel.	Quantitative; cross-sectional study.	Facilitators: Perceived smoking norms mediated the association between education and indoor smoking. Household smoking status and a worksite smoking ban also mediated this association via perceived norms, but only for fathers. Barriers: For both fathers and mothers who smoked, years of education was significantly negatively associated with indoor smoking behaviours.

Table 2. Studies that have assessed efforts to test smoke-free home interventions with a sample or sub-sample of men.

Reference	Country	Purpose	Population	Study Design	Key Findings of Relevance to Fathers
Baheiraei et al. 2011 [41]	Iran (Tehran)	To investigate whether counselling both mothers and fathers reduces their infants' exposure to SHS.	N = 130 (convenience sample of families with children less than 1 year old, exposed to SHS. In 97% of households only the father smoked. Families were recruited whilst attending a health centre for routine infant health checks).	Randomised controlled trial. Mothers in the intervention group each received 3 counselling sessions, one of which was face to face (location not specified) and two of which were by telephone, and fathers in the intervention group received 3 counselling sessions by telephone. The control group received usual care.	In the intervention group, the number of smoke-free homes increased significantly from 15% at baseline to 33.3% at the 3-month follow-up. The differences between the two groups were statistically significant ($p < 0.05$). The intervention was effective in reducing infant urinary cotinine levels ($p < 0.05$).
Chan et al. 2011 [42]	China (Hong Kong)	To study whether smoking fathers would smoke inside their homes owing to smoke-free legislation in public places.	Pre-legislation group (2005) comprised of 186 families and the 2006 group of 114 families Post legislation group (2007a) comprised of 742 non-smoking mothers and 608 fathers and the 2007b group of 189 mothers, 174 fathers.	Prospective survey of two cohorts of families recruited before legislation and a cross-sectional survey of families after legislation.	Significantly more fathers in the 2007a group than the 2006 group never smoked at home (26.7% vs. 14.0%, $p < 0.001$), and never smoked around their children (59.7% vs. 30.7%, $p < 0.001$). The differences remained significant after adjusting for the father's educational level and age. Regarding 60.6% of fathers who smoked at home and 45.3% of fathers who smoked around children in the 2007a group, they only smoked one to four cigarettes daily at home and around children, respectively.

Table 2. Cont.

Reference	Country	Purpose	Population	Study Design	Key Findings of Relevance to Fathers
Chan et al. 2014 [43]	China (Hong Kong)	To investigate the effect of maternal action to protect children from SHS and a 2007 public smoking ban, on children's exposure to SHS in the home.	333 families participated in surveys prior to the smoking ban and 742 families participated in surveys post smoking ban.	Quantitative study, comparing survey data and direct measurement of SHS exposure levels from previous studies conducted prior to a public smoking ban, with that from survey data and SHS exposure levels collected for the present study post smoking ban.	Fathers' smoking in the home decreased post-legislation. 29.3% of children post-legislation were exposed to SHS in the home, compared with 87.2% pre-legislation ($p < 0.01$). Hair nicotine level in mothers and children post-legislation was lower than pre-legislation. Over 90% of mothers pre-and post-legislation advised the fathers to reduce smoking, avoid smoking at home or avoid smoking near the children. This suggests that specific interventions for families should be expanded together with smoke-free legislation.
Nichter et al. 2015 [33] (see also Table 1)	India (Kerala)	To develop, refine and promote a community-based intervention to reduce SHS exposure among women and children at home.	Proof of concept study: N = 140 Pilot study 1: N = 95 Pilot study 2: N = 157 (husband wife pairs, where husband was a smoker).	Community based intervention including educational meetings, smoke free homes video, healthcare worker household visits, community meetings and community declarations of support for smoke-free homes.	At baseline, across the pilot studies, between 70–80% of men regularly smoked in their home, despite 80% of women having asked their husband not to. Six months post intervention between 34% and 59% of men who smoked no longer smoked in their home. The authors note that this represents a modest, but significant change in community smoking norms. No statistical tests of significance were applied to the data.
Yu et al. 2017 [44]	China (Changchun)	To investigate if interventions that incorporate traditional and mobile phone based education help create smoke-free homes for infants and increase quitting among fathers.	N = 342 (families: non-smoking mothers and their newborns currently exposed to SHS in the home by fathers' smoking).	Randomised controlled trial involving three groups: Intervention Group I-A received counselling on SHS harms to children, education on creating a smoke-free home, and posters to display in the home to encourage fathers and other visitors not to smoke. Intervention Group I-B received the same intervention as I-A, with additional text messages to the mother/father on harms of SHS to the mother and child. The father received additional text messages to quit smoking. Control Group: Received only standard care for their initial postnatal visits, which did not include any tobacco control or cessation counselling service.	Although no reduction of the self-reported exposure rate to SHS among surveyed mothers of newborns was found at 6 months, the rate at 12 months was significantly decreased in I-B compared to the control group. Participants in the I-B group were more likely to report "smoking never permitted inside home" compared to participants in control group at 12 months (1.17 vs. 4.71, $p < 0.05$). These findings suggest that the addition of an mHealth element to interventions with in-person counselling and provision of educational materials effectively aided in creating smoke-free homes among fathers of newborns.
Nacaroglu et al. 2017 [45]	Turkey (Izmir)	To determine whether informing families about their children's urinary cotinine levels curtailed the exposure of children to SHS.	N = 193 children (Intervention group 97, control group 96). Families of the children recruited via a local hospital. There was no report of the family make-up and gender differences in the sample.	Randomised controlled trial. Urinary cotinine levels were measured in all children. Parents in the intervention group were given education about SHS harms and were advised about their child's urinary cotinine levels by telephone. The control group were not informed about their child's urinary cotinine levels until the end of the study.	In the intervention group, significant decreases in the number of cigarettes that fathers smoked both daily (16.8 to 14.5) and at home (7.69 to 3.96) were evident ($p = 0.001$ and $p = 0.001$, respectively). Although the number of cigarettes smoked daily by mothers both at home and outside decreased, the decreases were not significant.

3.1. Facilitators and Barriers

Four of the seven studies identified that outlined fathers' views on facilitators and barriers associated with creating/maintaining a smoke-free home were conducted in Asian countries (two in China, one in India, and one in Japan) [33–35,40], and three were conducted in Canada [36–39] (with one study reported in two papers [37,38]. Four studies used qualitative methods (focus groups, semi-structured face to face interviews, and telephone interviews) to explore the fathers' views on creating/maintaining a smoke-free home [34–38]. Three of these studies had a wider study remit: to explore gender relations and masculinity in fathers who smoke [36]; fathers' smoking behaviours [40], and fathers' perspectives on stopping smoking [38]. One study used mixed methods (survey and focus groups) across different study phases [33], one was a quantitative study reporting findings from a cross-sectional survey [40], and one ethnographic study drew on interview transcripts, photographs that fathers had taken to document where their smoking took place both during and after their partner's pregnancy, and field notes [39]. Four studies included mother and fathers [33–35,40] and three studies comprised exclusively of fathers [36–39].

3.1.1. Beliefs and Knowledge

Beliefs and knowledge about SHS have the potential to enable or restrict the fathers' attempts to create and maintain a smoke-free home. Inaccurate or incomplete knowledge about the health risks of SHS exposure can contribute to SHS exposure in children. In a qualitative study conducted in China [34], where approximately 60% of men and 7% women smoke, nine males (fathers/grandfathers) who were current smokers and one female (mother or grandmother, not specified) who was a non-smoker had misconceptions about SHS at home, believing that smoking in the living room or in the toilet does not lead to children being exposed to SHS. Participants (eight males who smoked, one female who smoked and six male non-smokers) thought that younger children were particularly at risk from SHS-related health issues because they were still developing, and six participants (four male smokers, one female smoker, and one female non-smoker) believed that once the child is older, their organs have developed and the risks are reduced, meaning that smoking in front of them is less harmful. The authors suggest that a lack of SHS-related knowledge on the part of smokers, mixed with Chinese social and cultural norms that are pro-smoking (see Section 3.1.2), has contributed to SHS exposure in children.

In quantitative survey work conducted in Kerala, India [33], where approximately 25% of men and 3% of women smoke, seventy percent of mothers surveyed from 140 households reported that their husband regularly smoked inside the house. Survey findings also indicated that fathers underestimated the risks associated with SHS exposure to children more often than mothers; 65% of mothers considered that SHS exposure could cause serious childhood illness compared to only 32% of fathers, and 28% of mothers believed it could cause minor illness or was harmless, compared to 42% of fathers.

In contrast, a qualitative study investigating the smoking-related experiences of immigrant Chinese fathers in Canada [37] highlighted the enabling role that knowledge can have in conjunction with becoming a father in a country where the message that SHS is harmful to pregnant women and young children had become commonplace. The 22 Chinese Canadian fathers in the study who smoked or had recently quit smoking reported that they had dramatically changed their smoking patterns because of concerns for their children's health.

3.1.2. Cultural and Perceived Social Norms

The Canadian study above [37] highlights how Chinese fathers could conform to dominant Canadian smoking norms and extend the ban on indoor smoking in public places into homes. It is well established that parents (mothers and fathers) with less formal education are more likely to smoke indoors, contributing to the social inequalities in home-smoking rates [4]. A Japanese cross-sectional survey suggested that parents who smoke with less formal education are more likely to perceive pro-smoking norms, which in turn may be associated with smoking in the home [40]. However, this study also found that household smoking status and worksite smoking status mediated the association between education and indoor smoking behaviours for fathers only. On this basis, the authors suggest that discouraging pro-smoking norms in the home and work social networks could help to reduce fathers' smoking in the home.

3.1.3. Gender Power Relations

Gender power relations within the household can enable or restrict the change to a smoke-free home where fathers smoke indoors. Nichter et al. [33] recognized the difficulty for individual women in Kerala, India to effect change in their household, developing a community-level rather than household-based smoke-free home intervention to change fathers' smoking behaviour in the home as a result. Survey findings suggested that fathers were unwilling to change their smoking behaviour based on their wife's or children's requests not to smoke in the home. Findings from focus groups conducted with mothers suggested it was, in some circumstances, inappropriate but also potentially dangerous to challenge their husband's home-smoking behaviour. Mothers also experienced difficulties in asking guests not to smoke in the home, which might be interpreted as disrespectful, given that it is culturally appropriate for men to smoke. Similar findings came from a recent qualitative Chinese study of families [34]. All 15 fathers who were current smokers reported that they smoked at home. Home-smoking restrictions were not discussed by families because of the social acceptability of smoking and authoritarian attitudes of the father or father-in-law. Three fathers effectively resisted their wives wishes for a smoke-free family home, with one saying, *"Every time I lit a cigarette at home my wife would complain, but I pretended that I did not to hear that she was talking. I knew she would stop her noise after sometime."* [34] (p. 360) In contrast, findings from one qualitative study [35] with 13 fathers who were current smokers and 17 mothers who were non-smokers living in China with at least one child suggested that in most cases, mothers did have the authority to influence their husband's home-smoking behaviour, although in a minority of cases, this was a sensitive issue. Many participants who had a smoke-free home policy had adopted it early on in their relationship. This often coincided with what the authors consider to be an 'important opportunity' before beginning a family, when men might be particularly invested in the health of their family in the home.

3.1.4. Shifting Perceptions and Responsibilities Related to Fatherhood

In Canada, there is some evidence that changes in home-smoking patterns may be influenced by fatherhood. In one qualitative study [36] with 20 fathers, the majority described altering their home-smoking routines, with one reporting that smoking outside *"comes with the territory"* of fatherhood (p. 394). Gendered divisions of labour supported fathers' smoking behaviours outside of the home, using chores including mowing the lawn and walking the dog as opportunities to keep their smoking outside. In some cases, being at home and involved in childcare reduced the fathers' opportunities to smoke, a finding supported by the study of Chinese fathers who had moved to Canada [37]. The authors report that these fathers, conceding that their smoking could no longer be an autonomous decision, adopted a shift in masculine identity to that of 'protector', separating their smoking behaviours from family life to fulfil the contemporary role of the involved father. This was also the case in the Canadian study of new fathers [39], where fathers spoke of their preference to smoke at work rather than at home, as this gave them freedom to smoke without the surveillance from or risk to their child or partner. Some fathers linked the discussion of their outdoor smoking to notions of good fathering. Ten of the twenty participants had moved their smoking outdoors, although a minority reported that they broke house rules and secretly smoked indoors when the opportunity arose. Several participants were nostalgic for pre-fathering days when they had had the freedom to smoke inside the home.

3.2. Interventions

Of the six papers that assessed efforts to test smoke-free home interventions involving fathers, all but one were conducted in Asian countries (three in China, one in India, one in Iran) [33,41–44], with the remaining study conducted in Turkey [45]. Three were randomised controlled trials (RCT) assessing the feasibility of providing families with different counselling/educational interventions [41,44,45]. Two studies used a repeated cross-sectional design to assess the impacts of a ban on smoking in public places on home-smoking levels comparing pre-and post-ban survey data and home-smoking behaviour [42,43]. One study reported on assessing the feasibility of developing and delivering a community-based counselling/educational intervention across one proof of concept study and two pilot studies [33]. All six papers recruited both mothers and fathers to their sample. Three incorporated the objective assessment of SHS levels as an intervention component (two using infant urinary cotinine samples [41,45], and one using hair nicotine levels in mothers and children [43]).

3.2.1. Counselling and Education

An RCT [41] in Iran demonstrated that counselling both fathers and mothers, alongside the receipt of an educational pamphlet and a sticker depicting a smoke-free home where the father chooses to smoke outside to protect his child, led to a significant reduction in exposure to SHS in the home (measured by cotinine and parental report) at the three month follow up. In Iranian families, cigarette smoking is not the cultural norm for women, reflected in the study sample whereby in 97% of households, only the father smoked. Fathers were viewed as not likely to be comfortable receiving instructions from their wives about refraining from smoking in the home, therefore in this cultural context, developing an intervention that directly encourages fathers to protect their children was considered important. Study findings suggested that despite these gendered cultural norms, a brief counselling program has the potential to change fathers' home-smoking behaviour, at least in the short term. However, there was a lack of association between reported exposures and infant urinary cotinine levels, and the authors suggest that culture could play a role in the degree of accurate disclosure about smoking and SHS exposure.

3.2.2. Education and Objective Assessment of Second-hand Smoke Levels in the Home

Presenting families with objective evidence on child SHS exposure using urinary cotinine levels, in conjunction with education materials, was shown to be an effective means of reducing SHS in the home in an RCT in Turkey [45]. In the intervention group, there were significant reductions in the number of cigarettes that fathers, but not mothers, smoked both daily and at home. Again, there was no correlation between child urinary cotinine levels and parentally reported SHS levels, suggesting that parents consciously or unconsciously did not acknowledge SHS exposure, or reported incomplete information. Of the children involved in the study, 81.4% showed signs of SHS exposure, and urinary cotinine levels were also high in the children of parents who claimed they never smoked in the home with children nearby. The authors suggest that such high levels may be explained by a lack of parental awareness, with parents not understanding that smoking at home, even when children are not present, can still lead to SHS exposure.

3.2.3. Education and Mobile-Health Interventions

One RCT conducted in China (Changchun) [44] assessed whether an intervention that incorporated traditional and mobile-phone based education could assist families in creating a smoke-free home for infants. Non-smoking mothers of newborns and fathers received counselling at the same time, which facilitated spousal interaction and support, and encouraged the mothers to be the change agents. Mothers of the newborns in the intervention group reported reduced exposure to SHS at 12 months, suggesting that women have an important role to play in helping their spouses to change their smoking behaviour, as outlined in Section 3.1.3. However, the study relied on self-reporting to evaluate outcomes, which may be biased and inaccurate regarding SHS exposure levels in the home.

3.2.4. Community-Based Interventions

In India, a community-based smoke-free homes initiative was developed, refined, and promoted across the state of Kerala, with the aim of reducing SHS exposure among mothers and children at home [33]. The initiative used a combination of healthcare worker household visits, and an educational video with positive messages to support fathers' abstinence from smoking in the home as a sign of caring for women and children, and as a social value linked to the cultural value of male responsibility. The video also included testimonials from community members who had successfully created a smoke-free home as part of previous piloting of the initiative. At the baseline, across two pilot studies conducted in different communities, between 70–80% of fathers regularly smoked in the home, despite 80% of mothers having asked their husbands not to. Six months post intervention between 34% and 59% of fathers who smoked self-reported no longer smoking in the home. These observations were not validated by objective assessment of SHS levels.

3.2.5. Impact of Smoke-Free Public Places Legislation

Two related studies investigated the impact of introducing smoke-free legislation in public places in Hong Kong on parental home-smoking behaviour [42,43]. In the first study, survey findings from the pre-and post-legislation groups found that significantly more fathers never smoked at home post-legislation (27% vs. 14%) and these differences remained significant after adjusting for the fathers' educational level and age. The second study compared survey data with the assessment of SHS exposure levels, finding again that fathers smoking in the home significantly decreased post-legislation. Hair nicotine levels were lower in mothers and children post-legislation, and more mothers took action to protect their children from SHS including taking their children away from smoking and advising their husbands to quit. However, post-legislation, over 60% of the fathers reported that they still smoked at home when their children were not there, suggesting that more specific and effective smoke-free homes interventions are required in the future to assist fathers in changing their home-smoking behaviour.

4. Discussion

In this synthesis, we described studies that report on the role that beliefs/knowledge, cultural and perceived social norms, gender power relations and fatherhood play in fathers' views on the creation and maintenance of a smoke-free home. We also highlighted the findings of interventions that have been developed to assist fathers to create a smoke-free home.

To date, whilst published systematic reviews and thematic syntheses of the smoke-free homes literature have incorporated studies including fathers as participants [10,46,47], the focus in most studies is on mothers' experiences. Consequently, the barriers and facilitators that mothers face in creating/maintaining a smoke-free home are well documented, with gender imbalances visible through their lack of agency in effecting change in fathers' smoking behaviours in the home [10]. A minority of interventions have been shown to reduce children's exposure to SHS and improve children's health, but the features that differentiate the effective interventions from those without clear evidence of effectiveness remain unclear [46]. The quality of evidence has been suggested to range from low to very low, and several suggestions have been made to address this in future interventions, for example by including more participants, describing interventions in more detail [46] and ensuring that objective outcomes are measured at baseline, at the end of the intervention, and at longer-term follow-up [47]. None of these suggestions include addressing the current gender imbalance inherent in smoke-free homes research, and yet increasing the involvement of fathers specifically could enhance our understanding of which interventions work for whom, and why. This would likely assist in improving our knowledge and understanding of the challenges that mothers and fathers face in reducing children's exposure to SHS in the home, which could in turn lead to the development of interventions that more effectively engage all adult smoking household members.

The synthesis only identified 13 papers published over the last 10 years (written in the English language) that included findings on fathers' roles in creating a smoke-free home, either through qualitative studies exploring barriers and facilitators, or through the development of interventions aiming to reduce children's SHS exposure levels in the home. It is clear that cultural and gender norms play a significant role in shaping fathers' beliefs and knowledge regarding the health risks of SHS exposure to children, and the importance associated with creating a smoke-free home. The extent to which the interventions outlined take account of the barriers and facilitators identified in this review varied. All but one of the intervention studies were conducted in Asian countries where smoking is not the cultural norm for women, and children are largely exposed to SHS through the father. Mothers may feel powerless to change their husband's behaviour and fathers may not be willing to listen to requests to keep their smoking outside, due to the social acceptability of male smoking and/or authoritative attitudes. Most of the intervention studies conducted recognize this cultural context, and some acknowledge that it may lead to mothers over-reporting changes in fathers' smoking behaviour in the home. Given these challenges, and in this cultural context, Nichter et al.'s [33] move away from an individual household intervention to the promotion of a community-wide intervention, with the end goal of changing smoking norms, shows promise. Their formative research also suggests that not smoking in the home could be effectively promoted as an important cultural value linked to male responsibility to protect the health of women and children, which fits with our finding that shifting perceptions and responsibilities related to fatherhood, and the role of the male as 'protector' [37–39] may facilitate fathers creating a smoke-free home. However, given the paucity of research conducted on fathers' roles in creating a smoke-free home, further research is required to verify the utility of this approach.

A second approach that has shown initial promise is currently being trialled in Bangladesh to evaluate the effectiveness of a community-based intervention to reduce SHS exposure at home, primarily targeting men via mosques [48]. This cluster RCT is based on the findings of a pilot trial that concluded that a smoke-free home intervention was acceptable to Muslim communities, and feasible to deliver in mosques [49,50]. If found to be effective in changing smoking behaviour in the home, this approach could be generalizable to other communities with similar male smoking norms where faith-based settings (i.e., churches, mosques, synagogues) play an integral part in their lives [48].

Norms associated with male smoking differ significantly in Asian countries when compared to norms in the US, the UK, and other areas of Europe, where gender differences in smoking rates are less pronounced [51]. Little is known about the fathers' roles and experiences of creating/maintaining a smoke-free home in these areas of the world, where gender equality may be a collective aspiration, for example, through the championing of initiatives such as shared parental leave. As most of the studies included in this scoping review were conducted in countries where gender inequality often exists, we acknowledge that approaches that are acceptable within these countries may not be generalizable to countries with a greater emphasis on gender equality. Different approaches may be required in Western European countries, for example, compared to Asian countries, to support fathers to effectively create and maintain a smoke-free home.

We were unable to source published research that considered the implications of different family/household compositions on creating a smoke-free home including fathers' roles and experiences of negotiating smoke-free homes with an ex-partner to protect children who spend their time living between two parent's homes. In addition, our searches found no studies that explored the role that fathers might play as agents of change in households where mothers smoke and fathers are non-smokers. A better understanding of fathers' smoke-free home roles in different family compositions and smoking profiles, and the cultural context that their smoking behaviour operates within, could be considered as important to progress our understanding of the factors that lead to the creation and effective maintenance of a smoke-free family home. Despite the call for gender-sensitive and gender transformative approaches to tobacco control, these approaches have not been utilized in smoke-free homes research, which may have perpetuated the mothers' responsibility for health in the home in this context, doing little to shift gender norms. Most of the studies identified in this review have focused on fathers' individual roles and behaviours related to smoking in the home, without addressing some of the structural-level factors that shape masculinities (i.e., poverty, migration, racism, gender inequality) and give rise to smoking, and smoking in the home among fathers. The importance of structural interventions has been emphasized in relation to conducting gender-transformative work with men [52] because while men do have agency to make positive individual health changes, this agency sits in a wider social, economic, and cultural context that both constrains and enables individual choices [52,53]. Targeting this wider structural context could lead to more successful and fuller engagement with fathers in the future [52], which is key because effectively engaging fathers in the creation/maintenance of a smoke-free home has the potential to benefit the entire family, and improve gender equity as well as health.

Current smoke-free home intervention research involving fathers has been limited because of a lack of objective measurement of SHS exposure. One study conducted in China suggested that social desirability bias may affect some reporting of the prevalence of smoking in the home [34]. A study conducted in Iran has suggested that culture could play a role in the degree of accurate disclosure about smoking in the home [41]. A second Chinese study reported that even among participants (men and women with and without children) with a complete smoke-free home policy, 33% were exposed to SHS 'in the past week'. Older relatives and visitors who smoke were reported as the key barrier to creating a smoke-free home, reflecting the Chinese value system whereby elder generations and visitors to the home are highly respected [54]. This finding builds on those of an earlier Chinese study conducted in six counties that found that 42% of non-smokers would offer cigarettes to guests visiting the home [55].

Introducing smoke-free public places legislation is associated with multiple child health benefits [56] including reduced exposure to SHS via increased home-smoking restrictions [57]. Two of the studies included in this scoping review suggest that the introduction of smoke-free legislation in Hong Kong may have assisted in reducing paternal smoking in the home [42,43], although 60% of the fathers involved in the Chan et al. [43] study reported that they still smoked at home when their children were not present. The challenge of capturing this fluidity of home-smoking rules in survey questions aiming to measure smoke-free home prevalence has been highlighted in previous research [10], and the importance of exploring fluidity as well as including objective measures of SHS exposure where practical, has been recommended in future intervention studies [10]. Consideration should also be given to the importance of developing theory-based smoke-free home interventions, as none of the studies described in this review paper had an explicit theoretical basis, and yet interventions based on theory are likely to be more successful than those non-theory based [58].

A key strength of this study lies in our comprehensive approach to conducting the scoping review. Triangulation was achieved by involving multiple authors in extraction, analysis, and interpretation of the results. Limiting our included data to English language papers may have biased the findings, and in scoping only published studies, it is possible that we missed other relevant research available as 'grey' literature. In addition, we screened potentially relevant papers by title and abstract only in the initial stages of the review process, which may have resulted in some papers with relevant findings documented in the full text of the paper being excluded, although our supplementary searches may have mitigated this somewhat. We also acknowledge that widening our inclusion criteria to include studies with expectant fathers may have revealed additional findings of relevance related to the specific context of a 'teachable moment'. However, this was a small-scale review and our inclusion/exclusion criteria were agreed to on this basis. No quality appraisals were made of individual studies, as this was a rapid scoping review that adopted an inclusive approach.

5. Conclusions

Fathers have a central role to play in the creation and maintenance of a smoke-free family home. However, this scoping review highlights that very few published studies have (a) explored the barriers and facilitators associated with their role, or (b) developed and tested interventions designed to actively involve and appeal to fathers. The findings of this scoping review suggest that attitudes/knowledge, cultural and social norms, gender power relations. and shifting perceptions and responsibilities related to fatherhood could impact on the fathers' views of their role in relation to creating/maintaining a smoke-free home, but additional research is required to support these suggestions, given the limitations of the scoping review already discussed. There are too few published intervention study findings that have focused on fathers' roles in creating a smoke-free home to draw conclusions regarding effective approaches. However, in some Asian cultures where smoking is considered a social norm for men and not for women, a move away from individual household interventions to the promotion of a community-based intervention approach shows initial promise. However, research is also required in areas of the world where gender differences in smoking rates are less pronounced to begin to understand the fathers' roles, successes, and challenges in creating and maintaining a smoke-free home, as effectively engaging fathers in the creation/maintenance of a smoke-free homes has the potential to not only benefit the entire family, but also improve gender equity and health.

Supplementary Materials: The following are available online at http://www.mdpi.com/1660-4601/16/24/5164/s1, File S1: List of papers excluded at the full text screening stage.

Author Contributions: Conceptualization, R.O., S.S., A.A., and L.G.; Investigation, P.M., K.A., and R.O.; Writing–original draft preparation, R.O. and K.A.; Funding acquisition, R.O., S.S., and A.A.; Supervision, R.O., K.A., S.S. and A.A.; Methodology and formal analysis K.A., P.M., and R.O.; A.A., S.S.; Validation, P.M., R.O., and K.A.; Writing—review and editing, and visualization, all authors.

Funding: This research was funded by Cancer Research UK, grant number [C67395/A27911]. The APC (Article Processing Charge) was funded by the University of Stirling.

Conflicts of Interest: The authors declare no conflicts of interest. The funders had no role in the design of the study; in the collection, analyses, or interpretation of data; in the writing of the manuscript, or in the decision to publish the results.

Appendix A

Sample search strategy

Table A1. Web of Science Core Collection (SCI-EXPANDED Science Citation Index Expanded; SSCI Social Sciences Citation Index; A&HCI Arts and Humanities Citation Index).

No.	Search String [1]
#1	TS = (smok * OR tobacco OR cigarette * OR indoor * OR passive OR "ETS" OR "SHS" OR secondhand OR second-hand OR "second hand" OR antismoking OR "anti-smoking")
#2	TS = (home$ OR "at-home" OR hous * OR accommodation$ OR "private" OR "privacy" OR resid * OR cohabit * OR co-habit *)
#3	TS = (father * OR step-father * OR stepfather * OR paternal OR husband * OR "male partner" OR "male partners" OR masculine *)
#4	#3 AND #2 AND #1
#5	#4 AND LANGUAGE: (English) AND Timespan = 2008–2019

[1] TS searches the title, abstract, and keywords fields of a record; * represents any group of characters including no character; $ represents zero or one character.

Additional sources

When we compared our resulting list of included studies against those of other literature reviews on related topics ("The barriers and facilitators to smoking cessation experienced by women's partners during pregnancy and the post-partum period: a systematic review of qualitative research" (Flemming et al. 2015 [29]) and "Gender, smoking and tobacco reduction and cessation: a scoping review" (Bottorff et al. 2014 [19])), we were interested to see that the studies that passed our inclusion criteria did not overlap much with the included studies. By examining the academic database indexing for the studies included by Flemming et al. (2015) and Bottorff et al. (2014), we found that records for these studies (usually titles, abstracts, and keywords) did not include terms for the 'home' concept from our search strategy, and a few did not include terms for the 'fathers' concept from our strategy. As the studies, broadly speaking, included fathers as a population and investigated smoking behaviours, we added the studies included in the two reviews to our pool of studies for further assessment. Many of the studies were authored by one or both of two Canadian academics, therefore we also ran a search for papers authored by Dr Joan Bottorff or Professor John Oliffe published since January 2008 that mentioned smoking/tobacco (Web of Science Citation Indices search string run on 19 August 2019: AU = (Bottorff OR Oliffe) AND TS = (smok * OR tobacco)). These additional sources added one study to our final results (Oliffe et al. 2010 [39]).

References

1. Drope, J.; Schluger, N.; Cahn, Z.; Drope, J.; Hamill, S.; Islami, F.; Liber, A.; Nargis, N.; Stoklosa, M. *The Tobacco Atlas*; American Cancer Society and Vital Strategies: Atlanta, GA, USA, 2018.
2. Jones, L.L.; Atkinson, O.; Longman, J.; Coleman, T.; McNeill, A.; Lewis, S.A. The motivators and barriers to a smoke-free home among disadvantaged caregivers: Identifying the positive levers for change. *Nicotine Tob. Res.* **2011**, *13*, 479–486. [CrossRef]
3. Oberg, M.; Jaakkola, M.S.; Woodward, A.; Peruga, A.; Prüss-Ustün, A. Worldwide burden of disease from exposure to second-hand smoke: A retrospective analysis of data from 192 countries. *Lancet* **2011**, *337*, 139–146. [CrossRef]
4. Saito, J.; Tabuchi, T.; Shibanuma, A.; Yasuoka, J.; Nakamura, M.; Jimba, M. 'Only fathers' smoking' contributes the most to socioeconomic inequalities: Changes in socioeconomic inequalities in infants' exposure to second hand smoke over time in Japan. *PLoS ONE* **2015**, *10*, e0139512. [CrossRef] [PubMed]
5. Zhang, X.; Martinez-Donate, A.P.; Kuo, D.; Jones, N.R.; Palmersheim, K.A. Trends in home smoking bans in the U.S.A., 1995–2007: Prevalence, discrepancies and disparities. *Tob. Control* **2012**, *21*, 330–336. [CrossRef] [PubMed]
6. Pisinger, C.; Hammer-Helmich, L.; Andreasen, A.H.; Jorgensen, T.; Glumer, C. Social disparities in children's exposure to second hand smoke at home: A repeated cross-sectional survey. *Environ. Health* **2012**, *11*, 65. [CrossRef] [PubMed]
7. Kuntz, B.; Lampert, T. Social disparities in parental smoking and young children's exposure to secondhand smoke at home: A time-trend analysis of repeated cross-sectional data from the German KiGGS study between 2003–2006 and 2009–2012. *BMC Public Health* **2016**, *16*, 485. [CrossRef]
8. Gartner, C.E.; Hall, W.D. Is the socioeconomic gap in childhood exposure to secondhand smoke widening or narrowing? *Tob. Control* **2013**, *22*, 344–348. [CrossRef]
9. Scottish Government. The Scottish Health Survey 2015: Volume 1: Main Report. 2016. Available online: http://www.gov.scot/Publications/2016/09/2764 (accessed on 22 July 2019).
10. Passey, M.E.; Longman, J.M.; Robinson, J.; Wiggers, J.; Jones, L.L. Smoke-free homes: What are the barriers, motivators and enablers? A qualitative systematic review and thematic synthesis. *BMJ Open* **2016**, *6*, e010260. [CrossRef]
11. Ng, M.; Freeman, M.K.; Fleming, T.D.; Robinson, M.; Dwyer-Lindgren, L.; Thomson, B.; Wollum, A.; Sanman, E.; Wulf, S.; Lopez, A.D.; et al. Smoking prevalence and cigarette consumption in 187 countries, 1980–2012. *JAMA* **2014**, *311*, 183–192. [CrossRef] [PubMed]
12. World Health Organization. Global Health Observatory Data Repository 2019. Available online: https://blogs.worldbank.org/opendata/men-smoke-5-times-more-women (accessed on 22 July 2019).
13. Vitali, M.; Protano, C. How relevant are fathers who smoke at home to the passive smoking exposure of their children? *Acta Paediatr.* **2017**, *106*, 74. [CrossRef]
14. Semple, S.; Abidin, E.; Amos, A.; Hashim, Z.; Siddiqi, K.; Ismail, N.; On Behalf of the Participants of the Smoke-Free Homes Workshop (Kuala Lumpur, 7–9 May 2018). The Kuala Lumpur Charter on Smoke-Free Homes. Tobacco Control Weblog. Available online: https://blogs.bmj.com/tc/2018/06/25/the-kuala-lumpur-charter-on-smoke-free-homes (accessed on 22 July 2019).
15. Jacobson, B. *The Ladykillers: Why Smoking Is a Feminist Issue*; Pluto Press: London, UK, 1981.
16. Greaves, L. *Background Paper on Women and Tobacco*; Health Canada: Ottawa, ON, Canada, 1990.
17. Oliffe, J.L.; Bottorff, J.L.; Sarbit, G. Supporting fathers' efforts to be smoke-free: Program principles. *Can. J. Nurs. Res.* **2012**, *44*, 64–82. [PubMed]

18. Bottorff, J.L.; Oliffe, J.L.; Sarbit, G.; Huisken, A.; Caperchione, C.; Anand, A.; Howay, K. Evaluating the feasibility of a gender-sensitized smoking cessation program for fathers. *Psychol. Men Masc.* **2019**, *20*, 194–207. [CrossRef]
19. Bottorff, J.L.; Haines-Saah, R.; Kelly, M.T.; Oliffe, J.L.; Torchalla, I.; Poole, N.; Greaves, L.; Robinson, C.A.; Ensom, M.H.; Okoli, C.T.; et al. Gender, smoking and tobacco reduction and cessation: A scoping review. *Int. J. Equity Health* **2014**, *12*, 114. [CrossRef] [PubMed]
20. Greaves, L.; Pederson, A.; Poole, N. (Eds.) *Making It Better: Gender-Transformative Health Promotion*; Canadian Scholars Press: Toronto, ON, Canada, 2014; p. 22.
21. Greaves, L. Can tobacco control be transformative? Reducing gender inequity and tobacco use among vulnerable populations. *Int. J. Environ. Res. Public Health* **2014**, *11*, 792–803. [CrossRef] [PubMed]
22. Tricco, A.C.; Lillie, E.; Zarin, W.; O'Brien, K.; Colquhoun, H.; Kastner, M.; Levac, D.; Ng, C.; Sharpe, J.P.; Wilson, K.; et al. A scoping review on the conduct and reporting of scoping reviews. *BMC Med. Res. Methodol.* **2016**, *16*, 15. [CrossRef] [PubMed]
23. Tricco, A.C.; Lillie, E.; Zarin, W.; O'Brien, K.K.; Colquhoun, H.; Levac, D.; Moher, D.; Peters, M.D.J.; Horsley, T.; Weeks, L.; et al. PRISMA Extension for Scoping Reviews (PRISMA-ScR): Checklist and Explanation. *Ann. Intern. Med.* **2018**, *169*, 467–473. [CrossRef] [PubMed]
24. World Health Organization. Who Report on the Global Tobacco Epidemic. 2009. Implementing Smoke-Free Environments. Available online: https://www.who.int/tobacco/mpower/2009/GTCR_2009-web.pdf (accessed on 22 July 2019).
25. McBride, C.M.; Emmons, K.M.; Lipkus, I.M. Understanding the potential of teachable moments: The case of smoking cessation. *Health Educ. Res.* **2003**, *18*, 156–170. [CrossRef]
26. Gage, J.D.; Everett, K.D.; Bullock, L. A review of research literature addressing male partners and smoking during pregnancy. *J. Obstet. Gynecol. Neonatal Nurs.* **2007**, *36*, 574–580. [CrossRef]
27. Pollak, K.I.; Denman, S.; Gordon, K.C.; Lyna, P.; Rocha, P.; Brouwer, R.N.; Fish, L.; Baucom, D.H. Is pregnancy a teachable moment for smoking cessation among US Latino expectant fathers? A pilot study. *Ethn. Health* **2010**, *15*, 47–59. [CrossRef]
28. Yin, H.; Chen, X.; Zheng, P.; Kegler, M.; Shen, Q.; Xu, B. A neglected opportunity for China's tobacco control? Shift in smoking behaviour during and after wives' pregnancy. *Tob. Induc. Dis.* **2016**, *14*, 39. [CrossRef]
29. Bottorff, J.L.; Oliffe, J.; Kalaw, C.; Carey, J.; Mroz, L. Men's constructions of smoking in the context of women's tobacco reduction during pregnancy and postpartum. *Soc. Sci. Med.* **2006**, *62*, 3096–3108. [CrossRef] [PubMed]
30. Flemming, K.; Graham, H.; McCaughan, D.; Angus, K.; Bauld, L. The barriers and facilitators to smoking cessation experienced by women's partners during pregnancy and the post-partum period: A systematic review of qualitative research. *BMC Public Health* **2015**, *25*, 849. [CrossRef] [PubMed]
31. Munn, Z.; Peters, M.D.J.; Stern, C.; Tufanaru, C.; McArthur, A.; Aromataris, E. Systematic review or scoping review? Guidance for authors when choosing between a systematic or scoping review approach. *BMC Med. Res. Methodol.* **2018**, *18*, 143. [CrossRef] [PubMed]
32. Moher, D.; Liberati, A.; Tetzlaff, J.; Altman, D.G.; The PRISMA group. Preferred reporting items for systematic reviews and MetaAnalyses: The PRISMA statement. *PLoS Med.* **2009**, *6*, e1000097. [CrossRef] [PubMed]
33. Nichter, M.; Padmajam, S.; Nichter, M.; Sairu, P.; Aswathy, S.; Mini, G.K.; Bindu, V.C.; Pradeepkumar, A.S.; Thankappan, K.R. Developing a smoke free homes initiative in Kerala, India. *BMC Public Health* **2015**, *15*, 480. [CrossRef] [PubMed]
34. Abdullah, A.S.; Hua, F.; Xia, X.; Hurlburt, S.; Ng, P.; MacLeod, W.; Siegel, M.; Griffiths, S.; Zhang, Z. Second-hand smoke exposure and household smoking bans in Chinese families: A qualitative study. *Health Soc. Care Community* **2012**, *20*, 356–364. [CrossRef] [PubMed]
35. Berg, J.C.; Zheng, P.; Kegler, M.C. Perceived benefits of smoke-free homes, the process of establishing them, and enforcement challenges in Shanghai, China: A qualitative study. *BMC Public Health* **2015**, *15*, 89. [CrossRef]
36. Kwon, J.; Oliffe, J.L.; Bottorff, J.L.; Kelly, M.T. Heterosexual gender relations and masculinity in fathers who smoke. *Res. Nurs. Health* **2014**, *37*, 391–398. [CrossRef]
37. Mao, A.; Bottorff, J.L.; Oliffe, J.L.; Sarbit, G.; Kelly, M.T. A qualitative study of Chinese Canadian fathers' smoking behaviours: Intersecting cultures and masculinities. *BMC Public Health* **2015**, *15*, 286. [CrossRef]

38. Mao, A.; Bottorff, J.L.; Oliffe, J.L.; Sarbit, G.; Kelly, M.T. A qualitative study on Chinese Canadian male immigrants' perspectives on stopping smoking: Implications for tobacco control in China. *Am. J. Men's Health* **2018**, *12*, 812–818. [CrossRef]
39. Oliffe, J.L.; Bottorff, J.L.; Johnson, J.L.; Kelly, M.T.; LeBeau, K. Fathers: Locating smoking and masculinity in the postpartum. *Qual. Health Res.* **2010**, *20*, 330–339. [CrossRef] [PubMed]
40. Saito, J.; Shibanuma, A.; Yasuoka, J.; Kondo, N.; Takagim, D.; Jimba, M. Education and indoor smoking among parents who smoke: The mediating role of perceived social norms of smoking. *BMC Public Health* **2018**, *18*, 211. [CrossRef] [PubMed]
41. Baheiraei, A.; Kharaghani, R.; Mohsenifar, A.; Kazemnejad, A.; Alikhani, S.; Sharifi Milani, H.; Mota, A.; Hovell, M.F. Reduction of secondhand smoke exposure among healthy infants in Iran: Randomized controlled trial. *Nicotine Tob. Res.* **2011**, *13*, 840–847. [CrossRef] [PubMed]
42. Chan, S.S.C.; Leung, D.Y.P.; Mak, Y.W.; Leung, G.M.; Leung, S.; Lam, T.H. New anti-smoking legislation on second-hand smoke exposure of children in homes. *Hong Kong Med. J.* **2011**, *17*, S38–S42.
43. Chan, S.S.; Cheung, Y.T.; Leung, D.Y.; Mak, Y.W.; Leung, G.M.; Lam, T.H. Secondhand smoke exposure and maternal action to protect children from secondhand smoke: Pre- and post-smokefree legislation in Hong Kong. *PLoS ONE* **2014**, *9*, e15781. [CrossRef] [PubMed]
44. Yu, S.; Duan, Z.; Redmon, P.B.; Eriksen, M.P.; Koplan, J.P.; Huang, C. mHealth intervention is effective in creating smoke-free homes for newborns: A randomized controlled trial study in China. *Sci. Rep.* **2017**, *7*, 9276. [CrossRef]
45. Nacaroglu, H.T.; Can, D.; Gunay, I.; Karkiner, C.; Gunay, T.; Cimrin, D.; Nalcabasmaz, T. Does raising awareness in families reduce environmental tobacco smoke exposure in wheezy children? *Postepy Dermatol. Alergol.* **2017**, *34*, 350–356. [CrossRef]
46. Behbod, B.; Sharma, M.; Baxi, R.; Roseby, R.; Webster, P. Family and carer smoking control programmes for reducing children's exposure to environmental tobacco smoke. *Cochrane Database Syst. Rev.* **2018**, *31*, CD001746. [CrossRef]
47. Rosen, L.J.; Myers, V.; Winickoff, J.P.; Kott, J. Effectiveness of interventions to reduce tobacco smoke pollution in homes: A systematic review and meta-analysis. *Int. J. Environ. Res. Public Health* **2015**, *12*, 16043–16059. [CrossRef]
48. Mdege, N.; Fairhurst, C.; Ferdous, T.; Hewitt, C.; Huque, R.; Jackson, C.; Kellar, I.; Parrott, S.; Semple, S.; Sheikh, A.; et al. Muslim Communities Learning About Second-hand Smoke in Bangladesh (MCLASS II): Study protocol for a cluster randomised controlled trial of a community-based smoke-free homes intervention, with or without Indoor Air Quality feedback. *Trials* **2019**, *20*, 11. [CrossRef]
49. Shah, S.; Ainsworth, H.; Fairhurst, C.; Tilbrook, H.; Sheikh, A.; Amos, A.; Parrott, S.; Torgerson, D.; Thompson, H.; King, R.; et al. Muslim communities learning about second-hand smoke: A pilot cluster randomised controlled trial and cost-effectiveness analysis. *NPJ Prim. Care Respir. Med.* **2015**, *25*, 15052. [CrossRef] [PubMed]
50. King, R.; Warsi, S.; Amos, A.; Shah, S.; Mir, G.; Sheikh, A.; Siddiqi, K. Involving mosques in health promotion programmes: A qualitative exploration of the MCLASS intervention on smoking in the home. *Health Educ. Res.* **2017**, *32*, 293–305. [CrossRef] [PubMed]
51. Hitchman, S.C.; Fong, G.T. Gender empowerment and female-to-male smoking prevalence ratios. *Bull. World Health Organ.* **2011**, *89*, 195–202. [CrossRef] [PubMed]
52. Dworkin, S.L.; Fleming, P.L.; Colvin, C.J. The promises and limitations of gender-transformative health programming with men: Critical reflections from the field. *Cult. Health Sex.* **2015**, *17*, 128–143. [CrossRef] [PubMed]
53. Gupta, G.R.; Parkhurst, J.O.; Ogden, J.A.; Aggleton, P.; Mahal, A. Structural approaches to HIV prevention. *Lancet* **2008**, *372*, 764–775. [CrossRef]
54. Zheng, P.; Berg, C.J.; Kegler, M.C.; Fu, W.; Wang, J.; Zhou, X.; Liu, D.; Fu, H. Smoke-free homes and home exposure to secondhand smoke in Shanghai, China. *Int. J. Environ. Res. Public Health* **2014**, *11*, 12015–12028. [CrossRef]
55. Wang, C.P.; Ma, S.J.; Xu, X.F.; Wang, J.F.; Mei, C.Z.; Yang, G.H. The prevalence of household second-hand smoke exposure and its correlated factors in six counties of China. *Tob. Control* **2009**, *18*, 121–126. [CrossRef]
56. Been, J.V.; Nurmatov, U.V.; Cox, B.; Nawrot, T.S.; van Schayck, C.P.; Sheikh, A. Effect of smoke-free legislation on perinatal and child health: A systematic review and meta-analysis. *Lancet* **2014**, *383*, 1549–1560. [CrossRef]

57. Monson, E.; Arsenault, N. Effects of enactment of legislative (public) smoking bans on voluntary home smoking restrictions: A review. *Nicotine Tob. Res.* **2017**, *19*, 141–148. [CrossRef]
58. Prestwich, A.; Webb, T.; Conner, M. Using theory to develop and test interventions to promote changes in health behaviour: Evidence, issues, and recommendations. *Curr. Opin. Psychol.* **2015**, *5*, 1–5. [CrossRef]

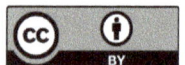

© 2019 by the authors. Licensee MDPI, Basel, Switzerland. This article is an open access article distributed under the terms and conditions of the Creative Commons Attribution (CC BY) license (http://creativecommons.org/licenses/by/4.0/).

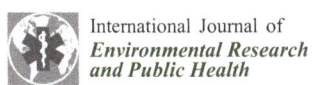

Review

Using a Developmental-Relational Approach to Understand the Impact of Interpersonal Violence in Women Who Struggle with Substance Use

Naomi C. Z. Andrews [1,*], Mary Motz [2], Bianca C. Bondi [3], Margaret Leslie [2] and Debra J. Pepler [3]

1. Department of Child and Youth Studies, Brock University,1812 Sir Isaac Brock Way, St. Catharines, ON L2S 3A1, Canada
2. Mothercraft, Early Intervention Department, 860 Richmond Street West, Toronto, ON M6J 1C9, Canada; mmotz@mothercraft.org (M.M.); mleslie@mothercraft.org (M.L.)
3. Department of Psychology, York University, 4700 Keele Street, Toronto, ON M3J 1P3, Canada; bbondi@yorku.ca (B.C.B.); pepler@yorku.ca (D.J.P.)
* Correspondence: nandrews@brocku.ca; Tel.: +1-905-688-5550 (ext. 4654)

Received: 27 September 2019; Accepted: 28 November 2019; Published: 3 December 2019

Abstract: Substance use among women is a major public health concern. This review article takes a developmental-relational approach to examine processes through which early relational trauma and violence in relationships may lead to substance use. We examine how early exposure to violence in relationships can impact neurological development, specifically through interference with physiological mechanisms (e.g., the hypothalamic-pituitary-adrenal axis), brain structure and functioning (e.g., the hippocampus and prefrontal cortex), and neuropsychological development (e.g., executive functioning and emotion regulation) across the lifespan. Further, we discuss the impact of exposure to violence on the development of relational capacity, including attachment, internal working models, and subsequent interpersonal relationships across the lifespan, and how these developmental pathways can lead to continued problematic substance use in women.

Keywords: interpersonal violence; domestic violence; substance use; intervention; women; developmental-relational; gender-specific approach

1. Introduction

Substance use among women is a major public health concern. There is recognition of the concurrent challenges associated with substance use and the barriers to reduce use for women (e.g., poverty, untreated mental health difficulties [1,2]). Another challenge is women's experiences with interpersonal violence. Interpersonal violence is commonly thought of as domestic violence or intimate partner violence. Though both women and men experience violence in partner relationships, women are more often victims of violence in relationships, experience more severe forms of violence, and are more afraid of the harm that abusers cause than are men (e.g., [3]). Importantly, experiences with violence in relationships often begin before women enter adulthood (e.g., via childhood maltreatment, witnessing violence between parents) and continue throughout adolescence and into early adulthood. It is for this reason that we use the term interpersonal violence (IPV), to highlight the developmental and intergenerational nature of violence in relationships and that violence in relationships is not exclusive to violence between partners. For many women, the struggle with substance use arises from their experiences of trauma and violence in relationships across development. Though there are many types of trauma for women, we will focus on interpersonal trauma, or trauma associated with violence in relationships. In this review paper, we discuss developmental mechanisms—neurological and relational—through which early and ongoing experiences with IPV can lead to substance use.

Though these developmental mechanisms may exist for both women and men, this paper will focus on what we know about these processes among women. That is, through clinical experience working with women who have substance use issues and a review of literature on women's substance use and relationships, this paper will explore the ways in which substance use may be a mechanism for coping with negative and traumatic relational experiences that many women have experienced since childhood and across development. Further, given that women are more often victims of interpersonal violence than are men [3], we focus on the pathways to substance use for women using a developmental-relational approach, and describe the importance of gender-specific programming for women who have experienced IPV and who use substances.

2. A Developmental-Relational Approach to Understand the Impact of IPV for Women

A developmental-relational approach is one in which the bidirectional associations between development and relationships are emphasized as important processes in understanding behavior and functioning. From a developmental perspective, we consider the individual and environmental contributions to development, and focus on how the transactional nature of these contributions changes and grows over time throughout childhood, adolescence, and adulthood [4]. From this perspective, developmental experiences are seen as contributing to cascading trauma and violence in relationships and future substance use, given their impact on neurological and relational mechanisms. In working with substance using women and their children, we recognize that negative developmental experiences must be attended to across the lifespan to promote optimal neurological and relational development. From a relational perspective, we consider development—growth within the individual, the environment, and within and across systems—as coming about through relationships with others [5,6]. Thus, the developmental-relational approach places individuals' behaviors (e.g., substance use) within a larger context that includes an understanding of their history and ongoing development over time, and a focus on how behavior is shaped through relationships within the broader systemic context.

This approach has been established through our research and clinical understanding of women attending a community-based prevention and early intervention program in Canada called Breaking the Cycle (BTC) [7,8]. Since 1995, Breaking the Cycle has provided comprehensive, integrated supports for mothers who are struggling with substance use issues, and their young children aged 0-6 years. Programming at BTC is directed towards women, their children, and the mother-child relationship. Over the past 25 years, we have come to understand that the vast majority of women who struggle with substance use issues in their adult lives have been traumatized in relationships since early childhood and across development. The lifelong struggle with trauma in relationships is often part of the experience faced by women with substance use issues. A developmental-relational approach can be used to more fully understand this link, as follows. (1) Experiences of interpersonal violence can be viewed as disruptions to normative developmental processes across the lifespan that can create and perpetuate lifelong trauma; (2) Interpersonal violence can begin in early childhood, including experiences of child maltreatment and neglect, and have enduring and compounding impacts, often continuing into adolescence and adulthood [9]; (3) Experiences of trauma in relationships can also involve witnessing violence between parents or caregivers, being manipulated by one caregiver to abuse the other, experiencing the aftermath of violence against a caregiver, and suffering the consequences of financial abuse, among others [10–12]; (4) Early traumatic experiences can also include household dysfunction, including conflictual parental divorce or separation, parental incarceration, as well as living with a parent experiencing mental health or substance use issues [13,14]. These adverse childhood experiences (ACEs) are consistently shown to relate to poor mental and physical health outcomes and wellbeing in adulthood [14–16]. All of these experiences are relational in nature, in that they disrupt positive bonds between caregivers and children, they damage a child's sense of safety in relationships, and they disrupt the development of secure attachment between children and their parents [17,18]. These disruptions can have long-term consequences across development and into adulthood [19,20]. As such, it is essential to understand developmental experiences of trauma in relationships as pervading beyond early childhood, contributing to a cascade of trauma and violence in relationships given their impact on adult life, including difficulties forming healthy relationships, difficulties in parenting, ineffective coping strategies, and problematic substance use. It is also vital to consider the potential underlying neurological and relational mechanisms that may contribute to these cascading effects.

These links are evident in our work with women who struggle with substance use at BTC. Women's initiation of substance use, problematic substance use, use of substances to cope, and inability or difficulty abstaining from substance use stem from the lifelong trauma of adverse relational experiences and their impact on development. For instance, in a sample of 160 women who had substance use issues and received services at BTC, the majority reported experiences of interpersonal violence in childhood (see [21] for a full description of the sample and methodology). Specifically, 88% of women reported a history of physical abuse, with almost half of those women (49%) reporting that the abuse began when they were 10 years or younger (see Table 1). Eighty-nine percent of women reported a history of emotional abuse, with over half of those women reporting that the abuse started before adolescence (12 years or younger). Finally, 76% of women reported a history of sexual abuse, with almost a quarter (22%) of those women reporting that the abuse began when they were five years old or younger. Almost half (43%) of women had involvement with the child welfare system when they were children.

Table 1. Percentage of Women Reporting Histories of Abuse Across Childhood.

Onset of Abuse	Physical Abuse (%)	Emotional Abuse (%)	Sexual Abuse (%)
Percentage of women reporting histories of abuse (total)	88	89	76
Onset (among women who reported abuse)			
"As long as I can remember"	5	10	0
Early childhood	9	7	22
Childhood	35	33	20
Late childhood	5	4	6
Early adolescence	6	6	13
Adolescence	15	24	12
Late adolescence	3	1	8
Adulthood	22	15	19

Early childhood = 0–5 years. Childhood = 6–10 years. Late childhood = 11–12 years. Early adolescence = 13–14 years. Adolescence = 15–16 years. Late adolescence = 17–18 years. Adulthood = 19 years or older.

The overwhelming majority of women at BTC have used or are currently using alcohol, and many reported that their alcohol use began at very young ages: 19% of women reported first using alcohol when they were 10 years old or younger (in the same sample of 160 women; [21]). Problematic alcohol use also began early: 7% reported that problematic use began in childhood, and an additional 56% reported that problematic use began in adolescence. Women also reported that they started to use other substances at very young ages (12 or younger), with 24% of those who used reporting early cannabis and 6% reporting early cocaine or crack cocaine use. Of the women who used, many reported that their use of these substances became problematic in adolescence (prior to age 19): 77% cannabis, 74% nicotine, 66% hallucinogens, 64% amphetamines, 43% barbiturates, 39% cocaine, 38% heroin, and 27% crack cocaine. As girls and teenagers, these women began using substances as a means of coping with the relational trauma that they were experiencing and/or had experienced. One BTC woman talked about her history of physical abuse at the hands of her mother, who was also a substance user:

> All of the things I witnessed at home really affected me in my early teenage years ... and at that point I became addicted myself. And so, even though I kind of had a realization that I was following in my mom's footsteps, I wasn't really able to do anything about it, and my own cycle of addiction kind of took over at that point. [22] (p. 98)

Another woman discussed how her early experiences of violence and trauma had lifelong consequences on her patterns of thought and behavior.

> *It creates a lifetime of fear because you've spent a lifetime like that, walking on eggshells, not knowing ... just expected to duck the next blow ... It's something that's been one of the hardest things in my life to challenge and attempt to change, because it's something that I've been formed like ... I have, you know, severe reactionary issues when it comes to safety, and conversely overreactive sense of safety.* [23] (p. 22)

Our research has also identified the developmental pathways leading to continued problematic substance use. These pathways have been discussed as dynamic cascades or developmental cascades: early risk factors increase exposure to more risk processes that develop across the lifespan [24–26]. From a developmental-relational perspective, we have begun to understand how early experiences of interpersonal violence can cascade to impact and impede development across development and into adulthood. Without healthy relationships, relationship capacity is delayed and relationship perspectives are skewed (e.g., women learn to expect violence as a part of close relationships; see Section 2). As one BTC woman reported:

> *There was all this violence in our house, and I thought that was normal, and I thought that's what I was supposed to be growing up. And I was receiving violence from whomever, and I just let that happen ...* [27] (p. 15)

The continued impact of these relationship challenges is also evident in women's ongoing experiences of violence, with 14% of women reporting that their current partner relationships have been abusive, and 13% of women reporting that their past partner relationships were violent (see [21] for sample details). Other close relationships appear to be impacted as well, as many women reported little to no contact with their families of origin (little to no contact with mothers, 31%; and fathers, 47%), or reported difficult and/or abusive relationships with their mothers (25%) and fathers (9%). One BTC woman talked about the effect of violence in her family:

> *[It] de-sensitized you a little bit ... my parents were so abusive towards each other, and there was no respect or love or affection, and there was always turmoil, turmoil, turmoil – we were moving, there was fighting, there was police, there was violence – that I found out even as an adult, because that was so normal for me, if my life was going along smoothly and calmly, it's like unfamiliar so I create this chaos, this craziness, because that feels more comfortable to me.* [27] (p. 16)

Through the work conducted at BTC, it is also evident that an intervention focusing on supporting healthy relationships can help to decrease women's problematic use of substances. For instance, in a comparison of BTC to a standard integrated treatment program that included a focus on addiction treatment but did not focus explicitly on supporting and enhancing relationship capacity, it was found that women attending BTC had improvements in relationship capacity, mental health symptoms, as well as addiction severity [28]. Indeed, improvements in relationship capacity among women at BTC further predicted decreases in addiction severity, even accounting for other improvements, including social support, mental health, and abstinence self-efficacy. In another study, it was found that the duration of service use at BTC was associated with improvements in women's substance use (as well as improvements in the parent-child relationship) [21]. Further, the earlier that woman began the relationship-based intervention (i.e., during pregnancy as opposed to postnatally), the more positive the outcomes. These studies provide further support for the critical link between relationship capacity and substance use issues, as evidenced by improvements based on attending a relationship-based and trauma-informed intervention program.

It should be noted that there are many co-occurring factors that compound the life challenges of women with substance use issues; these factors include poverty, low educational attainment, unstable housing, criminal involvement, and mental health difficulties (often untreated). Women at BTC reported high levels of depression and anxiety and a lack of social support from both family and friends [7]. These factors, as well as a host of other factors, are implicated in the complex interplay of, and challenges associated with, problematic substance use for women, particularly in the context of parenting. Though we won't address these factors in detail here, they are often present and play a critical role in women's continued substance use. Thus, we acknowledge the impact of these additional factors, but focus on using a developmental-relational approach to elucidate the role of prior trauma and experiences of relational violence across the lifespan in our understanding of women's substance use.

3. Origins of Substance Use in Women Exposed to IPV

Research offers converging evidence that exposure to IPV in childhood and across development contributes to future substance use issues. Robust effects are found specifically for females within the literature, with substance use issues persisting into middle adulthood for only female (and not male) victims of childhood maltreatment [29–32] and physical abuse [33]. Although there are a few studies on the mechanisms of the intergenerational pathway from IPV in childhood to subsequent substance use issues, several processes have been proposed. The disruptive effects of early experiences of IPV on psychosocial functioning, the stress response system, and the limbic system may lead to heightened risk-taking behaviors, such as the use of substances [34,35]. Substance use may also serve as an external mechanism to cope with, or escape from, the negative effects of trauma across development [36]. Several studies have indicated that maltreatment may result in greater risk for the development of internalizing symptoms in females than in males (e.g., [37–40]). This differential risk could account, in part, for the higher incidence of internalizing problems in females relative to males (e.g., [41,42]). Therefore, as an external coping mechanism, substance use is thought to be particularly notable in women given that they may be more prone than men to internalizing symptoms due to early experiences of IPV, which can elicit self-destructive behaviors (i.e., substance use) [43]. Because substance use does not directly address the negative effects of trauma, the need for substances may persist or increase over time, thus heightening the risk for substance use issues and dependence [30]. Given that women exposed to early IPV are also more likely to have low self-esteem or low perceived self-efficacy, substance use issues have been proposed as a means through which they enhance their self-esteem [30]. Chronic substance use may also arise from these women's low perceived self-efficacy in regards to maintaining abstinence [36]. In addition, substance use may be a means through which women are able to reduce feelings of isolation and loneliness, gain control over negative experiences, or engage in self-destructive behavior [43]. Externalizing behaviors, antisocial behaviors, and abuse-related posttraumatic stress disorder (PTSD) may mediate the relation between early experiences of IPV and future substance use issues [30]. In the following sections, we discuss the mechanisms that appear most significant in leading women to substance use within a developmental-relational perspective.

3.1. IPV and Neurological Development

Exposure to IPV can negatively impact neurological development, affecting physiological mechanisms, brain structure and functioning, as well as overall neuropsychological development. Although neurological development is most vulnerable to the effects of IPV during early childhood, these detrimental effects persist across the lifespan. Impairments in neurological development impact other developmental domains, including physical, cognitive, and social-emotional development. The literature highlighted in this section predominately captures studies on male and female victims of childhood maltreatment; however, some studies are specific to females with histories of childhood maltreatment or intimate partner violence (e.g., [44,45]).

3.1.1. Physiological Mechanisms

Exposure to IPV can interfere with the sympathetic nervous system and the hypothalamic-pituitary-adrenal (HPA) axis. Exposure to IPV can induce chronic psychological stress that results in repeated activation of the HPA axis and subsequent HPA axis dysfunction [44,46,47].

Children exposed to IPV often have elevated baseline cortisol (stress hormone) levels, as well as a faster increase and slower decline of cortisol following stress exposures [48]. At chronically elevated levels, cortisol can have neurotoxic effects on "nonessential" brain regions during the stress response [44]. Neurotoxic effects have subsequent consequences on brain structure and functioning [49], which can persist into adulthood [44,46]. Chronic cortisol elevation also leads to increased arousal, anxiety, aggression, hypervigilance, sympathetic nervous system stimulation, depression, and PTSD [50].

3.1.2. Brain Structure and Functioning

Many areas of the brain undergo neurobiological changes upon exposure to chronic stress via IPV across development. Research has identified the effects of IPV on brain structure and functioning in the midbrain, sensory cortices and fiber tracts, corpus callosum, and dopaminergic reward circuit (e.g., [51]). There is also a substantial body of research on the structural and functional effects of IPV on the stress response system through the HPA axis, which is expanded upon below.

The plasticity of the fetal, infant, and early childhood brain creates a heightened sensitivity to chemical influences of chronic stress exposure [52]. Many glucocorticoid receptors exist within the amygdala, hippocampus, and prefrontal cortex (PFC), which are part of a network of connected regions involved in the stress response. Exposure to early stressful experiences alters the size and neuronal architecture of these regions, contributing to functional differences in learning, memory, and executive functioning [46,53]. Chronic exposure to stress is associated with overactivity in the amygdala and orbitofrontal cortex, as well as the loss of neurons and neuronal connections in the hippocampus and medial PFC [53]. Functionally, these structural changes result in more fear and anxiety due to the hyperactivation of the amygdala, alongside lower higher-order PFC control [54].

The hippocampus is involved in the HPA axis and modulates cortisol levels; however, chronic stress diminishes this capacity due to hippocampal volume loss, which is linked to memory and mood-related impairments [53,54]. Chronic stress exposure can lead to impairments in memory encoding and contextual learning, which are vital for discriminating conditions of danger from safety [44,53]. Decreased neuronal volume in the PFC impairs executive and cognitive functioning; the loss of neuronal connections between the hippocampus and the PFC hinders the PFC's regulation of heightened cortisol levels and the regulation of autonomic balance between sympathetic and parasympathetic nervous system responses [46,53]. Chronic stress also induces architectural and connection changes within and between the hippocampus, PFC, and amygdala, potentially contributing to variability in stress-responsiveness [55]. These structural changes can functionally heighten reactivity to mild levels of stress and impair coping abilities during future stress both in childhood and across the lifespan (e.g., [52]).

3.1.3. Neuropsychological Development

Although research has only begun to address the structural and related functional impairments in brain development due to exposure to IPV, there is a substantial body of research on the resulting neuropsychological impairments in executive functioning and emotion regulation. Executive functioning enables flexible, context-appropriate, goal-oriented emotional and behavioral responses and is largely localized in the PFC [56]. Exposure to IPV during childhood is associated with the development of impairments in executive functioning processes, which, in turn, are associated with increased risk for PTSD and depression [46]. Deficits in executive functioning due to trauma in relationships may accumulate across development, persisting through adolescence and into adulthood; more pronounced deficits have been found with an earlier onset of trauma (e.g., [57]). Deficits in executive functioning pose heightened risk for future substance use issues; therefore, executive functioning deficits may represent a mechanism in the intergenerational pathway between IPV and substance use [58].

Differences in the structure, function, and connectivity of prefrontal regions underlying executive functioning processes are also associated with impairments in emotion regulation in adults with

PTSD due to IPV [45,59]. Emotion regulation involves strategies to manage cognitive, behavioral, and physiological responses to emotions [46] and is largely localized to the anterior cingulate cortex within the PFC [44]. Children exposed to IPV often have persisting deficits in emotion regulation, including attentional biases to negative or threatening stimuli, trouble recognizing emotions, and difficulty effectively modulating or reappraising distress [46]. Problems with emotion regulation are also correlated with lower levels of social competence, difficulties with peer relationships, aggressiveness, and disruptive behaviors that can impact functioning into adulthood [47]. Additionally, emotion dysregulation contributes to mental health problems, including PTSD and depression [60]. Children exposed to IPV may struggle with emotional awareness, understanding, and regulation because such capacities are developed, in part, through interactions with supportive caregivers and adults (e.g., [61]). Children who experience IPV often receive less positive modeling of emotional labeling, expression, and regulation behaviors, which leads to deficits in appropriate emotion regulation capacities [46]. Exposure to childhood IPV is linked to emotion regulation deficits across the lifespan; however, emotion regulation is most impacted by chronic trauma in early development [46]. Given that deficits in emotion regulation pose heightened risk for future substance use issues, emotion dysregulation may represent a critical mechanism in the pathway between IPV and substance use [62,63].

3.2. IPV and the Development of Relational Capacity

Exposure to IPV can negatively impact the development of relational capacity across various levels, affecting attachment, internal working models, and subsequent interpersonal relationships. The impact of IPV on the development of relational capacity contributes to future substance use issues. In fact, the link between difficulties in relationships and substance use may be particularly strong for women. Relationships are important to women, and women who use substances may have less social support and are more likely than men to have important people in their lives who also struggle with substance use issues (e.g., families of origin, partners) [64–67]. Further, male partners with substance use issues may be resistant to and unsupportive of their female partners' attempts to access treatment [68]; women may, therefore, be hesitant and fear damaging these relationships by engaging in substance use treatment. Thus, women's initiation and continuation of substance use (including relapse) may often occur in the context of relationships, or as a result of challenges in relationships. We will describe the pathways through which early and enduring experiences of violence in relationships can affect ongoing relationship challenges into adulthood, which in turn can impact women's substance use.

3.2.1. Attachment

Attachment theory postulates that children are predisposed to seek and sustain relationships that satisfy their intrinsic need for security [69]. The failure to develop secure attachment reverberates across the lifespan in the form of difficulties with relationships, self-esteem, and the regulation of emotions and impulses [70]. Predictable, sensitive, and responsive caregiving during times of stress is crucial for healthy child development [47]; however, for children exposed to IPV, chronic stress often occurs within the context of the caregiving relationship. Research has consistently demonstrated that maltreated children have higher rates of insecure attachment, namely disorganized attachment, relative to non-maltreated children, even when compared to other high-risk children (e.g., [71]). Similarly, maltreated children have been consistently found to be at heightened risk for future substance use issues [72–74], with effects persisting into middle adulthood for females only [29–32]. Children classified as having disorganized attachment often vacillate between avoidant and anxious parent-child behaviors due to conflicting and unpredictable caregiver responses; these children often have poor outcomes across many domains, including lower academic achievement and self-esteem, poor peer interactions, atypical classroom behaviors, cognitive immaturity, and externalizing behavioral concerns (e.g., [70]). Disorganized attachment is further associated with poor mental health outcomes in adulthood, including borderline personality disorder and dissociative identity disorder [75]. Although much research has indicated the relationship between maltreatment and future substance use issues, a growing body of literature has begun to address attachment as a key mechanism in this relationship [74]. Attachment insecurity with caregivers poses a heightened risk for future substance use issues in adolescence and adulthood [76–80]. There is also strong evidence for the temporal precedent of attachment issues, with insecure attachment predating the onset or increased use of substances across time [81].

3.2.2. Internal Working Models

The characteristic patterns of caregivers' responses to children's expression of attachment behavior accumulate over time [82]. These patterns are organized into schematic cognitive representations of the parent-child relationship, theorized as internal working models of attachment [69,83]. Children use their internal working models of attachment to perceive and appraise attachment-related information and to plan future action [83]. Based on the internal working model of attachment, children develop expectations about the self and others: the self as worthy or unworthy of care and protection and others as available or unavailable to provide care and protection when needed [69]. Children exposed to IPV develop negative models of themselves as unworthy of care and protection, and models of their caregivers as rejecting and unreliable [71]. Although internal working models of attachment develop across the lifespan alongside changes in cognitive capacity and attachment relationships, the models show great stability throughout life [84].

Children who experience IPV early in life may transfer their negative internal working models of attachment to future relationships, thus expecting the same abuse in adult relationships and viewing such abuse as normative [85,86]. Therefore, according to attachment theories, IPV in early caregiving relationships initiates a developmental cascade in which insecure attachments continue to occur across the lifespan, due to existing insecure internal working models [87]. In addition to impacting attachment in future relationships, internal working models contribute to one's ability to regulate emotions autonomously in the absence of an attachment figure [77]. As discussed above, deficits in emotion regulation contribute to future substance use issues, thus representing a mechanism in the pathway between IPV and substance use given the impact on attachment and internal working models [62,63]. Furthermore, IPV and insecure attachment are more common in children whose parents also experienced IPV and insecure attachment [88]. Therefore, there is intergenerational transmission of both attachment styles and IPV (e.g., [89–91]). Attachment styles and the development of internal working models have a putative mediating role in the intergenerational transmission of IPV and subsequent substance use issues, given that IPV becomes a frame through which people come to understand relationships, and substance use becomes a means through which people regulate emotions in the absence of secure attachment and positive internal working models [76,77,87]. This may be particularly problematic for women, given the importance women place on relationships and the lack of social support that substance using women often face (in comparison to men) [64,65].

3.3. A Model of IPV and Substance Use Across the Lifespan

Overall, early and enduring experiences of IPV negatively impact neurological development, namely physiological mechanisms, brain structure and functioning, as well as neuropsychological development (i.e., executive functioning and emotion regulation). Experiences of IPV across development are traumatic and disrupt the development of relational capacity, specifically attachment and internal working models that affect relationships characterized by IPV across the lifespan [71]. IPV negatively impacts executive functioning [46] and emotion regulation [44,46,47], which are also impaired through substance use issues [92]. There is a strong relationship between childhood IPV and future substance use issues [30], thus compounding the negative effects that both factors have on executive functioning and emotion regulation. These neuropsychological deficits interact to divert development onto a pathway toward unhealthy relationships. At the same time, these deficits elicit substance use as a necessary means of coping (see Figure 1 for an illustrative model).

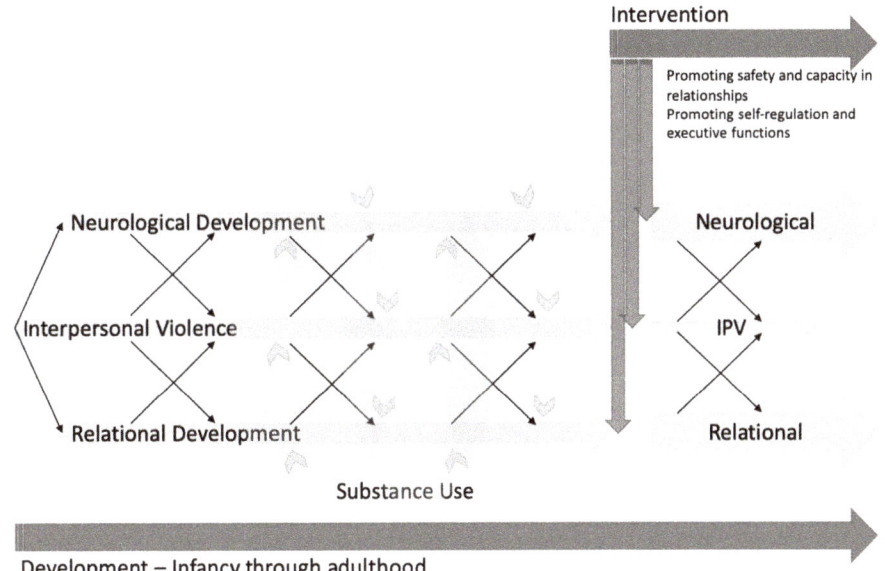

Figure 1. A model of interpersonal violence (IPV) and substance use (SU) across the lifespan, highlighting the bidirectional effects of IPV on neurological and relational development.

4. Conclusions

In this review paper, we have outlined how a developmental-relational approach helps us understand the link between women's experiences of violence in relationships across development and later substance use issues. Potential mechanisms that underly this pathway include impairments to neurological development, namely physiological mechanisms, brain structure and functioning, and neuropsychological development (i.e., executive functioning and emotion regulation), as well as impairment to the development of relational capacity (i.e., attachment and internal working models). Though there is a paucity of research specifically examining differences in these links between women and men (particularly regarding the neurological effects of childhood maltreatment), there is some evidence that early experiences of IPV may be particularly problematic for women and may lead to enduring substance use into adulthood. For instance, women may internalize trauma and turn to substances as a coping mechanism more so than men [43], and women's initiation and continuation of substance use seems to occur often in the context of relationships [66,67], which are negatively impacted by early experiences of IPV.

Through this review, we have highlighted that IPV is a lifelong disrupting force on women's neurological development and capacity for relationships, which can lead women to use substances, as well as to further developmental and relational impairments. These factors can perpetuate the pathway of IPV across the lifespan, while reinforcing substance use as a necessary means of coping. A developmental-relational approach to understanding substance use, therefore, has important implications for clinical practice. In a recent review, we outlined specific strategies that can be used to promote women's self-regulation and executive functions (e.g., supporting time management through reminder phone calls and predictable appointments), and promoting safety and capacity in relationships (e.g., staff training in trauma-informed practice) [93]. Attention should also be paid to strategies that may be uniquely important for women (e.g., including a buzzer entry system; not allowing male partners in the center) and mothers (e.g., providing child-minding and child development programming in the same program location). As such, by using a developmental-relational approach to understand women's pathways to substance use, we can begin to engage in a process of reparation and reintegration for women whose neurological development, sense of self, and capacity to form relationships has been significantly impacted by experiences of violence in relationships.

Author Contributions: For this article, several authors gave their individual contributions as follows: Conceptualization, N.C.Z.A., M.M., M.L., and D.J.P.; investigation, N.C.Z.A. and B.C.B.; writing—original draft preparation, N.C.Z.A., M.M., and B.C.B; writing—review and editing, M.L. and D.J.P; supervision, M.L. and D.J.P.

Funding: This research received no external funding.

Conflicts of Interest: The authors declare no conflict of interest.

References

1. Mandavia, A.; Robinson, G.G.N.; Bradley, B.; Ressler, K.J.; Power, A. Exposure to Childhood Abuse and Later Substance Use: Indirect Effects of Emotion Dysregulation and Exposure to Trauma. *J. Trauma. Stress* **2016**, *29*, 422–429. [CrossRef] [PubMed]
2. Wong, S.; Ordean, A.; Kahan, M. Substance Use in Pregnancy. *Int. J. Gynecol. Obstet.* **2011**, *114*, 190–202. [CrossRef]
3. Canadian Centre for Justice Statistics. *Family Violence in Canada: A Statistical Profile*; Minister of Industry: Ottawa, ON, Canada, 2014.
4. Sameroff, A. The Transactional Model. In *The Transactional Model of Development: How Children and Contexts Shape Each Other*; Sameroff, A., Ed.; American Psychological Association: Washington, DC, USA, 2009; pp. 3–21. [CrossRef]
5. Jordan, J.V.; Walker, M.; Hartling, L.M. (Eds.) *The Complexity of Connection*; The Guildford Press: New York, NY, USA, 2004.
6. Walker, M.; Rosen, W.B. (Eds.) *How Connections Heal: Stories from Relational-Cultural Therapy*; Guilford Press: New York, NY, USA, 2004.
7. Motz, M.; Leslie, M.; Pepler, D.; Moore, T.; Freeman, P. Breaking the Cycle: Measures of Progress 1995–2005. *J. Fas Int.* **2006**, *4*, 1–134.
8. Motz, M.; Leslie, M.; Pepler, D.J. Breaking the Cycle: A Comprehensive, Early Intervention Program Supporting Substance-Exposed Infants, Young Children, and Their Mothers. In *Healthy Development, Healthy Communities*; Pepler, D.J., Cummings, J., Craig, W.M., Eds.; PREVNet Series Volume IV: Kingston, ON, Canada, 2016; pp. 115–134.
9. Van der Kolk, B.A. This Issue: Child Abuse and Victimization. *Psychiatr. Ann.* **2005**, *35*, 374–379. [CrossRef]
10. Leslie, M.; Reynolds, W.; Motz, M.; Pepler, D.J. *Building Connections: Supporting Community-Based Programs to Address Interpersonal Violence and Child Maltreatment*; Mothercraft Press: Toronto, ON, Canada, 2016.
11. Katz, E. Beyond the Physical Incident Model: How Children Living with Domestic Violence Are Harmed by and Resist Regimes of Coercive Control. *Child Abus. Rev.* **2016**, *25*, 46–59. [CrossRef]
12. McTavish, J.R.; MacGregor, J.C.D.; Wathen, C.N.; MacMillan, H.L. Children's Exposure to Intimate Partner Violence: An Overview. *Int. Rev. Psychiatry* **2016**, *28*, 504–518. [CrossRef]
13. Crouch, E.; Probst, J.C.; Radcliff, E.; Bennett, K.J.; McKinney, S.H. Prevalence of Adverse Childhood Experiences (ACEs) among US Children. *Child Abus. Negl.* **2019**, *92*, 209–218. [CrossRef]
14. Felitti, V.J.; Anda, R.F.; Nordenberg, D.; Williamson, D.F.; Spitz, A.M.; Edwards, V.; Koss, M.P.; Marks, J.S. Relationship of Childhood Abuse and Household Dysfunction to Many of the Leading Causes of Death in Adults: The Adverse Childhood Experiences (ACE) Study. *Am. J. Prev. Med.* **1998**, *14*, 245–258. [CrossRef]
15. Fuller-Thomson, E.; Baird, S.L.; Dhrodia, R.; Brennenstuhl, S. The Association between Adverse Childhood Experiences (ACEs) and Suicide Attempts in a Population-Based Study. *Child Care Health Dev.* **2016**, *42*, 725–734. [CrossRef]
16. Kalmakis, K.A.; Chandler, G.E. Health Consequences of Adverse Childhood Experiences: A Systematic Review. *J. Am. Assoc. Nurse Pract.* **2015**, *27*, 457–465. [CrossRef]
17. Fusco, R.A. Socioemotional Problems in Children Exposed to Intimate Partner Violence: Mediating Effects of Attachment and Family Supports. *J. Interpers. Violence* **2017**, *32*, 2515–2532. [CrossRef] [PubMed]

18. Gustafsson, H.C.; Brown, G.L.; Mills-Koonce, W.R.; Cox, M.J. Intimate Partner Violence and Children's Attachment Representations during Middle Childhood. *J. Marriage Fam.* **2017**, *79*, 865–878. [CrossRef] [PubMed]
19. Oshri, A.; Sutton, T.E.; Clay-Warner, J.; Miller, J.D. Child Maltreatment Types and Risk Behaviors: Associations with Attachment Style and Emotion Regulation Dimensions. *Pers. Individ. Dif.* **2015**, *73*, 127–133. [CrossRef]
20. Widom, C.S.; Czaja, S.J.; Kozakowski, S.S.; Chauhan, P. Does Adult Attachment Style Mediate the Relationship between Childhood Maltreatment and Mental and Physical Health Outcomes? *Child Abus. Negl.* **2018**, *76*, 533–545. [CrossRef]
21. Leslie, M.; DeMarchi, G.; Motz, M. Breaking the Cycle: An Essay in Three Voices. In *With Child—Substance Use During Pregnancy: A Woman-Centered Approach*; Boyd, S., Marcellus, L., Eds.; Fernwood Publishing: Peterborough, UK, 2007; pp. 91–104.
22. BTC Client; Toronto, ON, Canada. Personal Communication, 2006.
23. Dodge, K.A.; Malone, P.S.; Lansford, J.E.; Miller, S.; Pettit, G.S.; Bates, J.E. A Dynamic Cascade Model of the Development of Substance-Use Onset. *Monogr. Soc. Res. Child Dev.* **2009**, *74*. [CrossRef]
24. Eiden, R.D.; Lessard, J.; Colder, C.R.; Livingston, J.; Casey, M.; Leonard, K.E. Developmental Cascade Model for Adolescent Substance Use from Infancy to Late Adolescence. *Dev. Psychol.* **2016**, *52*, 1619–1633. [CrossRef]
25. Otten, R.; Mun, C.J.; Shaw, D.S.; Wilson, M.N.; Dishion, T.J. A Developmental Cascade Model for Early Adolescent- Onset Substance Use: The Role of Early Childhood Stress. *Addiction* **2018**, *114*, 326–334. [CrossRef]
26. Breaking the Cycle. *Connections: A Group Intervention for Mothers and Children Experiencing Violence in Relationships*; Mothercraft Press: Toronto, ON, Canada, 2014.
27. Espinet, S.D.; Motz, M.; Jeong, J.J.; Jenkins, J.M.; Pepler, D. 'Breaking the Cycle' of Maternal Substance Use through Relationships: A Comparison of Integrated Approaches. *Addict. Res. Theory* **2016**, *24*, 375–388. [CrossRef]
28. Andrews, N.C.Z.; Motz, M.; Pepler, D.J.; Jeong, J.J.; Khoury, J. Engaging Mothers with Substance Use Issues and Their Children in Early Intervention: Understanding Use of Service and Outcomes. *Child Abus. Negl.* **2018**, *83*, 10–20. [CrossRef]
29. Appleyard, K.; Berlin, L.J.; Rosanbalm, K.D.; Dodge, K.A. Preventing Early Child Maltreatment: Implications from a Longitudinal Study of Maternal Abuse History, Substance Use Problems, and Offspring Victimization. *Prev. Sci.* **2011**, *12*, 139–149. [CrossRef]
30. Widom, C.; Hiller-Sturmhofel, S. Alcohol Abuse as a Risk Factor for and Consequence of Child Abuse. *Alcohol Res. Heal.* **2001**, *25*, 52. [CrossRef]
31. Widom, C.; Marmorstein, N.; White, R. Childhood Victimization and Illicit Drug Use in Middle Adulthood. *Psychol. Addict. Behav.* **2006**, *20*, 394. [CrossRef] [PubMed]
32. Widom, C.; White, H.; Czaja, S.; Marmorstein, N. Long-Term Effects of Child Abuse and Neglect on Alcohol Use and Excessive Drinking in Middle Adulthood. *J. Stud. Alcohol Drugs* **2007**, *68*, 317–326. [CrossRef]
33. Lansford, J.E.; Dodge, K.A.; Pettit, G.S.; Bates, J.E. Does Physical Abuse in Early Childhood Predict Substance Use in Adolescence and Early Adulthood? *Child Maltreat.* **2010**, *15*, 190–194. [CrossRef] [PubMed]
34. Anderson, C.M.; Teicher, M.H.; Polcari, A.; Renshaw, P.F. Abnormal T2 Relaxation Time in the Cerebellar Vermis of Adults Sexually Abused in Childhood: Potential Role of the Vermis in Stress Enhanced Risk for Drug Abuse. *Psychoneuroendocrinology* **2002**, *27*, 231–244. [CrossRef]
35. Repetti, R.L.; Taylor, S.E.; Seeman, T.E. Risky Families: Family Social Environments and the Mental and Physical Health of Offspring. *Psychol. Bull.* **2002**, *128*, 330. [CrossRef] [PubMed]
36. Latuskie, K.A.; Andrews, N.C.Z.; Motz, M.; Leibson, T.; Austin, Z.; Ito, S.; Pepler, D.J. Reasons for Substance Use Continuation and Discontinuation during Pregnancy: A Qualitative Study. *Women Birth* **2019**, *32*, e57–e64. [CrossRef]
37. McGee, R.A.; Wolfe, D.A.; Wilson, S.K. Multiple Maltreatment Experiences and Adolescent Behavior Problems: Adolescents' Perspectives. *Dev. Psychopathol.* **1997**, *9*, 131–149. [CrossRef]
38. Lansford, J.E.; Dodge, K.A.; Pettit, G.S.; Bates, J.E.; Crozier, J.; Kaplow, J. A 12-Year Prospective Study of the Long-Term Effects of Early Child Physical Maltreatment on Psychological, Behavioral, and Academic Problems in Adolescence. *Arch. Pediatr. Adolesc. Med.* **2002**, *156*, 824–830. [CrossRef]

39. Macmillan, H.L.; Fleming, J.E.; Streiner, D.L.; Lin, E.; Boyle, M.H.; Jamieson, E.; Duku, E.K.; Walsh, C.A.; Wong, M.Y.Y.; Beardslee, W.R. Childhood Abuse and Lifetime Psychopathology in a Community Sample. *Am. J. Psychiatry* **2001**, *158*, 1878–1883. [CrossRef]
40. Herringa, R.J.; Birn, R.M.; Ruttle, P.L.; Burghy, C.A.; Stodola, D.E.; Davidson, R.J.; Essex, M.J. Childhood Maltreatment Is Associated with Altered Fear Circuitry and Increased Internalizing Symptoms by Late Adolescence. *Proc. Natl. Acad. Sci. USA* **2013**, *110*, 19119–19124. [CrossRef] [PubMed]
41. Kessler, R.C.; Berglund, P.; Demler, O.; Jin, R.; Merikangas, K.R.; Walters, E.E. Lifetime Prevalence and Age-of-Onset Distributions of DSM-IV Disorders in the National Comorbidity Survey Replication. *Arch. Gen. Psychiatry* **2005**, *62*, 593–602. [CrossRef] [PubMed]
42. Cahill, L. Why Sex Matters for Neuroscience. *Nat. Rev. Neurosci.* **2006**, *7*, 477. [CrossRef] [PubMed]
43. Widom, C.; Ireland, T.; Glynn, P.J. Alcohol Abuse in Abused and Neglected Children Followed-up: Are They at Increased Risk? *J. Stud. Alcohol* **1995**, *56*, 207–217. [CrossRef] [PubMed]
44. Wong, J.Y.H.; Fong, D.Y.T.; Lai, V.; Tiwari, A. Bridging Intimate Partner Violence and the Human Brain: A Literature Review. *Traumaviolenceabus.* **2014**, *15*, 22–33. [CrossRef]
45. Thomaes, K.; Dorrepaal, E.; Draijer, N.; De Ruiter, M.B.; Van Balkom, A.J.; Smit, J.H.; Veltman, D.J. Reduced Anterior Cingulate and Orbitofrontal Volumes in Child Abuse-Related Complex PTSD. *J. Clin. Psychiatry* **2010**, *71*, 1636–1644. [CrossRef]
46. Cross, D.; Fani, N.; Powers, A.; Bradley, B. Neurobiological Development in the Context of Childhood Trauma. *Clin. Psychol. Sci. Pract.* **2017**, *24*, 111–124. [CrossRef]
47. Carpenter, G.L.; Stacks, A.M. Developmental Effects of Exposure to Intimate Partner Violence in Early Childhood: A Review of the Literature. *Child. Youth Serv. Rev.* **2009**, *31*, 831–839. [CrossRef]
48. Tarullo, A.R.; Gunnar, M.R. Child Maltreatment and the Developing HPA Axis. *Horm. Behav.* **2006**, *50*, 632–639. [CrossRef]
49. Lupien, S.J.; Ouellet-Morin, I.; Herba, C.M.; Juster, R.; McEwen, B.S. From Vulnerability to Neurotoxicity: A Developmental Approach to the Effects of Stress on the Brain and Behavior. In *Epigenetics and Neuroendocrinology*; Springer: Cham, Switzerland, 2016. [CrossRef]
50. De Bellis, M.D.; Zisk, A. The Biological Effects of Childhood Trauma. *Child Adolesc. Psychiatr. Clin. North Am.* **2014**, *23*, 185–222. [CrossRef]
51. Teicher, M.H. Wounds That Time Won't Heal: The Neurobiology of Child Abuse. *Cerebrum* **2000**, *2*, 50–67.
52. National Scientific Council on the Developing Child. Excessive Stress Disrupts the Architecture of the Developing Brain. *Cent. Dev. Child Harv. Univ.* **2005**. [CrossRef]
53. Shonkoff, J.P.; Garner, A.S. The Lifelong Effects of Early Childhood Adversity and Toxic Stress. *Pediatrics* **2012**, *129*, e232–e246. [CrossRef]
54. McEwen, B.S.; Gianaros, P.J. Stress- and Allostasis-Induced Brain Plasticity. *Annu. Rev. Med.* **2010**, *62*, 431–445. [CrossRef] [PubMed]
55. Boyce, W.T.; Ellis, B.J. Biological Sensitivity to Context: I. An Evolutionary-Developmental Theory of the Origins and Functions of Stress Reactivity. *Dev. Psychopathol.* **2005**, *17*, 271–301. [CrossRef] [PubMed]
56. Miyake, A.; Friedman, N.P.; Emerson, M.J.; Witzki, A.H.; Howerter, A.; Wager, T.D. The Unity and Diversity of Executive Functions and Their Contributions to Complex "Frontal Lobe" Tasks: A Latent Variable Analysis. *Cogn. Psychol.* **2000**, *41*, 49–100. [CrossRef]
57. Cowell, R.A.; Cicchetti, D.; Rogosch, F.A.; Toth, S.L. Childhood Maltreatment and Its Effect on Neurocognitive Functioning: Timing and Chronicity Matter. *Dev. Psychopathol.* **2015**, *27*, 521–533. [CrossRef]
58. Tarter, R.E.; Kirisci, L.; Mezzich, A.; Cornelius, J.R.; Pajer, K.; Vanyukov, M.; Gardner, W.; Blackson, T.; Clark, D. Neurobehavioral Disinhibition in Childhood Predicts Early Age at Onset of Substance Use Disorder. *Am. J. Psychiatry* **2003**, *160*, 1078–1085. [CrossRef]
59. Van Harmelen, A.L.; Van Tol, M.J.; Dalgleish, T.; Van der Wee, N.J.A.; Veltman, D.J.; Aleman, A.; Spinhoven, P.; Penninx, B.W.J.H.; Elzinga, B.M. Hypoactive Medial Prefrontal Cortex Functioning in Adults Reporting Childhood Emotional Maltreatment. *Soc. Cogn. Affect. Neurosci.* **2013**, *9*, 2026–2033. [CrossRef]
60. Werner, K.; Gross, J.J. Emotion Regulation and Psychopathology: A Conceptual Framework. In *Emotion Regulation and Psychopathology: A Transdiagnostic Approach to Etiology and Treatment*; Guilford Press: New York, NY, USA, 2010. [CrossRef]
61. Bariola, E.; Gullone, E.; Hughes, E.K. Child and Adolescent Emotion Regulation: The Role of Parental Emotion Regulation and Expression. *Clin. Child Fam. Psychol. Rev.* **2011**, *14*, 198. [CrossRef]

62. Kober, H. Emotion Regulation in Substance Use Disorders. In *Handbook of Emotion Regulation*, 2nd ed.; Gross, J.J., Ed.; Guilford Press: New York, NY, USA, 2014.
63. Wilcox, C.E.; Pommy, J.M.; Adinoff, B. Neural Circuitry of Impaired Emotion Regulation in Substance Use Disorders. *Am. J. Psychiatry* **2016**, *173*, 344–361. [CrossRef] [PubMed]
64. Publications Office of the European Union. *A Gender Perspective on Drug Use and Responding to Drug Problems*; Publications Office of the European Union: Luxembourg, 2006.
65. Arsova Netzelmann, T.; Dan, M.; Dreezens-Fuhrke, J.; Kalikov, J.; Karnite, A.; Kucharova, B.; Musat, G. *Women Using Drugs: A Qualitative Situation and Needs Analysis. Cross-Country Rapid Assessment and Response (RAR Report)*; SPI Forschung gGmbH: Berlin, Germany, 2015.
66. Jones, A.; Weston, S.; Moody, A.; Millar, T.; Dollin, L.; Anderson, T.; Donmall, M. *The Drug Treatment Outcomes Research Study (DTORS): Baseline Report*; Home Office: London, UK, 2007.
67. Tuchman, E. Women and Addiction: The Importance of Gender Issues in Substance Abuse Research. *J. Addict. Dis.* **2010**, *29*, 127–138. [CrossRef] [PubMed]
68. United Nations Office on Drugs and Crime (UNODC). *World Drug Report 2016*; United Nations Office on Drugs and Crime: Vienna, Austria, 2016.
69. Bowlby, J. *Attachment and Loss. Volume II: Separation*; Basic Books: New York, NY, USA, 1973.
70. Putnam, F.W. The Impact of Trauma on Child Development. *Juv. Fam. Court J.* **2006**, *57*, 1–11. [CrossRef]
71. Stronach, E.P.; Toth, S.L.; Rogosch, F.; Oshri, A.; Manly, J.T.; Cicchetti, D. Child Maltreatment, Attachment Security, and Internal Representations of Mother and Mother-Child Relationships. *Child Maltreat.* **2011**, *16*, 137–145. [CrossRef] [PubMed]
72. Gabrielli, J.; Jackson, Y.; Huffhines, L.; Stone, K. Maltreatment, Coping, and Substance Use in Youth in Foster Care: Examination of Moderation Models. *Child Maltreat.* **2018**, *23*, 175–185. [CrossRef]
73. Greger, H.K.; Myhre, A.K.; Klöckner, C.A.; Jozefiak, T. Childhood Maltreatment, Psychopathology and Well-Being: The Mediator Role of Global Self-Esteem, Attachment Difficulties and Substance Use. *Child Abus. Negl.* **2017**, *70*, 122–133. [CrossRef]
74. Hayre, R.S.; Goulter, N.; Moretti, M.M. Maltreatment, Attachment, and Substance Use in Adolescence: Direct and Indirect Pathways. *Addict. Behav.* **2019**, *90*, 196–203. [CrossRef]
75. Lyons-Ruth, K. Contributions of the Mother–Infant Relationship to Dissociative, Borderline, and Conduct Symptoms in Young Adulthood. *Infant Ment. Health J.* **2008**, *29*, 203–218. [CrossRef]
76. Lindberg, M.A.; Zeid, D. Interactive Pathways to Substance Abuse. *Addict. Behav.* **2017**, *66*, 76–82. [CrossRef]
77. Schindler, A.; Bröning, S. A Review on Attachment and Adolescent Substance Abuse: Empirical Evidence and Implications for Prevention and Treatment. *Subst. Abus.* **2015**, *36*, 304–313. [CrossRef]
78. Schindler, A.; Thomasius, R.; Sack, P.M.; Gemeinhardt, B.; Küstner, U.; Eckert, J. Attachment and Substance Use Disorders: A Review of the Literature and a Study in a Drug Dependent Adolescents. *Attach. Hum. Dev.* **2005**, *7*, 207–228. [CrossRef] [PubMed]
79. Becoña Iglesias, E.; Del Río, E.F.; Calafat, A.; Fernández-Hermida, J.R. Attachment and Substance Use in Adolescence: A Review of Conceptual and Methodological Aspects. *Adicciones* **2014**, *26*, 77–86. [CrossRef]
80. Unterrainer, H.F.; Hiebler-Ragger, M.; Rogen, L.; Kapfhammer, H.P. Addiction as an Attachment Disorder. *Nervenarzt* **2018**, *89*, 1043–1048. [CrossRef] [PubMed]
81. Fairbairn, C.E.; Briley, D.A.; Kang, D.; Fraley, R.C.; Hankin, B.L.; Ariss, T. A Meta-Analysis of Longitudinal Associations between Substance Use and Interpersonal Attachment Security. *Psychol. Bull.* **2018**, *144*, 532. [CrossRef]
82. Page, T. The Attachment Partnership as Conceptual Base for Exploring the Impact of Child Maltreatment. *Child Adolesc. Soc. Work J.* **1999**, *16*, 419–437. [CrossRef]
83. Bretherton, I.; Munholland, K.A. Internal Working Models in Attachment Relationships: A Construct Revisited. In *Handbook of Attachment: Theory, Research, and Clinical Applications*; Cassidy, J., Shaver, P.R., Eds.; Guilford Press: New York, NY, USA, 1999.
84. Creeden, K. The Neurodevelopment Impact of Early Trauma and Insecure Attachment: Re-Thinking Our Understanding and Treatment of Sexual Behavior. *Sex. Addict. Compulsivity* **2004**, *11*, 223–247. [CrossRef]
85. Cicchetti, D.; Cummings, E.M.; Greenberg, M.T.; Marvin, R. *An Organizational Perspective on Attachment beyond Infancy: Implications for Theory, Measurement, and Research*; University of Chicago Press: Chicago, IL, USA, 1990; pp. 3–49.

86. Feeney, B.C.; Cassidy, J.; Ramos-Marcuse, F. The Generalization of Attachment Representations to New Social Situations: Predicting Behavior during Initial Interactions with Strangers. *J. Pers. Soc. Psychol.* **2008**, *95*, 1481. [CrossRef]
87. Özcan, N.K.; Boyacioğlu, N.E.; Enginkaya, S.; Bilgin, H.; Tomruk, N.B. The Relationship between Attachment Styles and Childhood Trauma: A Transgenerational Perspective—A Controlled Study of Patients with Psychiatric Disorders. *J. Clin. Nurs.* **2016**, *25*, 2357–2366. [CrossRef]
88. Sitko, K.; Bentall, R.P.; Shevlin, M.; O'Sullivan, N.; Sellwood, W. Associations between Specific Psychotic Symptoms and Specific Childhood Adversities Are Mediated by Attachment Styles: An Analysis of the National Comorbidity Survey. *Psychiatry Res.* **2014**, *217*, 202–209. [CrossRef]
89. Finzi-Dottan, R.; Harel, G. Parents' Potential for Child Abuse: An Intergenerational Perspective. *J. Fam. Violence* **2014**, *29*, 397–408. [CrossRef]
90. Rada, C. Violence against Women by Male Partners and against Children within the Family: Prevalence, Associated Factors, and Intergenerational Transmission in Romania, a Cross-Sectional Study. *BMC Public Health* **2014**, *14*, 129. [CrossRef] [PubMed]
91. Fowler, J.C.; Allen, J.G.; Oldham, J.M.; Frueh, B.C. Exposure to Interpersonal Trauma, Attachment Insecurity, and Depression Severity. *J. Affect. Disord.* **2013**, *149*, 313–318. [CrossRef] [PubMed]
92. Milligan, K.; Usher, A.M.; Urbanoski, K.A. Supporting Pregnant and Parenting Women with Substance-Related Problems by Addressing Emotion Regulation and Executive Function Needs. *Addict. Res. Theory* **2017**, *25*, 251–261. [CrossRef]
93. Motz, M.; Andrews, N.; Bondi, B.; Leslie, M.; Pepler, D. Addressing the Impact of Interpersonal Violence in Women Who Struggle with Substance Use through Developmental-Relational Strategies in a Community Program. *Int. J. Environ. Res. Public Health* **2019**, *16*, 4197. [CrossRef]

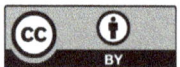

© 2019 by the authors. Licensee MDPI, Basel, Switzerland. This article is an open access article distributed under the terms and conditions of the Creative Commons Attribution (CC BY) license (http://creativecommons.org/licenses/by/4.0/).

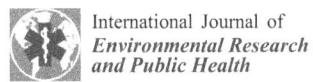

Review

Addressing the Impact of Interpersonal Violence in Women Who Struggle with Substance Use Through Developmental-Relational Strategies in a Community Program

Mary Motz [1], Naomi C. Z. Andrews [2,*], Bianca C. Bondi [3], Margaret Leslie [1] and Debra J. Pepler [3]

1. Early Intervention Department, Mothercraft, 860 Richmond Street West, Toronto, ON M6J 1C9, Canada; mmotz@mothercraft.org (M.M.); mleslie@mothercraft.org (M.L.)
2. Department of Child and Youth Studies, Brock University, 1812 Sir Isaac Brock Way, St. Catharines, ON L2S 3A1, Canada
3. Department of Psychology, York University, 4700 Keele Street, Toronto, ON M3J 1P3, Canada; bbondi@yorku.ca (B.C.B.); pepler@yorku.ca (D.J.P.)
* Correspondence: nandrews@brocku.ca

Received: 27 September 2019; Accepted: 26 October 2019; Published: 30 October 2019

Abstract: From a developmental–relational framework, substance use in women can be understood as relating to early experiences of violence in relationships and across development. This article uses a developmental-relational approach to outline specific strategies that can be used by service providers and to guide interventions for women with substance use issues. By reviewing research and clinical work with women attending a community-based prevention and early intervention program, we describe how specific components of programming can target the developmental and intergenerational pathway between experiences of violence in relationships and substance use. We include the voices of women who attended the program to support the strategies discussed. Specifically, these strategies address the impact of interpersonal violence on substance use by promoting the process of repair and reintegration for women whose neurological development, sense of self, and capacity to form relationships have been significantly impacted by experiences of violence in relationships.

Keywords: interpersonal violence; domestic violence; substance use; intervention; women; developmental–relational; gender-specific approach

1. Introduction

Many women who struggle with substance use have had a history of violent and traumatic experiences in relationships, often beginning in childhood [1]. These early experiences of interpersonal violence can negatively impact both neuropsychological development (e.g., executive functioning and emotion regulation) and the development of relational capacity (e.g., attachment and internal working models) [2]. Some refer to interpersonal violence (IPV) as domestic violence, family violence, or intimate partner violence; we use the term IPV to highlight the intergenerational nature of violence in relationships and that violence in relationships is often not exclusive to violence between partners. A developmental-relational approach is one in which the bidirectional associations between development and relationships are emphasized as important processes in understanding behaviour and functioning. A developmental perspective emphasizes the transactional links between the individual and the environment, and the effect of each on the other over time [3]. From a relational perspective, we consider that people, institutions, and systems grow through relationships with others [4,5]. This perspective helps us understand the link between women's experiences of violence in relationships across development and their later substance use issues. That is, through a developmental–relational approach, individuals' behaviour (e.g., substance use) can be understood within a context that includes their history and development, with a particular focus on how behaviour is shaped through relationships. To be effective in supporting women to make changes and achieve their addiction recovery goals, interventions need to address the impact of disruptions to women's development of self-regulation, executive functions, and relationship capacity as a result of their lifelong experiences with IPV [2]. Interventions need to be direct, purposeful, gender-specific, and trauma-informed, as well as grounded in attachment, developmental, and relational theory. With these theoretical and treatment foundations, it is possible to promote repair and reintegration for women whose neurological development, sense of self, and capacity to form healthy relationships have been significantly impacted by IPV.

Over the past 25 years, our research and clinical work with women attending a community-based prevention and early intervention program in Canada called Breaking the Cycle (BTC) have illuminated several specific strategies necessary to address the impact of IPV. Since 1995, BTC has provided comprehensive, integrated supports for mothers who are struggling with substance use issues, and their young children aged 0 to 6 years [6,7]. Programming at BTC is directed towards women, their children, and the mother–child relationship. BTC was developed through extensive community consultations that included street-based, community-based, and institutionally-based service providers who worked with women with substance use issues and substance-exposed children [8]. Interviews with members of the potential service population were also conducted. These consultations formed the basis of BTC's design and philosophy. BTC operates under formal partnership with nine agencies that include services relating to addiction treatment, health, and child development and protection. The development of BTC has been an evolving and emergent process, and research and program evaluation have been built into BTC since its inception. Through evaluation and listening to the voices of the women and children served by BTC, the program has expanded its range of services as well as its methods of service delivery.

Research has identified components of intervention programming and the therapeutic relationship that women with substance use issues find supportive [9]. There is research pointing to how therapeutic relationships promote emotion regulation and executive functioning [10]. With research as an integral component of BTC, we have confirmed the efficacy of gender-specific interventions based on a developmental-relational approach for women with a history of IPV and substance use. We have demonstrated successful engagement of, and enduring service relationships with, this marginalized population of women [11,12] to achieve outcomes related to substance use recovery, mental health functioning, and relationship capacity [13]. The following section describes some key intervention strategies used at BTC to (1) promote self-regulation and executive functions and (2) promote safety and capacity in relationships. Focus groups and interviews are regularly conducted with women at BTC for program evaluation and research purposes. The quotes that follow are drawn from previous BTC program evaluations [6,8] and other interviews completed for research and program evaluation, as indicated. These quotes are provided to highlight the voices and perspectives of the women who attend BTC. All women provided consent for their words to be used in publication.

2. Promoting Self-Regulation and Executive Functions

IPV and early experiences of trauma and violence in relationships can have a profound impact on the development of self-regulation and executive functioning strategies [14,15]. Deficits in executive functions also pose a heightened risk for future substance use issues [16]. As such, from a developmental-relational perspective, promoting self-regulation and executive functions is an essential part of programming at BTC, particularly given that women who use substances as a result of lifelong experiences with IPV struggle to regulate their behaviour and emotions, which ultimately impacts their psychosocial functioning. To do this, programming at BTC focuses on: (1) supporting time management, (2) monitoring the organization and ambiance of the program space, (3) encouraging regulated interactions, and (4) paying attention to readiness and internal processes.

2.1. Supporting Time Management

> I like that she'll meet me, just because it motivates you ... For myself, being an addict, sometimes you need somebody to come to you, and help you ... sometimes you'll make appointments and cancel. And I'm fresh into recovery, and can't wait to meet her there, it's like she's going to be there, she's going to be there, which is really helpful because it's motivating. [6] (p. 53)

When a woman makes the decision (whether assisted or unassisted) to call and access services for her substance use, it can be frustrating, disempowering, and demotivating to encounter an answering service or to be told that no one is available to meet with her for a number of weeks or months. During open hours at BTC, the telephone is always answered by a staff member and as soon as basic referral information is gathered, an initial appointment is scheduled within two weeks (two business days for pregnant women). Beginning with that first appointment, approaches and strategies are introduced to support women to be successful in accessing BTC services. For example, women with impaired executive functioning may struggle with organization and time management. Staff use appointment cards and/or provide women with calendars as tools to remind them of their next appointment. In scheduling appointments, BTC staff support women to consider a date and time that will work for them in the context of other priorities in their lives, which may include appointments with mandated services (e.g., probation or parole appointments, child welfare appointments), medical and mental health services, access visits with children, as well as child care/school drop-off and pick-up for children. In the early engagement phase of service, women are assured that their appointment time is reserved for them on a weekly basis and, even if they forget or are unable to attend, that appointment slot will be held for them in the following week.

Throughout the entire time that a woman accesses service at BTC, there is predictability, not only with her own appointments, but also in the overall structure in which programming is delivered. Women are provided with reminder telephone calls about upcoming individual and group meetings as a means of supporting their time management, as well as helping them to recognize that staff are thinking about them and anticipating their presence at the centre. There is consistency and predictability in program scheduling. Groups are offered at the same day and time each week, year after year, and are wrapped around food services (daily breakfast and lunch); group interventions complement times when individual appointment sessions are offered and co-occur with child-minding hours. This service structure supports women to anticipate programming at BTC, to schedule their own time accordingly, and ultimately to increase the probability of them attending and achieving service plan goals.

2.2. Monitoring the Organization and Ambiance of the Program Space

> The whole package ... (The Parent-Infant Therapist) still comes to our home on a bi-weekly basis, we have (the paediatrician/toxicologist) for any medical problems, we have (the public health nurse) for any questions on how to breastfeed ... You don't have to go to different locations all over the place, it's all under one roof, so a lot of the information you can access here. And knowing that (the child development counsellors) are always there. Because you don't have anyone else. [6] (p. 84)

The organization of the physical space at BTC has been carefully and deliberately planned. The integrated, single-access program is located in a downtown Toronto neighborhood which is accessible by public transportation. It is close to other services that BTC women access regularly, including withdrawal management and treatment services, community hospitals where there are physicians with expertise in addictions medicine, community housing and shelters, supplemental food programming, services for Indigenous peoples, and community healthcare.

BTC itself offers a wide range of programming so women can access many of the services that they need in one location. These services are offered at times that complement each other so that women do not have to participate in only one of two services that they need. Programming includes individual counselling and group interventions (e.g., addictions, mental health, interpersonal relationship, and trauma), intensive case management, daily breakfast and lunch, food and clothing donations, tokens for public transportation, prenatal street outreach, probation and parole appointments, parenting and early intervention programs for children ages 0 to 6 years, including weekly home visitation and child-minding.

The centre itself has a calm and home-like ambiance, which is often a contrast to the institutional settings where the women have accessed services previously. The main area of the centre is a spacious kitchen and living room where women are able to relax and attend to their own and their children's needs. The sizable playroom enables women to participate in mother–child group programming and play with their children. It has natural lighting and a large internal window so women can observe their children. The centre has been designed to be comfortable and inviting, without being overstimulating for women (and children) who require support with self-regulation and executive functioning. Staff engage with the women and their children through friendly conversations in the main area of the centre. At the same time, BTC staff are conscientious about confidentiality and hold private counselling discussions in appropriate private spaces. BTC staff gently redirect conversation, when required, which models and promotes women's self-regulation and boundary setting. BTC staff guide the women in a humble, relational, and positive way, without ever being punitive or shaming.

A significant component of supporting women with histories of IPV to develop a sense of trust in relationships is to provide safe and welcoming environments for them and for their children. At BTC, particular focus is given to ensuring that the environment feels safe to everyone who is in the centre. Programs are structured and drop-in services are not available; BTC staff know everyone who uses the space. Women who access programming at BTC know that staff are aware of and are familiar with everyone in the space. There is a buzzer-entry system to gain access to the suite which helps us monitor the flow of people into the centre. There is a receptionist who greets anyone who enters the centre. Although BTC follows a harm reduction model, women are not permitted to be actively using substances on-site or to be impaired as a result of substance use. Male partners are not allowed to wait inside the centre for women while they access programming. These safety guidelines around safety were developed based on feedback received directly from women during the early stages of the program. Women were pleased to be asked their opinions about how the program could help them to feel safe. Over the years, women continue to comment and agree that these features are integral to their feelings of safety, trust, and confidence in working towards their intervention goals.

Finally, BTC programming is directed towards women who are mothers; therefore, the physical environment is designed for the children, aged 0 to 6 years, who are in the centre and accessing services. Although it is beyond the scope of this paper to describe how parenting and early intervention services are integrated into treatment for each family, supporting women in their maternal role, while also recognizing and treating them as women, is an important contributor to the success of the program. As women experience modeling and scaffolding to repair, reintegrate, and promote their neurological development, sense of self, and relationship capacity, they become aware of and are able to provide teachings around these factors with their young children. In this way, the intergenerational cycles of IPV and substance use, which have pervaded their own lives, are broken.

2.3. Encouraging Regulated Interactions

> The flexibility of this group is that we all get to learn things but also, there are times when women come in here and they're up to here, ready to cry, and if it's another group, there's no way everyone would stop for them, they wouldn't just stop for that one person, they would keep going. But here you can stop, just for that one person...each person is understanding. Like that's the whole thing about being an addict and understanding that, not just as pregnant women but as addicts you need to come in here and express yourself when you need to. [6] (p. 54)

Self-regulation is promoted as women interact with other clients and with staff at the centre. During the orientation process, women meet with a counsellor who describes the environment of safety and respect at BTC, including the expectations about how everyone in the program is to be treated.

For instance, women are asked not to refer to themselves, or others, by "street" names; bullying and gossiping are not tolerated. There are visual reminders in the form of inconspicuous but well-placed signs which remind women to respect the confidentiality of others.

At BTC, staff are conscious of and careful to model regulated interactions with women, other staff members, and external community service providers. Women have frequently commented on how they experience warm and caring relationships with their counsellors, which are different than those they have experienced before, even with family and friends. At the same time, women are given a clear understanding that these are professional and not personal relationships. Women at BTC typically have many other service relationships to maintain, including those with mandated sectors. Having the ability to draw upon the style of regulated behaviour that they observe, as well as the support of their counsellors, is an important part of managing difficult relationships, specifically when those interactions trigger traumatic feelings from their past. Eventually, with support and practice, women are able to navigate personal and professional relationships outside of BTC in a healthy manner that promotes the achievement of their goals. The following quote was obtained from an interview with a BTC client for the purposes of program evaluation in 2014. Informed consent was provided by the client:

> *I try to get everybody on the same page. Like here, I learned that from here. Everybody knows. The workers here have their meetings on Friday and it's a team ... everybody is a team. So I got used to that. Everybody's on the same page. I like the daycare to be on the same page as the school. I like the resource centre to be on the same page as everybody ... children's aid ... everybody has to be on the same page for the kids.*

At BTC, case conferences are often held with a woman and representatives from all of the agencies that provide services to her family. These services may include her parole officer and/or her child protection worker. Typically, the first time a case conference is held, the woman is understandably nervous and hesitant to share her opinions or to speak during the meeting. Through the support and example of her BTC counsellor, the woman is able to see the benefit of describing, not only her challenges, but also her own personal goals and successes with all service providers. Over the course of a few meetings, she may be able to see the benefit of a shared view of her family situation and eventually become comfortable enough to chair the meeting herself.

2.4. Attention to Readiness and Internal Processes

> *They didn't force anything upon you like "Okay you have to go to twelve step meetings, or you have to go to (detox), or you have to look at it this way". They give you, here's your five options, check every one out if you want, or you can choose which one, which path you want to go, but everyone's an individual and everyone's different, and one way may work for me that doesn't work for (another client) ... Everybody's an individual, it's not like "Here's how you've got to do it, and everyone's got to do it this way, and if you don't do it this way you're going to fail ... " or they didn't ever put it that way. It was always, "Here's your options, and try which ways you would like to do it in", not someone telling you "You have to do this".* [6] (p. 84)

At BTC, the Transtheoretical Model of the Stages of Change [17] is used to support women to consider change, not only in regard to their substance use, but also in other areas where they have developed goals, including interpersonal relationships, education or vocational aspirations, parenting and/or their children's development and well-being. The model recognizes that women require different types and levels of support based on their readiness to work towards their goals of making change. Programs and services at BTC are mapped onto the stages of change (precontemplation, contemplation, preparation, action, maintenance, and relapse) that women are demonstrating in different areas. For example, when women enter the program, they are typically very early in their consideration of making change in their substance use. Even if they are no longer regularly using their identified primary substance, there may be other substances that they are using in a problematic manner. The *Relapse Prevention Group* is recommended for women who are in the precontemplation or contemplation stage of change with their substance use. Women who are closer to the action stage often participate in the *Connections* group, which is a program developed at BTC to address IPV and its connection to substance use and parenting [18], and women in the maintenance stage can participate in the *Recovery* group. Understanding and assessing women's readiness for change is critical in engaging women in the process of change.

Counsellors at BTC use diverse strategies to support women in developing their capacity to regulate and meet their intervention goals. Self-regulation is supported through attention to and identification of feelings and internal states. Counsellors support women to identify, name, and reflect on internal emotional states, which may be their first experience in being helped to understand and cope with feelings. Noticing and reinforcing when a woman is able to regulate in challenging situations is as important as providing strategies when she is having difficulty. Grounding and mindfulness strategies are also used to support regulation and recovery. Milligan and colleagues [10] have outlined a similar range of treatment strategies for substance using women, including helping women to develop action-oriented recovery goals, supporting the navigation of community resources and systems, as well as understanding and orienting supports to a woman's own learning style.

3. Promoting Safety and Capacity in Relationships

Not only can early exposure to IPV negatively impact the development of self-regulation, but IPV also affects the development of relational capacity. From a developmental-relational perspective, early experiences of violence in relationships can disrupt the positive bonds between children and their caregivers, and damage children's sense of safety in relationships [19,20]. These relational disruptions can have long-term consequences, including developmental cascades that impact adults' difficulties forming healthy relationships, difficulties in parenting, ineffective coping strategies, and problematic substance use. As such, forming trust with women who have a history of IPV in order to promote safety and enhance ongoing relationship capacity requires systemic and relational considerations in service provision, as well as attention to an open and welcoming therapeutic environment. In this section, we will discuss two specific ways in which safety and relationship capacity are supported at BTC: (1) engagement and building trust in relationships, and (2) maintaining relationships.

3.1. Engagement: Building Trust in Relationships

> There is obvious communication between all the workers here ... a real open, honest, communication, so you know I can talk to anyone of the women here and feel that same sort of support and you know that if it's necessary they'll probably pass on that information to someone else so everyone's on the same page as to where I'm at. [6] (p. 86)

At BTC, the formation of that trust begins in the very first appointments with the intake counsellor. Women are welcomed into the centre and given a tour that includes access to food and transportation costs, components which have become important for early engagement. Ensuring informed consent is a foundational part of the relationship development. There is transparency around service partnerships and practices, the voluntary nature of the program, the role of research at BTC, expectations that women should have around privacy and confidentiality, as well as the limitations of our services. At the beginning of the therapeutic relationship, having open and honest discussions with women creates a foundation of trust and provides an opportunity for repair in relationships when challenges arise.

Other systemic considerations that promote safe relationships include a requirement that staff at BTC are trained in trauma-informed practice [21]. Efforts are made to reduce the barriers that women experience in accessing services to meet their own needs, such as providing child-minding and instrumental supports. Finally, women experience a comprehensive and community-based approach to services, with providers from different programs and sectors forming effective and collaborative relationships to support women in reaching their goals.

3.2. Maintaining Relationships

> I've been with her (BTC counsellor) when I was clean, when I relapsed, when I went through treatment ... she's loving, she's caring, she's compassionate, she's understanding, she's patient, she's challenging when need be. She has no bias, she has no judgement, she has resources. [6] (p. 53)

> Like she really does listen to you. She listens to what you say. And she remembers. And I assume that she probably talks to all of us, but when she comes to talk to you, she remembers what you said last week and it's not written down in a book. She knows you as a person. [6] (p. 53)

When women who use substances experience programming and therapeutic relationships that are congruent with their needs, it can be a transformative experience that promotes enhanced capacity for relating. Women have described elements of their relationships with BTC counsellors that they felt were facilitative for them. These elements included respect, understanding, authenticity, mutual empathy, and reciprocity [8].

Staff at BTC recognize that attending to women's emotional safety sometimes requires crisis management—meeting the woman where she is at and managing her immediate needs and concerns before turning the focus to intake forms and assessments. Pacing the collection of current and historical information about a family is critical as well. Some women who use substances can be mistrustful of service providers and are not willing to disclose meaningful information until they have established a sense of trust with a counsellor. Other women seem less able to keep themselves safe and may disclose information too quickly, which can leave them feeling exposed and vulnerable after the appointment. This may trigger service avoidance or substance use as a coping mechanism. Supporting a woman to provide information at a slow pace can help her to stay emotionally safe and understood. Similarly, BTC staff members do not view the intake assessment as a process to uncover the "truth" about a woman's life. A woman's story unfolds over time and she should not be required or encouraged to disclose more than she is ready to, especially related to her history of trauma. For this reason, counsellors at BTC use a narrative approach when they are establishing relationships with women and learning about their story, as opposed to sitting with an intake questionnaire or going through a chart in a prescribed manner.

Motivational interviewing approaches are designed to support women to build commitment towards the changes they need to make to reach their stated goals; it also promotes understanding of their own ambivalence to these changes [22]. Through a therapeutic relationship with a counsellor who is empathic, accepting, and non-judgmental, external barriers to change are identified and the benefits to making change are explored and highlighted. Motivation and ultimately success in making change are determined by the interaction between the woman and her counsellor; however, the locus of control for change belongs to the woman and not to program staff. This approach is a key feature of the work that occurs at BTC. Through this relational intervention strategy with women, staff recognize and reflect that the experience of interactions within BTC may feel significantly different than those that women have had previously in both service and personal relationships. With that in mind, BTC staff are patient and supportive as women attempt to make changes in their interaction styles and in their ability to trust in relationships. BTC becomes a place where women practice a new style of behaving and relating, often for the first time. BTC staff are aware that women are constantly observing interactions that staff have with other clients, between each other, and with external community service providers as a model of healthy relationships; women look to staff to support the scaffolding of positive interaction styles. Finally, through their experiences of healthy interactions with staff, women who attend programming at BTC eventually begin to trust and depend on the knowledge that their stories will be held and remembered, even between counselling sessions. Women's awareness that they are kept in the mind of their therapists supports the repair and reintegration of a healthy sense of self and promotes a positive capacity for relationships for women who have been impacted by IPV and who use substances.

4. Conclusions

In this paper, we outlined specific strategies used at BTC, which promote self-regulation, executive functions, safety, and relationship capacity, in the context of a community-based prevention and early intervention program. A large part of the success of BTC has been based on the fact that it is a small, community-based, relational program. That being said, one challenge has been balancing the importance of the scale of the service model with the scope of issues faced by women with substance use issues, trauma, and histories of interpersonal violence. Similarly, women at BTC have indicated that there is a need for more services like BTC in other neighborhoods and communities, and that BTC should have more outreach and promotion in the community. In the future, it will be important to consider replications of the model described in this paper across jurisdictions, that are based in each individual community and that would maintain the fidelity of the developmental-relational aspects of the program.

Using a developmental–relational approach helps us understand the link between experiences of violence in relationships across development and later substance use issues. These factors can perpetuate the pathway of IPV across development, while reinforcing substance use as a necessary means of coping. At BTC, we are learning that it is possible to engage in a process of reparation and reintegration for those who have experienced IPV across development, by using a developmental-relational approach to guide care for women. Supporting a multi-generational response to issues of women's substance use recognizes the fact that women who misuse substances were once (often) children who experienced trauma within relationships, and that many women are also mothers striving to break this cycle in order to make their children's lives different. As women at BTC have shared, breaking the cycle of substance use involves listening to children who are abused or neglected, as that is where their problematic trajectories of substance use began. This quote was obtained from an interview with a BTC client as part of a research study in 2016. Informed consent was provided by the client:

> As amazing as it is to have these programs when we're 25, 26 ... if we can get the girls even younger. In my experience talking to women who have been raped [as children], there was nobody there to listen to them. Nobody believed them ... I think if we can try to have a voice for the younger generation we can somewhat break the cycle of it not turning into a 10 year issue of drug use or abuse.

Author Contributions: Conceptualization, M.M., N.C.Z.A., M.L., and D.J.P.; investigation, M.M.; writing—original draft preparation, M.M., N.C.Z.A., and B.C.B.; writing—review and editing, M.L. and D.J.P.; supervision, M.L. and D.J.P.

Funding: This research received no external funding.

Conflicts of Interest: The authors declare no conflict of interest.

References

1. Appleyard, K.; Berlin, L.J.; Rosanbalm, K.D.; Dodge, K.A. Preventing Early Child Maltreatment: Implications from a Longitudinal Study of Maternal Abuse History, Substance Use Problems, and Offspring Victimization. *Prev. Sci.* **2011**, *12*, 139–149. [CrossRef] [PubMed]
2. Andrews, N.C.Z.; Motz, M.; Bondi, B.; Leslie, M.; Pepler, D.J. Using a Developmental-Relational Approach to Understand the Impact of Interpersonal Violence in Women Who Struggle with Substance Use. Under review.
3. Sameroff, A. The Transactional Model. In *The Transactional Model of Development: How Children and Contexts Shape Each Other*; Sameroff, A., Ed.; American Psychological Association: Washington, DC, USA, 2009; pp. 3–21. [CrossRef]
4. Jordan, J.V.; Walker, M.; Hartling, L.M. (Eds.) *The Complexity of Connection*; The Guildford Press: New York, NY, USA, 2004.
5. Walker, M.; Rosen, W.B. (Eds.) *How Connections Heal. Stories from Relational-Cultural Therapy*; Guilford Press: New York, NY, USA, 2004.

6. Motz, M.; Leslie, M.; Pepler, D.; Moore, T.; Freeman, P. Breaking the Cycle: Measures of Progress 1995–2005. *J. FAS Int.* **2006**, *4*, 1–134.
7. Motz, M.; Leslie, M.; Pepler, D.J. Breaking the Cycle: A Comprehensive, Early Intervention Program Supporting Substance-Exposed Infants, Young Children, and Their Mothers. In *Healthy Development, Healthy Communities*; Pepler, D.J., Cummings, J., Craig, W.M., Eds.; PREVNet Series; PREVNet: Kingston, ON, Canada, 2016; Volume IV, pp. 115–134.
8. Leslie, M. (Ed.) *The Breaking the Cycle Compendium Vol. 1: The Roots of Relationships*; The Mothercraft Press: Toronto, ON, Canada, 2011.
9. Rutman, D.; Hubberstey, C. National Evaluation of Canadian Multi-Service FASD Prevention Programs: Interim Findings from the Co-Creating Evidence Study. *Int. J. Environ. Res. Public Health* **2019**, *16*, 1767. [CrossRef] [PubMed]
10. Milligan, K.; Usher, A.M.; Urbanoski, K.A. Supporting Pregnant and Parenting Women with Substance-Related Problems by Addressing Emotion Regulation and Executive Function Needs. *Addict. Res. Theory* **2017**, *25*, 251–261. [CrossRef]
11. Andrews, N.C.Z.; Motz, M.; Pepler, D.J.; Jeong, J.J.; Khoury, J. Engaging Mothers with Substance Use Issues and Their Children in Early Intervention: Understanding Use of Service and Outcomes. *Child. Abus. Negl.* **2018**, *83*, 10–20. [CrossRef] [PubMed]
12. Racine, N.; Motz, M.; Leslie, M.; Pepler, D.J. Breaking the Cycle Pregnancy Outreach Program. *J. Assoc. Res. Mothering* **2009**, *11*, 279–290.
13. Espinet, S.D.; Motz, M.; Jeong, J.J.; Jenkins, J.M.; Pepler, D. 'Breaking the Cycle' of Maternal Substance Use through Relationships: A Comparison of Integrated Approaches. *Addict. Res. Theory* **2016**, *24*, 375–388. [CrossRef]
14. Cross, D.; Fani, N.; Powers, A.; Bradley, B. Neurobiological Development in the Context of Childhood Trauma. *Clin. Psychol. Sci. Pract.* **2017**, *24*, 111–124. [CrossRef] [PubMed]
15. Cowell, R.A.; Cicchetti, D.; Rogosch, F.A.; Toth, S.L. Childhood Maltreatment and Its Effect on Neurocognitive Functioning: Timing and Chronicity Matter. *Dev. Psychopathol.* **2015**, *27*, 521–533. [CrossRef] [PubMed]
16. Tarter, R.E.; Kirisci, L.; Mezzich, A.; Cornelius, J.R.; Pajer, K.; Vanyukov, M.; Gardner, W.; Blackson, T.; Clark, D. Neurobehavioral Disinhibition in Childhood Predicts Early Age at Onset of Substance Use Disorder. *Am. J. Psychiatry* **2003**, *160*, 1078–1085. [CrossRef] [PubMed]
17. Prochaska, J.O.; DiClemente, C.C. Stages and Processes of Self-Change of Smoking: Toward an Integrative Model of Change. *J. Consult. Clin. Psychol.* **1983**, *51*, 390–395. [CrossRef] [PubMed]
18. Breaking the Cycle. *Connections: A Group Intervention for Mothers and Children Experiencing Violence in Relationships*; Mothercraft Press: Toronto, ON, Canada, 2014.
19. Fusco, R.A. Socioemotional Problems in Children Exposed to Intimate Partner Violence: Mediating Effects of Attachment and Family Supports. *J. Interpers. Violence* **2017**, *32*, 2515–2532. [CrossRef] [PubMed]
20. Gustafsson, H.C.; Brown, G.L.; Mills-Koonce, W.R.; Cox, M.J. Intimate Partner Violence and Children's Attachment Representations during Middle Childhood. *J. Marriage Fam.* **2017**, *79*, 865–878. [CrossRef] [PubMed]
21. Leslie, M.; Reynolds, W.; Motz, M.; Pepler, D.J. *Building Connections: Supporting Community-Based Programs to Address Interpersonal Violence and Child. Maltreatment*; Mothercraft Press: Toronto, ON, Canada, 2016.
22. Miller, W.R.; Rollnick, S. *Motivational Interviewing: Preparing People to Change Addictive Behavior*; Guilford Press: New York, NY, USA, 1991.

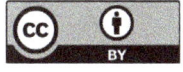

© 2019 by the authors. Licensee MDPI, Basel, Switzerland. This article is an open access article distributed under the terms and conditions of the Creative Commons Attribution (CC BY) license (http://creativecommons.org/licenses/by/4.0/).

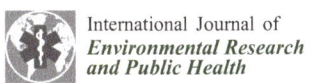

Commentary

The Presence and Consequences of Abortion Aversion in Scientific Research Related to Alcohol Use during Pregnancy

Sarah C.M. Roberts

Advancing New Standards in Reproductive Health (ANSIRH), Department of Obstetrics, Gynecology, and Reproductive Sciences, University of California, San Francisco, Oakland, CA 94143, USA; sarah.roberts@ucsf.edu; Tel.: +1-510-986-8962

Received: 13 June 2019; Accepted: 8 August 2019; Published: 13 August 2019

Abstract: Recent research has found that most U.S. state policies related to alcohol use during pregnancy adversely impact health. Other studies indicate that state policymaking around substance use in pregnancy—especially in the U.S.—appears to be influenced by an anti-abortion agenda rather than by public health motivations. This commentary explores the ways that scientists' aversion to abortion appear to influence science and thus policymaking around alcohol and pregnancy. The three main ways abortion aversion shows up in the literature related to alcohol use during pregnancy include: (1) a shift from the recommendation of abortion for "severely chronic alcoholic women" to the non-acknowledgment of abortion as an outcome of an alcohol-exposed pregnancy; (2) the concern that recommendations of abstinence from alcohol use during pregnancy lead to terminations of otherwise wanted pregnancies; and (3) the presumption of abortion as a negative pregnancy outcome. Thus, abortion aversion appears to influence the science related to alcohol use during pregnancy, and thus policymaking—to the detriment of developing and adopting policies that reduce the harms from alcohol during pregnancy.

Keywords: alcohol; pregnancy; abortion; policy

1. Background

Alcohol is a known teratogen that causes fetal alcohol syndrome (FAS) and a range of other harms to fetuses [1–5]. As many as 14.6 per 10,000 people worldwide may have FAS [6]. Alcohol use during pregnancy is common, with about 10% of pregnant women worldwide reporting any alcohol use [7]. In the U.S., 15% of pregnant women report any alcohol use and approximately 3% report binge drinking in the past month [8]. Rates of alcohol use during pregnancy are higher in some regions, such as Europe, and lower in others, such as the eastern Mediterranean, and Southeast Asia [7]. In the U.S., while there have been some minor fluctuations, rates of alcohol use during pregnancy have remained steady since the 1990s [9–13]. This means that alcohol use during pregnancy has remained common for decades in the U.S., despite considerable governmental and clinical attention in the U.S. and other countries.

To address drinking in pregnancy, many U.S. states have passed laws related to alcohol use in pregnancy. In the U.S., most states have at least one policy focusing on alcohol use during pregnancy (alcohol/pregnancy policies), and the number of alcohol/pregnancy policies has increased dramatically over the past 40 years [14]. However, until recently, there has been little quantitative research about the impacts of these policies. A recent comprehensive legal epidemiology [15] study found that, in the U.S., a few state alcohol/pregnancy policies may be associated with less self-reported drinking during pregnancy [16]. This legal epidemiology study also found that most state alcohol/pregnancy policies, at best, have no relationship to birth outcomes (such as low birth weight and preterm birth) or prenatal care use [17]. At worst, using methods that allow for causal inference, this study found that multiple state alcohol/pregnancy policies lead to increases in low birth weight and preterm birth, and decreases in prenatal care use [17]—leading to thousands of babies born with low birth weight, or preterm each year, due to the policies [18].

A recent study of state legislators in three U.S. states found that while state legislators are aware that drinking during pregnancy is harmful, they also believe (inaccurately) that "nobody does that any more" due to public health efforts [19]. Despite these beliefs and the lack of research evidence about the effectiveness of alcohol/pregnancy policies, these states have multiple alcohol/pregnancy policies and have recently adopted new alcohol/pregnancy policies [14]. This suggests a strong disconnect between research evidence and policy related to alcohol use during pregnancy.

One explanation for this disconnect is that U.S. policymaking related to alcohol as well as drug use during pregnancy has been influenced by an anti-abortion political agenda, having to do with treating the fetus as a separate person from the pregnant woman [20,21] rather than being driven by public health efforts designed to reduce harms from alcohol use during pregnancy [14]. For context, over the same 40-year time period that the number of state alcohol/pregnancy policies increased, there has also been a dramatic increase in the number of state-level policies restricting abortion in the U.S. [22]. While other countries where abortion is legal also have some restrictive abortion policies and limited availability of abortion services [23], politics related to abortion in the U.S. have been more ever present than in many other countries [24]. In the U.S., anti-abortion activism and politics emerged as a strong political force in the early 1980s [24,25], and has remained a major issue in U.S. politics since then [26]. However, the terms of the U.S. political debate are narrowly framed. While politicians opposed to abortion directly state their opposition, abortion rights supporters do not typically frame abortion or even the availability of abortion services as positive. Instead, they largely frame abortion as something to be avoided as much as possible, using the slogan of "safe, legal, and rare" to describe a vision for abortion [27]. Essentially, even abortion rights supporters in the U.S. use language that indicates an aversion to abortion.

This same aversion to abortion that is present in U.S. politics in general is also present in the scientific research related to alcohol use during pregnancy. The Merriam–Webster dictionary defines aversion as a feeling of repugnance toward something, with a desire to avoid or turn away from it, and as a tendency to extinguish a behavior or to avoid a thing or situation [28]. In this commentary, using this definition of aversion as a guide, I trace three main ways aversion to abortion appears to influence scientific questions asked and thus perhaps policy options scholars and other health professionals imagine related to alcohol (and drug) use during pregnancy. The three main ways that abortion aversion shows up in this literature include: "Shift from recommendation of abortion to non-acknowledgement of abortion as an outcome of alcohol or drug-exposed pregnancy," "Concern that abstinence messages lead to terminations of otherwise wanted pregnancies," and "Presumption of abortion as negative pregnancy outcome." This commentary describes each aspect of abortion aversion and argues that abortion aversion appears to influence science related to alcohol use during pregnancy, and thus policymaking—to the detriment of developing and adopting policies that reduce harms from alcohol during pregnancy.

2. Shift from Recommendation of Abortion to Non-Acknowledgement of Abortion as an Outcome of Alcohol-Exposed Pregnancy

2.1. Early Recommendation of Abortion

FAS had been identified multiple times in past centuries and earlier in the 1900s, before the diagnosis publicly and medically "stuck" in the 1970s [29,30]. Historian Janet Golden and sociologist Elizabeth Armstrong argued that experiences with thalidomide in the 1950s that allowed the imagining of the fetus as a separate being that could be harmed by a pregnant woman's behavior, contributed to the diagnosis sticking in the 1970s [29,31]. Golden also argued that the new availability of legal abortion services in 1973 that resulted from the U.S. Supreme Court Decision (Roe v. Wade) that legalized abortion throughout the U.S. was a key component of making the diagnosis of FAS stick during the 1970s. Essentially, legal abortion was a medical solution to the problem of FAS [29,31].

In fact, multiple peer-reviewed manuscripts published in the 1970s recommended or suggested abortion as a possible "solution" to (heavier) alcohol use during pregnancy, and to FAS [32–34]. This recommendation of abortion as a "solution" was made in one of the first manuscripts about FAS published by the medical researchers who "discovered" FAS in the U.S. in the 1970s [32]. In the manuscript, Jones and Smith concluded, "The frequency (43%) of adverse outcome of pregnancy for chronic alcoholic women suggests that serious consideration be given to early termination of pregnancy in severely chronic alcoholic women" (p. 1).

2.2. Disappearance of Abortion Recommendation

This focus on abortion as a "solution" to FAS essentially disappeared from the literature in the 1980s. There are a few possible explanations. First, Armstrong and Abel [35] argued that this abortion recommendation, which they characterized as "extreme," was one aspect of the "moral panic" that emerged related to alcohol use during pregnancy in the 1970s and 1980s. They suggested that the abortion recommendation disappeared due to newer studies finding that FAS was a rarer outcome of alcohol use during pregnancy than in earlier studies, and thus that such an "extreme" solution was no longer necessary. The idea of abortion as an "extreme" solution can also be viewed as an element of abortion aversion—i.e., that abortion is to be avoided if at all possible.

Second, during the 1980s and 1990s, the War on Drugs and the emergence of anti-abortion politics in the U.S. shifted visual images and framing in broadcast news stories about women who drink during pregnancy [20]. Specifically, the images and framing shifted from portrayals of how government warnings about drinking during pregnancy might benefit primarily white, middle class women, and their children, to images of women who drink during pregnancy as women of color, who are deviant and are causing irreversible damage to their fetuses. With this shift to the idea of maternal substance use as causing fetal harm, came larger societal efforts to control pregnant women's behavior more broadly—including both substance use during pregnancy and abortion [20].

Third, scientists in the 1980s and 1990s could have been influenced by a similar abortion aversion as that in U.S. politics. It is also possible that scientists, even if they did not share this aversion, were loath to stir controversy by directly addressing abortion in their work. They may also have been influenced by prohibitions in the U.S. on researching abortion provision using federal dollars [36].

2.3. Non-Acknowledgment of Abortion as a Possible Outcome

There are multiple instances in scientific literature where abortion is not acknowledged as a possible outcome of an alcohol-exposed pregnancy. For example, in the late 1990s, U.S. Centers for Disease Control and Prevention (CDC, the U.S. federal health agency) scientists started a body of research and interventions into what are now referred to as alcohol-exposed pregnancies, focusing on (often unintended) pregnancies in which women drank prior to discovering they were pregnant [37]. That some women who drink prior to discovering their pregnancy might have abortions (instead of giving birth) is absent from key highly cited studies—these studies created the idea of and set the research, policy, and intervention agendas for alcohol-exposed pregnancies (e.g., [37]).

A recent case illustrates how non-acknowledgement of abortion as a possible outcome influences the science about public health impacts of alcohol-exposed pregnancies. In 2016, scientists at the U.S. CDC used data about past month sexual behavior, contraception use, and alcohol use from a national survey to estimate the number of U.S. women at risk for an alcohol-exposed pregnancy [38]. The CDC produced multiple publicity materials to go along with their scientific report of this estimate [39,40]. The CDC publicity materials appeared to tell women of reproductive age that they should not drink unless they were using contraception [41]. There was a considerable pushback and, in fact, public ridicule and arguments to dismiss the entire premise of alcohol-exposed pregnancies [42–44]. Rather than have a public conversation about the harms related to alcohol use during pregnancy, communicate the importance of limiting drinking during pregnancy, and focus on solutions that might reduce harmful drinking [44], the conversation was mocking and dismissive of the CDC and their authority regarding harms from alcohol use during pregnancy. Importantly, abortion aversion appears present in this (seemingly counterproductive) effort. In their estimate, the CDC scientists used non-evidence-based assumptions related to abortion and abortion politics to draw inferences from the data available in the survey. First, they assumed pregnancies occur immediately after unprotected sex, i.e., prior to implantation. According to the American College of Obstetricians and Gynecologists and to U.S. government regulations, pregnancy occurs only after implantation [45,46], which takes place multiple days after fertilization [46]. Arguing that a pregnancy exists from the moment of fertilization is core to anti-abortion organizing in the U.S. [47]. The CDC authors also failed to acknowledge that not all alcohol-exposed pregnancies result in births, that some end in miscarriages and abortions. Along with these and other assumptions, their failure to acknowledge abortion as a possible outcome dramatically inflated the estimate of alcohol exposed pregnancies [48]. These inflated estimates are an element of and can contribute to moral panic related to alcohol use during pregnancy [35], and possibly influence the adoption of more harmful and stigmatizing policies.

As a second example, this non-acknowledgement of abortion as a possible outcome appears in clinical practice literature. Another highly cited study related to alcohol and pregnancy that was published in 2000, around the same time as the initial alcohol-exposed pregnancy article, and also by U.S. CDC scientists, explored what obstetricians and gynecologists need regarding their patients' alcohol use during pregnancy [49]. In this manuscript, there is also no mention of abortion. The lack of acknowledgement of abortion as a possible outcome is especially surprising in this manuscript, as more than 80% of the obstetricians and gynecologists surveyed said that they wanted information on thresholds of alcohol consumption that cause reproductive harm [49]. Thresholds that cause reproductive harm (as well as information which may modify the risk of harm, such as nutrition and socioeconomic status [50–53]) are highly relevant to whether a pregnant woman who consumed alcohol during pregnancy might want to consider abortion. To spell this out, providing information about differences in the rates of harms at different levels of consumption (or under different conditions) might provide what appears to be justification for counseling on, or the suggestion of, abortion as an option for women drinking at certain levels or under certain other conditions during pregnancy. The failure to assess provider practices or information needs related to abortion in what appears to be an agenda-setting study essentially precludes development of a research agenda that might include this abortion-related topic.

Certainly, factors other than abortion aversion may have influenced the disappearance of abortion as a possible outcome for an alcohol-exposed pregnancy or as a "solution" for FAS. In relation to FAS and more so in relation to drug use during pregnancy, there is a deeply problematic legacy of efforts to use state and other forms of power to coerce and control the reproduction of women who use alcohol and drugs [54–56]. The one article that focuses on abortion as a possible outcome of alcohol and drug-exposed pregnancies is a case study of two psychiatric patients with substance use disorders who want to terminate their pregnancies; the authors of this case study carefully explain and detail the ethics process they went through to allow these women to obtain their wanted abortions [57]. There is no question that awareness of the potential for coercion, and engaging in intentional efforts to avoid contributing toward any justification for coercion, is warranted. However, such intense and seemingly overpowering concern about not contributing to coercion may also contribute to the non-acknowledgement of abortion as a possible outcome, and thus limit research questions asked and policies imagined.

3. Concern that Abstinence Messages Lead to Terminations of Otherwise Wanted Pregnancies

In the 1980s, U.S. government official recommendations regarding alcohol use in pregnancy shifted from focusing on FAS and high levels of drinking during pregnancy to official recommendations of complete abstinence. Similar shifts—to either abstinence or to no more than low levels of drinking during pregnancy—occurred in other English speaking countries [58]. In relation to these shifted recommendations and associated health messages, new abortion-related concerns emerged. Specifically, a concern emerged that recommending complete abstinence from alcohol use during pregnancy would lead women to terminate otherwise wanted pregnancies [35,59–62]. This concern also appears in obstetrics and gynecology professional association guidelines, which state that low levels of drinking in early pregnancy are not indications for terminating pregnancies [63,64]. Connecting back to the lack of research about whether there is a threshold of drinking during pregnancy at which providers might recommend consideration of abortion, these guidelines do not state whether there is a level of drinking that is an indication for abortion.

One Australian study has documented the alcohol industry as a source of expressed concerns that health messages about alcohol and pregnancy (such as on warning labels) lead women to terminate pregnancies [65]. The alcohol industry has engaged in persistent efforts to manipulate scientists as well as policymakers to avoid policies that reduce overall alcohol consumption and thus their commercial interests [66,67]. The fact that the alcohol industry appears to be a source of this type of abortion aversion raises questions about the purpose of raising these concerns, and whether these concerns are distractions from other policy approaches that might hurt alcohol industry profits.

This type of abortion aversion is not innocuous. It appears to prioritize avoiding abortion over strategies that might help improve the health of women and fetuses in relation to alcohol. For example, a 2012 paper found no evidence for the argument that recommending abstinence from alcohol during pregnancy would lead women to terminate otherwise wanted pregnancies [68]. Alongside this paper, the journal published a commentary arguing that policymakers (in Australia) could feel comfortable recommending abstinence from alcohol during pregnancy, as they no longer had to worry that this recommendation would lead women to have abortions [69]. What the commentary failed to acknowledge was that there was no evidence or recent change in evidence about whether recommending abstinence actually translated into reduced alcohol use during pregnancy compared to no recommendation, or to a no more than low-level recommendation. More recent research has not found a difference in alcohol consumption during pregnancy between abstinence recommendations versus previous recommendations [70], which is consistent with individual-level counseling message research [71]. Essentially, though, the commentary argued that we should base alcohol/pregnancy policies on whether they lead women to have abortions, rather than whether they effectively reduce alcohol use during pregnancy or related harms. Effective public health policies are not created by only arguing that they do not have unintended effects—rather, they should be evaluated on whether they have intended effects and then whether they also have unintended effects. In this case, abortion aversion affected policy arguments related to alcohol use during pregnancy, and has likely affected the types of policies related to alcohol use during pregnancy that are imagined and thus implemented.

4. Presumption of Abortion as Negative Pregnancy Outcome

There is clear evidence that denying women abortions leads to more economic insecurity, worse short term physical health, and to violence from the man involved in the pregnancy, and that abortion is safer than childbirth [72–75]. Despite this evidence, public health agencies [76] and public health researchers often treat abortion as a negative outcome that should be prevented [77,78].

This same theme of abortion as a negative outcome exists in the literature regarding alcohol (and drug) use during pregnancy. A common way that this appears is within articles examining factors (including or focused explicitly on alcohol and drug use) associated with having an abortion (compared to birth) or multiple abortions (compared to one) [79–84]. While often not stated explicitly, the logic is that (heavier levels of) alcohol use among women of reproductive age leads to unintended pregnancy, which then leads to abortion (framed as a negative outcome), and to multiple abortions (framed as even more negative outcomes).

5. Implications

The role of abortion aversion in influencing alcohol/pregnancy policies matters from a public health perspective. Despite more than 40 years of policymaking related to alcohol use during pregnancy, alcohol use during pregnancy has remained relatively steady in the U.S. since the 1990s [9–13]. Combined with the evidence that extant alcohol/pregnancy policies do not effectively reduce the harms from alcohol use during pregnancy, and that they may increase these harms [16–18], that alcohol use during pregnancy has remained steady indicates that new policy approaches are needed. As a first step in developing policies that can effectively reduce alcohol use and related harms during pregnancy, scientists, health professionals, and public health professionals need to explore how our own explicit or implicit abortion aversion has influenced the types of scientific questions we ask, and the ways in which we frame policy conversations. Only after coming to terms with how abortion aversion has influenced our science and policymaking to date can we move forward in crafting new questions and new possible solutions.

Removing abortion aversion from the science related to alcohol use during pregnancy might allow us to pursue research questions such as: What policies, structures, and services are necessary to ensure that women with alcohol and drug use disorders are able to obtain wanted abortions? What is the rate of adverse outcomes at different levels and patterns of alcohol use during pregnancy when combined with different social and nutritional characteristics? Which, if any, health messages and guidelines around drinking during pregnancy reduce alcohol consumption during pregnancy, as well as the related harms?

6. Conclusions

Abortion aversion appears to influence science and thus policymaking related to alcohol use during pregnancy, which is to the detriment of developing and adopting policies that reduce harms from alcohol use during pregnancy. To conceptualize and then develop and enact policies that may be more likely to reduce alcohol use during pregnancy and related harms, scientists, clinicians, and policy influencers need to become aware of how aversion to abortion has influenced science and policymaking to date, and engage in intentional practices to avoid being influenced by abortion aversion moving forward.

Funding: Authors received support from a core grant to ANSIRH, the research group at UCSF in which author is housed, for the time spent researching and writing this manuscript.

Acknowledgments: The author would like to thank Laurie Drabble, Diana Greene Foster, Sue Thomas, and Katie Woodruff for providing helpful and constructive feedback on earlier drafts of the manuscript.

Conflicts of Interest: The authors declare no conflict of interest. The sponsor had no role in study design; in the collection, analyses, or interpretation of data; in the writing of the manuscript; or in the decision to publish the results.

References

1. Sokol, R.J.; Delaney-Black, V.; Nordstrom, B. Fetal alcohol spectrum disorder. *JAMA* **2003**, *290*, 2996–2999. [CrossRef]
2. O'Leary, C.M.; Bower, C. Guidelines for pregnancy: What's an acceptable risk, and how is the evidence (finally) shaping up? *Drug Alcohol Rev.* **2012**, *31*, 170–183. [CrossRef]
3. Sayal, K.; Heron, J.; Golding, J.; Alati, R.; Smith, G.D.; Gray, R.; Emond, A. Binge pattern of alcohol consumption during pregnancy and childhood mental health outcomes: Longitudinal population-based study. *Pediatrics* **2009**, *123*, e289–e296. [CrossRef]
4. May, P.A.; Gossage, J.P.; Marais, A.S.; Hendricks, L.S.; Snell, C.L.; Tabachnick, B.G.; Stellavato, C.; Buckley, D.G.; Brooke, L.E.; Viljoen, D.L. Maternal risk factors for fetal alcohol syndrome and partial fetal alcohol syndrome in South Africa: A third study. *Alcohol Clin. Exp. Res.* **2008**, *32*, 738–753. [CrossRef]
5. Strandberg-Larsen, K.; Gronboek, M.; Andersen, A.M.; Andersen, P.K.; Olsen, J. Alcohol drinking pattern during pregnancy and risk of infant mortality. *Epidemiology* **2009**, *20*, 884–891. [CrossRef]

6. Popova, S.; Lange, S.; Probst, C.; Gmel, G.; Rehm, J. Global prevalence of alcohol use and binge drinking during pregnancy, and fetal alcohol spectrum disorder. *Biochem. Cell Biol.* **2018**, *96*, 237–240. [CrossRef]
7. Popova, S.; Lange, S.; Probst, C.; Gmel, G.; Rehm, J. Estimation of national, regional, and global prevalence of alcohol use during pregnancy and fetal alcohol syndrome: A systematic review and meta-analysis. *Lancet Glob. Health* **2017**, *5*, e290–e299. [CrossRef]
8. Popova, S.; Lange, S.; Probst, C.; Parunashvili, N.; Rehm, J. Prevalence of alcohol consumption during pregnancy and Fetal Alcohol Spectrum Disorders among the general and Aboriginal populations in Canada and the United States. *Eur. J. Med. Genet.* **2017**, *60*, 32–48. [CrossRef]
9. Centers for Disease Control and Prevention Prevention. Alcohol consumption among pregnant and childbearing-aged women—United States, 1991 and 1995. *MMWR Morb. Mortal. Wkly. Rep.* **1997**, *46*, 346–350.
10. Centers for Disease Control and Prevention. Alcohol use among women of childbearing age—United States, 1991–1999. *MMWR Morb. Mortal. Wkly. Rep.* **2002**, *51*, 273.
11. Centers for Disease Control and Prevention. Alcohol use among pregnant and nonpregnant women of childbearing age—United States, 1991–2005. *MMWR Morb. Mortal. Wkly. Rep.* **2009**, *58*, 529–532.
12. Zhao, G.; Ford, E.S.; Tsai, J.; Li, C.; Ahluwalia, I.B.; Pearson, W.S.; Balluz, L.S.; Croft, J.B. Trends in health-related behavioral risk factors among pregnant women in the United States: 2001–2009. *J. Womens Health* **2012**, *21*, 255–263. [CrossRef]
13. Denny, C.H.; Acero, C.S.; Naimi, T.S.; Kim, S.Y. Consumption of alcohol beverages and binge drinking among pregnant women aged 18–44 years—United States, 2015–2017. *MMWR Morb. Mortal. Wkly. Rep.* **2019**, *68*, 365–368. [CrossRef]
14. Roberts, S.C.M.; Thomas, S.; Treffers, R.; Drabble, L. Forty years of state alcohol and pregnancy policies in the USA: Best practices for public health or efforts to restrict women's reproductive rights? *Alcohol Alcohol.* **2017**, *52*, 715–721. [CrossRef]
15. Burris, S.; Ashe, M.; Levin, D.; Penn, M.; Larkin, M. A transdisciplinary approach to public health law: The emerging practice of legal epidemiology. *Annu. Rev. Public Health* **2016**, *37*, 135–148. [CrossRef]
16. Roberts, S.; Mericle, A.; Subbaraman, M.; Thomas, S.; Treffers, R.; Delucchi, K.; Kerr, W. State policies targeting alcohol use during pregnancy and alcohol use among pregnant women 1985–2016: Evidence from the Behavioral Risk Factor Surveillance System. *Women Health Issues* **2019**, *29*, 213–221. [CrossRef]
17. Subbaraman, M.S.; Thomas, S.; Treffers, R.; Delucchi, K.; Kerr, W.C.; Martinez, P.; Roberts, S.C.M. Associations between state-level policies regarding alcohol use among pregnant women, adverse birth outcomes, and prenatal care utilization: Results from 1972 to 2013 Vital Statistics. *Alcohol. Clin. Exp. Res.* **2018**, *42*, 1511–1517. [CrossRef]
18. Subbaraman, M.S.; Roberts, S.C.M. Costs associated with policies regarding alcohol use during pregnancy: Results from 1972–2015 Vital Statistics. *PLoS ONE* **2019**, *14*, e0215670. [CrossRef]
19. Woodruff, K.; Roberts, S.C.M. "Alcohol during pregnancy? Nobody does that any more": State legislators' use of evidence in making policy on alcohol use in pregnancy. *J. Stud. Alcohol Drugs* **2019**, *80*, 380–388. [CrossRef]
20. Golden, J. "A tempest in a cocktail glass": Mothers, alcohol, and television, 1977–1996. *J. Health Politics Policy Law* **2000**, *25*, 473–498. [CrossRef]
21. Paltrow, L.M. The war on drugs and the war on abortion: Some initial thoughts on the connections, intersections and effects. *Reprod. Health Matters* **2002**, *10*, 162–170. [CrossRef]
22. Guttmacher Institute. *Last Five Years Account for More than One-Quarter of All Abortion Restrictions Enacted Since Roe*; Guttmacher Institute: New York, NY, USA, 2016.
23. Levels, M.; Sluiter, R.; Need, A. A review of abortion laws in Western-European countries. A cross-national comparison of legal developments between 1960 and 2010. *Health Policy* **2014**, *118*, 95–104. [CrossRef]
24. Abortion USA. Available online: https://doi.org/10.1016/S0140-6736(89)92869-9 (accessed on 4 May 2019).
25. McKeegan, M. The politics of abortion: A historical perspective. *Womens Health Issues* **1993**, *3*, 127–131. [CrossRef]
26. Joffe, C. What will become of reproductive issues in Trump's America? *Reprod. Health Matters* **2017**, *25*, 1287826. [CrossRef]
27. Weitz, T.A. Rethinking the mantra that abortion should be "safe, legal, and rare". *J Womens Hist.* **2010**, *22*, 161–172. [CrossRef]

28. Merriam-Webster. *Definition of Aversion*; Merriam-Webster: Springfield, MA, USA, 2019.
29. Armstrong, E.M. *Conceiving Risk, Bearing Responsibility: Fetal Alcohol Syndrome and the Diagnosis of Moral Disorder*; The Johns Hopkins University Press: Baltimore, MD, USA, 2003; p. 277.
30. Warren, K.R.; Hewitt, B.G. Fetal alcohol spectrum disorders: When science, medicine, public policy, and laws collide. *Dev. Disabil. Res. Rev.* **2009**, *15*, 170–175. [CrossRef]
31. Golden, J.L. *Message in a Bottle: The Making of Fetal Alcohol Syndrome*; Harvard University Press: Cambridge, MA, USA, 2005; p. 232.
32. Jones, K.L.; Smith, D.W. The fetal alcohol syndrome. *Teratology* **1975**, *12*, 1–10. [CrossRef]
33. Beyers, N.; Moosa, A. The Fetal Alcohol Syndrome. *S. Afr. Med. J.* **1978**, *54*, 575–578.
34. Majewski, F.; Fischbach, H.; Peiffer, J.; Bierich, J.R. Interruption of pregnancy in alcoholic women (author's transl). *Dtsch. Med. Wochenschr.* **1978**, *103*, 895–898. [CrossRef]
35. Armstrong, E.M.; Abel, E.L. Fetal alcohol syndrome: The origins of a moral panic. *Alcohol Alcohol.* **2000**, *35*, 276–282. [CrossRef]
36. CFR. *Electronic Code of Federal Regulations*; CFR: New York, NY, USA, 2018; CFR 45, Part 46, Subpart B, 46.204.
37. Floyd, R.L.; Decoufle, P.; Hungerford, D.W. Alcohol use prior to pregnancy recognition. *Am. J. Prev. Med.* **1999**, *17*, 101–107. [CrossRef]
38. Green, P.P.; McKnight-Eily, L.R.; Tan, C.H.; Mejia, R.; Denny, C.H. Vital Signs: Alcohol-Exposed Pregnancies—United States, 2011–2013. *MMWR. Morb. Mortal. Wkly. Rep.* **2016**, *65*, 91–97. [CrossRef]
39. Centers for Disease Control and Prevention. *More than 3 Million US Women at Risk for Alcohol-Exposed Pregnancy*; Centers for Disease Control and Prevention: Atlanta, GA, USA, 2016.
40. Centers for Disease Control and Prevention. *Alcohol and Pregnancy: Why Take the Risk?* Centers for Disease Control and Prevention: Atlanta, GA, USA, 2016.
41. Crawford, C. *Dissecting the CDC's Advice to Avoid Alcohol-Exposed Pregnancies*; AAFP News: Leawood, KS, USA, 2016.
42. Cunha, D. *The CDC's Alcohol Warning Shames and Discriminates Against Women*; Time Magazine: New York, NY, USA, 2016.
43. Donnelly, T. The CDC's New Alcohol Guidelines for Women, Updated for Men. Available online: http://brokelyn.com/cdc-alcohol-guidelines-for-a-violent-man/ (accessed on 13 June 2019).
44. Golden, J. Women and Alcohol: Let's Talk About the Real Problem. Available online: http://nursingclio.org/2016/02/06/women-and-alcohol-lets-talk-about-the-real-problem/ (accessed on 29 March 2017).
45. ACOG. *Prenatal Development: How Your Baby Grows During Pregnancy*; ACOG: Washington, DC, USA, 2018.
46. CFR 45, Part 46, Subpart B, 46.202. Electronic Code of Federal Regulations. Available online: https://www.ecfr.gov/cgi-bin/retrieveECFR?gp=&SID=83cd09e1c0f5c6937cd9d7513160fc3f&pitd=20180719&n=pt45.1.46&r=PART&ty=HTML#se45.1.46_1201 (accessed on 13 June 2019).
47. National Right to Life. *When does Life Begin?* National Right to Life: Washington, DC, USA, 2019.
48. Roberts, S.C.M.; Thompson, K.M. Estimating the Prevalence of United States Women with Alcohol-exposed Pregnancies and Births. *Womens Health Issues* **2019**, *29*, 188–193. [CrossRef]
49. Diekman, S.T.; Floyd, R.L.; Decoufle, P.; Schulkin, J.; Ebrahim, S.H.; Sokol, R.J. A survey of obstetrician-gynecologists on their patients' alcohol use during pregnancy. *Obstet. Gynecol.* **2000**, *95*, 756–763. [CrossRef]
50. Ammon Avalos, L.; Kaskutas, L.A.; Block, G.; Li, D.K. Do multivitamin supplements modify the relationship between prenatal alcohol intake and miscarriage? *Am. J. Obstet. Gynecol.* **2009**, *201*, 563.e1–563.e9. [CrossRef]
51. Jacobson, S.W.; Carter, R.C.; Molteno, C.D.; Stanton, M.E.; Herbert, J.S.; Lindinger, N.M.; Lewis, C.E.; Dodge, N.C.; Hoyme, H.E.; Zeisel, S.H.; et al. Efficacy of maternal choline supplementation during pregnancy in mitigating adverse effects of prenatal alcohol exposure on growth and cognitive function: A randomized, double-blind, placebo-controlled clinical trial. *Alcohol Clin. Exp. Res.* **2018**, *42*, 1327–1341. [CrossRef]
52. May, P.A.; Gossage, J.P. Maternal risk factors for fetal alcohol spectrum disorders: Not as simple as it might seem. *Alcohol Res. Health* **2011**, *34*, 15–26.
53. May, P.A.; Hamrick, K.J.; Corbin, K.D.; Hasken, J.M.; Marais, A.S.; Blankenship, J.; Hoyme, H.E.; Gossage, J.P. Maternal nutritional status as a contributing factor for the risk of fetal alcohol spectrum disorders. *Reprod. Toxicol.* **2016**, *59*, 101–108. [CrossRef]
54. Roberts, D.E. *Killing the Black Body: Race, Reproduction, and the Meaning of Liberty*; Vintage: New York, NY, USA, 1999.

55. Schedler, G. Does society have the right to force pregnant drug addicts to abort their fetuses? *Soc. Theory Pract.* **1991**, *17*, 369–384. [CrossRef]
56. Kolata, G. Woman in abortion dispute ends her pregnancy. *N. Y. Times Web.* **1992**, A10.
57. Hennelly, M.; Yi, J.; Batkis, M.; Chisolm, M.S. Termination of pregnancy in two patients during psychiatric hospitalization for depressive symptoms and substance dependence. *Psychosomatics* **2011**, *52*, 482–485. [CrossRef]
58. O'Leary, C.M.; Heuzenroeder, L.; Elliott, E.J.; Bower, C. A review of policies on alcohol use during pregnancy in Australia and other English-speaking countries, 2006. *Med. J. Aust.* **2007**, *186*, 466–471.
59. Lipson, A.H.; Webster, W.S. Response to letters dealing with warning labels on alcoholic beverages. *Teratology* **1990**, *41*, 479–489. [CrossRef]
60. Koren, G. Drinking and pregnancy. *CMAJ* **1991**, *145*, 1552–1554.
61. Koren, G.; Koren, T.; Gladstone, J. Mild maternal drinking and pregnancy outcome: Perceived versus true risks. *Clin. Chim. Acta* **1996**, *246*, 155–162. [CrossRef]
62. Todorow, M.; Moore, T.E.; Koren, G. Investigating the effects of low to moderate levels of prenatal alcohol exposure on child behaviour: A critical review. *J. Popul. Ther. Clin. Pharmacol.* **2010**, *17*, e323–e330.
63. Carson, G.; Cox, L.V.; Crane, J.; Croteau, P.; Graves, L.; Kluka, S.; Koren, G.; Martel, M.J.; Midmer, D.; Nulman, I.; et al. Alcohol use and pregnancy consensus clinical guidelines. *J. Obstet. Gynaecol. Can.* **2010**, *32*, S1–S2. [CrossRef]
64. ACOG. Committee opinion no. 473: Substance abuse reporting and pregnancy: The role of the obstetrician-gynecologist. *Obstet. Gynecol.* **2011**, *117*, 200–201. [CrossRef]
65. Avery, M.R.; Droste, N.; Giorgi, C.; Ferguson, A.; Martino, F.; Coomber, K.; Miller, P. Mechanisms of influence: Alcohol industry submissions to the inquiry into fetal alcohol spectrum disorders. *Drug Alcohol Rev.* **2016**, *35*, 665–672. [CrossRef]
66. McCambridge, J.; Mialon, M. Alcohol industry involvement in science: A systematic review of the perspectives of the alcohol research community. *Drug Alcohol Rev.* **2018**, *37*, 565–579. [CrossRef]
67. McCambridge, J.; Mialon, M.; Hawkins, B. Alcohol industry involvement in policymaking: A systematic review. *Addiction* **2018**, *113*, 1571–1584. [CrossRef]
68. Roberts, S.C.M.; Avalos, L.A.; Sinkford, D.; Foster, D.G. Alcohol, tobacco and drug use as reasons for abortion. *Alcohol Alcohol.* **2012**, *47*, 640–648. [CrossRef]
69. O'Leary, C.M. Alcohol and Pregnancy: Do Abstinence Policies Have Unintended Consequences? *Alcohol Alcohol.* **2012**, *47*, 638–639. [CrossRef]
70. Kesmodel, U.S.; Urbute, A. Changes in drinking patterns, attitudes towards and knowledge about alcohol consumption during pregnancy in a population of pregnant Danish women. *Alcohol Clin. Exp. Res.* **2019**, *43*, 1213–1219. [CrossRef]
71. Armstrong, M.A.; Kaskutas, L.A.; Witbrodt, J.; Taillac, C.J.; Hung, Y.Y.; Osejo, V.M.; Escobar, G.J. Using drink size to talk about drinking during pregnancy: A randomized clinical trial of Early Start Plus. *Soc. Work Health Care* **2009**, *48*, 90–103. [CrossRef]
72. Gerdts, C.; Dobkin, L.; Foster, D.G.; Schwarz, E.B. Side effects, physical health consequences, and mortality associated with abortion and birth after an unwanted pregnancy. *Womens Health Issues* **2016**, *26*, 55–59. [CrossRef]
73. Foster, D.G.; Biggs, M.A.; Ralph, L.; Gerdts, C.; Roberts, S.; Glymour, M.M. Socioeconomic outcomes of women who receive and women who are denied wanted abortions in the United States. *Am. J. Public Health* **2018**, *108*, 407–413. [CrossRef]
74. Roberts, S.C.M.; Biggs, M.A.; Chibber, K.S.; Gould, H.; Rocca, C.H.; Foster, D.G. Risk of violence from the man involved in the pregnancy after receiving or being denied an abortion. *BMC Med.* **2014**, *12*, 144. [CrossRef]
75. Raymond, E.G.; Grimes, D.A. The comparative safety of legal induced abortion and childbirth in the United States. *Obstet. Gynecol.* **2012**, *119*, 215–219. [CrossRef]
76. Berglas, N.F.; Johns, N.E.; Rosenzweig, C.; Hunter, L.A.; Roberts, S.C.M. State and local health department activities related to abortion: A web site content analysis. *J. Public Health Manag. Pract.* **2018**, *24*, 255–262. [CrossRef]
77. Zhang, B.; Nian, Y.; Palmer, M.; Chen, Q.; Wellings, K.; Oniffrey, T.M.; Yu, T.; Huang, L.; Fan, S.; Du, Y.; et al. An ecological perspective on risk factors for repeat induced abortion in China. *Sex. Reprod. Healthc.* **2018**, *18*, 43–47. [CrossRef]

78. Taft, A.J.; Powell, R.L.; Watson, L.F.; Lucke, J.C.; Mazza, D.; McNamee, K. Factors associated with induced abortion over time: Secondary data analysis of five waves of the Australian Longitudinal Study on Women's Health. *Aust. N. Z. J. Public Health* **2019**, *43*, 137–142. [CrossRef]
79. Martino, S.C.; Collins, R.L.; Ellickson, P.L.; Klein, D.J. Exploring the link between substance abuse and abortion: The roles of unconventionality and unplanned pregnancy. *Perspect. Sex. Reprod. Health* **2006**, *38*, 66–75. [CrossRef]
80. Massaro, L.T.S.; Abdalla, R.R.; Laranjeira, R.; Caetano, R.; Pinsky, I.; Madruga, C.S. Alcohol misuse among women in Brazil: Recent trends and associations with unprotected sex, early pregnancy, and abortion. *Braz. J. Psychiatry* **2019**, *41*, 131–137. [CrossRef]
81. Tran, N.T.; Clavarino, A.; Williams, G.M.; Najman, J.M. Life course outcomes for women with different alcohol consumption trajectories: A population-based longitudinal study. *Drug Alcohol Rev.* **2016**, *35*, 763–771. [CrossRef]
82. Dong, Y.; Zhang, H.; Wang, Y.; Tao, H.; Xu, S.; Xia, J.; Huang, W.; He, H.; Zaller, N.; Operario, D. Multiple abortions and sexually transmitted infections among young migrant women working in entertainment venues in China. *Women Health* **2015**, *55*, 580–594. [CrossRef]
83. Keenan, K.; Grundy, E.; Kenward, M.G.; Leon, D.A. Women's risk of repeat abortions is strongly associated with alcohol consumption: A longitudinal analysis of a Russian national panel study, 1994–2009. *PLoS ONE* **2014**, *9*, e90316. [CrossRef]
84. Abdala, N.; Zhan, W.; Shaboltas, A.V.; Skochilov, R.V.; Kozlov, A.P.; Krasnoselskikh, T.V. Correlates of abortions and condom use among high risk women attending an STD clinic in St. Petersburg, Russia. *Reprod. Health* **2011**, *8*, 28. [CrossRef]

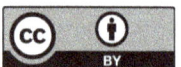

© 2019 by the author. Licensee MDPI, Basel, Switzerland. This article is an open access article distributed under the terms and conditions of the Creative Commons Attribution (CC BY) license (http://creativecommons.org/licenses/by/4.0/).

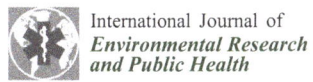 International Journal of
*Environmental Research
and Public Health*

Article

Gender Equality, Drinking Cultures and Second-Hand Harms from Alcohol in the 50 US States

Katherine J. Karriker-Jaffe [1,*], **Christina C. Tam** [1], **Won Kim Cook** [1], **Thomas K. Greenfield** [1] and **Sarah C.M. Roberts** [2]

1. Alcohol Research Group, Public Health Institute, Emeryville, CA 94608, USA; ctam@arg.org (C.C.T.); wcook@arg.org (W.K.C.); tgreenfield@arg.org (T.K.G.)
2. Advancing New Standards in Reproductive Health (ANSIRH), Department of Obstetrics, Gynecology & Reproductive Sciences, University of California, San Francisco, Oakland, CA 94612, USA; sarah.roberts@ucsf.edu
* Correspondence: kkarrikerjaffe@arg.org

Received: 13 September 2019; Accepted: 19 November 2019; Published: 21 November 2019

Abstract: Background: Gender inequality and cultures of binge drinking may increase the risk of second-hand harms from alcohol. Methods: Using the 2014–2015 National Alcohol Survey and 2015 National Alcohol's Harm to Others Survey (N = 7792), we examine associations of state-level gender equality measures (contraceptive access, abortion rights, women's economic equality) and binge drinking cultures (rates of men's and women's binge drinking) with individual-level indicators of second-hand harms by drinking strangers and partners/spouses. Results: In main effects models, only male binge drinking was associated with greater odds of harms from drinking strangers. There were significant interactions of gender equality with male binge drinking: High male binge drinking rates were more strongly associated with stranger-perpetrated harms in states low on contraceptive access or abortion rights compared to states high on these measures. Conversely, male binge drinking was more strongly associated with spouse/partner-perpetrated second-hand harms in states with more economic equality, compared to states lower on this measure. Conclusions: Detrimental effects of high male binge drinking rates may be modified by gender equality. Targeted interventions may reduce alcohol-related harms experienced by women in states with high rates of male binge drinking. Restrictions in access to contraception and abortion may exacerbate harms due to men's drinking.

Keywords: alcohol's harms to others; gender equality; drinking cultures

1. Introduction

Gender equality refers to the parity of women and men (an absence of inequity or bias) on key economic, social and political indicators [1]. Gender inequality is rooted in the power structures in a society that allocates resources and opportunities differentially to men [2]. Globally and in the United States (US), gender (in)equality has been linked to many health outcomes, particularly for women [3,4] and children [5,6], but also for men [4,7]. For example, in the US, greater state-level gender equality is associated with better mental health for women [3], reduced teen pregnancy [6], better birth outcomes [6], reduced infant mortality [5] and lower mortality rates for both men [4,7] and women [4]. Gender equality encompasses dimensions of economic participation and opportunity (such as the proportion of women engaging in paid labor), educational attainment (such as the proportion of women with a university education), political participation and empowerment (such as the proportion of women who voted in a recent election or the proportion of women in state-wide elected office), and reproductive rights (such as access to abortion services) [8–12], and each of these dimensions may contribute to better health.

Greater gender equality may be associated with increases in some health risk behaviors among women [2]. This could be due to a combination of changes in social norms, industry tactics to increase market share [13] and a variety of other factors such as women's disposable income and leisure time [14]. There is some concern that greater gender equality may be associated with increased alcohol consumption among women [15,16]. In the US, data do not appear to support concerns about greater gender equality leading to increased drinking by women, however. One US study found women's drinking was either negatively or not significantly associated with state-level gender equality measures including reproductive rights, women's political participation and gender equality in socioeconomic status (SES) [12]. In fact, findings suggested that increased gender equality was associated with lower levels of risky drinking by both women and men [12]. The current study examines associations between gender equality and second-hand harms from alcohol, including an investigation of the moderating effects of men's and women's drinking cultures.

Second-hand harms due to alcohol—which also are called alcohol's harm to others, externalities and collateral damage from drinking [17]—range in severity from complaints, such as being kept awake at night by drunken noise in the streets, or being harassed or bothered by someone who had been drinking, to more severe concerns, such as being assaulted by someone who had been drinking or being in a drink-driving accident [18]. These second-hand effects of alcohol are prevalent. US general population survey data suggest almost 20% of adults report at least one harm caused by someone who had been drinking in the prior year [19], and lifetime estimates of these harms approach 60% [20]. Rates of harm are even higher in other countries such as Canada [17] and Australia [21], as well as in some low- and middle-income countries [22]. There also is notable geographic variability within societies in the prevalence of second-hand harms from alcohol [22], as well as in the social patterning of these harms [23]. For example, recent US data show that women report more harms from drinking spouses/partners compared to men [19,24,25], with an elevated risk of physical aggression from such perpetrators [25]. These second-hand effects of alcohol have serious consequences for mental health [19,26–29], particularly if the harms were caused by someone close to the victim, such as a drinking spouse or family member [19,27,28].

Many studies have examined the relationship between gender equality and violence against women (see, for example [30] and the review by Roberts [8]), but fewer have looked specifically at alcohol-related harms. A US study using neighborhood (small area) data found greater gender equality was associated with reduced rates of violence perpetrated by young men, with no increases in violence perpetrated by young women [31]. An international study found gender equality was associated with smaller differences between women's and men's drinking in public places, such as bars [32]. Those authors speculated that an increased presence of women in these public drinking venues could put them at increased risk of alcohol-related harm. They also posited, alternatively, that the increased presence of women also could change the culture of public drinking venues by making the places less masculine, thus perhaps reducing alcohol-associated harms, such as fights or other violent events that often occur in such locales. They actually found the opposite in a subsequent paper [33], with a decreased presence of women in bars in some countries appearing to be protective for men in terms of reducing fights. However, this study focused only on the proportion of men and women drinking in bars as the key predictor, and it included a range of countries that varied in terms of drinking culture (including rules and norms about the acceptability of drinking) and other factors, such as rates of violence, that could not be adequately controlled in analyses. Here, we focus on whether state-level indicators of gender equality in the US are associated with second-hand harms due to someone else's drinking, as well as the ways in which drinking cultures may affect this association.

Significant differences across cultures in people's attitudes, norms and behaviors related to drinking have been noted [34]. In addition to varying in gender equality, the 50 US states also vary in men's and women's drinking patterns [35,36], foretelling variability in drinking cultures by gender. In the US, each state has unique characteristics relevant to the determination of a drinking culture and to corresponding alcohol consumption patterns and alcohol-related problems.

Factors that may underlie or influence drinking culture include a state's demographic make-up in terms of age, gender, race/ethnicity groups, and socioeconomic status; a state's mix of religions with differing perspectives on alcohol use; historical and cultural practices related to drinking (or not drinking); and state alcohol policies and regulatory regimes [35]. There are indications that state binge drinking rates are a reasonable proxy for drinking culture, and that these may influence drinking behaviors, as well as the second-hand effects of drinking. For example, a US study found the state binge drinking rate was an independent predictor of binge drinking among students who attended college in the same state [37]. To date, we are unaware of any published studies that have examined state binge drinking rates in relation to second-hand harms from drinking, although one study found proximity to colleges with high levels of binge drinking was related to greater reports of second-hand harms by community members living in nearby neighborhoods [38]. This suggests that risks for second-hand harms perpetrated by drinking strangers may be elevated in states with high rates of binge drinking. Second-hand harms caused by known drinkers also may be elevated in such states. This may be particularly true for female victims, as women are more likely than men to report being close to a male heavy drinker [39] (e.g., a spouse/partner) and women in many countries—including the US, Australia and New Zealand—are more likely than men to experience harm caused by a known drinker [23].

Based on the extant literature showing associations between gender equality, alcohol consumption and violence, we hypothesize that harms due to someone else's drinking would be more common in states with lower gender equality (Hypothesis 1a) and in states with high rates of binge drinking (Hypothesis 1b), especially binge drinking by men. We also examined whether these contexts had synergistic effects, anticipating that the combination of low gender equality with higher rates of men's binge drinking would be associated with particularly elevated levels of second-hand harms from alcohol. That is, we hypothesize that the expected relationship between a culture of binge drinking by men in the state and second-hand harms due to drinking would be exacerbated by gender inequality (Hypothesis 2). Given gender differences in the social patterning of second-hand alcohol harms, we also expected the interaction of gender inequality and drinking culture to emerge for alcohol-related harms reported by women rather than for harms reported by men (Hypothesis 3). For men, we instead anticipated that higher rates of binge drinking would be associated with more harms, regardless of the level of gender equality in the state. Because we were not sure how these associations might differ by perpetrator type, we examined an overall indicator of harms, and then used separate indicators for stranger- and spouse/partner-perpetrated harms.

2. Materials and Methods

2.1. Survey Datasets

We used pooled cross-sectional data from the 2014–2015 National Alcohol Survey (NAS) and 2015 National Alcohol's Harm to Others Survey (NAHTOS). These surveys incorporated the same dual-frame landline and mobile telephone sampling design that also included Black/African American and Hispanic/Latino oversamples (hereafter Black and Hispanic, respectively). One eligible respondent from each household was randomly selected, and computer-assisted interviews were administered in either English or Spanish. The overall cooperation rates for the NAS and NAHTOS were 45.4% and 47.3%, respectively (averaged across landline and cell phone surveys). The Institutional Review Boards of the Public Health Institute in Oakland, CA, and of the fieldwork agency (ICF, Inc., Fairfax, VA, USA) approved all survey protocols. The human subjects' protections for the 2015 US National Alcohol Survey were approved on 6 September 2013 (IRB#I13-019). The protocol was subsequently included in an overarching approval (with ongoing, yearly oversight) for the National Alcohol Survey Series (IRB#I16-028). The human subjects protections for the 2015 US National Alcohol's Harm to Others Survey were approved on 18 December 2014 (IRB#I13-018). For more details on the NAS, see Karriker-Jaffe et al. [19], and for more information on the NAHTOS, see Kaplan et al. [40].

For both surveys, respondent addresses were geocoded and linked with the state-level predictors described below. Due to missing data on some state-level indicators, respondents living in Washington, DC (n = 49) were not included in the analyses.

The analytic sample (N = 7792) was restricted to respondents who had no missing data on key dependent variables, and who had location identifiers at the state level. In the weighted sample, 52.6% of respondents were female (n = 4636), the average age was 47.1 years old (SD = 17.8) and the majority was non-Hispanic White (66.3%), followed by Hispanics (14.1%), Blacks (11.9%) and respondents of other or missing race/ethnicity (7.7%).

2.2. Measures

2.2.1. Outcome Variables

Respondents reported whether they experienced any of eight harms due to someone else's drinking in the past year. Second-hand harms included: (a) having family problems or marriage difficulties; (b) being pushed, hit or assaulted; (c) having house, car or other property vandalized; (d) having financial trouble; (e) being in a traffic accident; (f) being harassed, bothered, called names or otherwise insulted; (g) feeling threatened or afraid; and (h) being physically harmed. These items have been used on prior US [19,20,41], Canadian [42] and multi-national surveys [43]. As previously detailed [19], each harm was attributed to specific perpetrators, including intimate partners (spouses as well as boyfriends/girlfriends) and/or strangers (someone not known by name). In the analytic sample, 19.2% had experienced one or more of these harms in the past year, with 4.0% reporting harm due to the drinking of intimate partners and 8.8% reporting second-hand harm from strangers.

2.2.2. State-Level Predictors

Gender equality measures. In the present study, indicators for state policies related to gender equality included two indicators of reproductive rights (contraceptive access, abortion rights) and one indicator of economic equality between men and women.

Reproductive rights. Reproductive rights/autonomy measures often incorporate indicators such as birth outcomes or life expectancy or adolescent birth rates [10,11] that could plausibly be related to the outcomes under consideration in this analysis. To avoid this potential limitation, we use two indicators of reproductive rights—indicators of the extent to which state policies facilitate or restrict contraceptive access and abortion rights—that more explicitly measure the extent to which women have control over their own reproductive lives [44].

Contraceptive access is a dichotomous measure indicating whether the state offered or required insurance coverage of contraception and/or low-income access to family planning, versus neither [44]. Of all respondents, 80.4% lived in states with some form of subsidized contraceptive access. States with restricted coverage of contraception were Alaska, Idaho, Kansas, Kentucky, Nebraska, North and South Dakota, Tennessee, Texas, Utah and Virginia.

Abortion rights scores from the year 2015 were derived from NARAL, a national pro-choice organization that tracks abortion and contraception policies in each state [44]. Each of the 50 states was assigned a grade from A+ to F. For the present analysis, states were dichotomized to reflect having more abortion rights (i.e., grade B− or higher) or fewer abortion rights. When women's access to abortion is restricted, they may be at increased risk of intimate partner violence from a man involved in an unwanted pregnancy [45]. Of all respondents, just 43.7% lived in states with more abortion rights for women. States with more restricted access to abortion were Alabama, Arizona, Arkansas, Florida, Georgia, Idaho, Indiana, Kansas, Kentucky, Louisiana, Michigan, Mississippi, Missouri, Nebraska, North and South Carolina, North and South Dakota, Ohio, Oklahoma, Pennsylvania, Tennessee, Texas, Utah and Virginia.

Economic equality. We used an existing measure of state-level economic equality between men and women that operationalizes economic equality using median annual earnings for women employed full-time year round, the earnings ratio between women and men employed full-time year round, percent of women in the labor force and percent of all women employed in managerial or professional occupations [46]. States were assigned a grade from A+ to F that reflected policies supporting economic equality between men and women. This measure was dichotomized into those states that support economic equality (i.e., grades ranging from A to C) versus not. Of all respondents, 78.7% lived in states supporting economic equality. States that scored poorly on this measure were Alabama, Arkansas, Florida, Idaho, Indiana, Kentucky, Louisiana, Mississippi, Montana, Nevada, Oklahoma, South Carolina, South Dakota, Utah and West Virginia.

Drinking culture, by gender. To operationalize drinking cultures, we used 2013 data from the Behavioral Risk Factors Surveillance System [47] on the percentage of men, and separately, women, in each state reporting binge drinking in the past 30 days. Binge drinking was defined as having four or five (or more) drinks on one occasion for women and men, respectively. The average state-level binge drinking rates across the US were 23.0% for men (SD = 2.2%) and 11.1% for women (SD = 2.2%). These data were centered on the overall US averages for the multivariate models. Higher rates of binge drinking indicate state drinking cultures more supportive of binge drinking. In the weighted analysis sample, state-level binge drinking rates for men and women were highly correlated ($r = 0.87$, $p < 0.01$).

Median income. Data on each state's annual median household income came from the US American Community Survey, which is administered by the US Census Bureau [48]. The weighted average state-level median income for the analytic sample was US$54,006 (SD = $7768); the variable was transformed to represent increments of US$10,000. Median income was moderately positively correlated with men's ($r = 0.33$, $p < 0.01$) and women's ($r = 0.44$, $p < 0.01$) binge drinking rates, as well as with the measures of gender equality, with the weakest association being with the indicator of contraceptive access ($r = 0.08$, $p < 0.01$) and stronger associations with the indicators for abortion rights ($r = 0.68$, $p < 0.01$) and economic equality ($r = 0.51$, $p < 0.01$).

2.2.3. Individual-Level Predictors

Drinking status. Each respondent's past-year drinking status was derived from the National Institute on Alcohol Abuse and Alcoholism's (NIAAA) stated guidelines for at-risk or heavy drinking. At-risk drinking is defined as consuming more than three or four drinks on a single day, or more than seven or 14 drinks per week, for women and men, respectively. Of the weighted analytic sample, 33.3% were non-drinkers, 38.9% were drinkers who did not exceed the recommended guidelines, and 27.8% were at-risk drinkers in the past year.

Demographic covariates. Models also adjusted for respondents' gender, age, marital status (separated, divorced, widowed, and never married, versus married or living with a partner), race/ethnicity (using mutually-exclusive indicators for Hispanic, Black and other race/ethnicity, versus non-Hispanic White), education (less than a college degree versus a 4-year college degree or more), and income in the past year (classified into categories: "up to $20,000", "$20,001–60,000", "$60,001–$100,000", "$100,001 or more", and missing income, 11.6% of sample).

2.3. Analyses

The data consisted of a two-level hierarchy with individuals nested within states, and therefore we tested associations using multilevel logistic regression. We estimated main effects and interaction models using the state-level gender equality indicators and binge drinking rates by gender using the full sample, followed by gender-stratified analyses. For significant interactions, we also report Wald chi-square tests of the difference between the main effects and interaction models. Interactions were graphed using values of continuous variables at +/− 1 standard deviation from the mean. Data were weighted to adjust for the sampling strategy and nonresponse; all analyses were conducted using Stata version 15 [49].

3. Results

Descriptive statistics overall and for the gender-stratified samples are shown in Table 1. Women were older than men, and they also were more likely than men to be unmarried, Black and low-income. Women were more likely than men to be non-drinkers, and they were less likely than men to be at-risk drinkers. There were no differences by gender in any of the state-level variables.

Table 1. Sample descriptives and weighted bivariate comparisons by gender (N = 7792).

Variables	Full Sample N = 7792	Men n = 3156	Women n = 4636	p
Unmarried (%)	42.3	40.1	44.3	*
Race/Ethnicity (%)				***
White	66.4	67.2	65.8	
Black	11.9	10.7	13.0	
Hispanic	14.1	15.0	13.3	
Other/Missing	7.5	7.1	7.9	
Less than College Degree	70.2	69.1	71.2	
Income (%)				***
Up to $20,000	20.9	18.0	23.6	
$20,000–$60,000	32.6	33.7	31.7	
$60,001–$100,000	20.3	21.0	19.7	
$100,001 or more	14.9	18.0	12.1	
Missing Income	11.3	9.3	13.0	
Age, M (SD)	52.6 (17.7)	51.3 (17.6)	53.5 (17.6)	†
Drinking Status (%)				***
Non-Drinker	33.3	29.7	36.7	
Drinker, Does not Exceed Guidelines [a]	38.8	37.4	40.0	
At-risk Drinker, Exceeds Guidelines	28.0	32.9	23.3	
State Median Income (by $10k), M (SD)	5.4 (0.8)	5.5 (0.8)	5.5 (0.8)	
State Male Binge Drinking %, M (SD)	23.1 (2.9)	23.0 (2.9)	23.0 (2.9)	
State Female Binge Drinking %, M (SD)	11.1 (2.1)	11.1 (2.1)	11.0 (2.1)	
State Gender Equality Indicators (%)				
Contraceptive Access	80.5	80.3	80.6	
Reproductive Rights	43.6	44.2	43.1	
Economic Equality	78.7	79.0	78.4	

*** $p < 0.001$ * $p < 0.05$ † $p < 0.10$; [a] U.S. National Institute on Alcohol Abuse and Alcoholism's (NIAAA) guidelines define at-risk drinking as consuming more than 3 or 4 drinks on a single day, or more than 7 or 14 drinks per week, for women and men, respectively.

3.1. Main Effects Models

In simultaneous main effects models testing the first hypothesis (1a), none of the gender equality measures were significantly associated with the second-hand harms due to alcohol overall, nor for men or women separately. These models also provide tests of the second hypothesis (1b): Adjusting for measures of gender equality and other state-level variables, the state rate of binge drinking by men was associated with increased odds of harms perpetrated by strangers overall (OR (95% CI) = 1.11 (1.00, 1.23)), although associations were not statistically significant in the gender-stratified models (OR (95% CI) = 1.12 (0.96, 1.31) for women; 1.09 (0.94, 1.26) for men). In the full sample, the association of male binge drinking rates with stranger-perpetrated harms persisted once individual-level covariates were added to the simultaneous model (OR (95% CI) = 1.12 (1.00, 1.24)). The male binge drinking rate was not significantly associated with the indicator of any past-year second-hand harm from alcohol, and it also was not significantly associated with spouse/partner-perpetrated harms. State rates of binge drinking by women and the state-level median household income were not significantly associated with second-hand harms from alcohol in any of the models.

3.2. Moderation Models

As expected (Hypothesis 2), there were some statistically significant interactions between indicators of gender equality and state male binge drinking rates. The findings for any past-year harm and for stranger-perpetrated harms suggested that the association between male binge drinking and second-hand harms was exacerbated by gender inequality.

3.2.1. Any Past-Year Second-Hand Harm

As shown in Table 2, in the full sample, there was a statistically significant interaction (OR = 0.92) between a state's male binge drinking rate and contraceptive access in relation to any past-year second-hand harm due to someone else's drinking (Wald chi-square (df = 18) = 441.69, $p < 0.001$). The marginal predicted probabilities showed a significant association of states' male binge drinking rates with past-year harm due to someone else's drinking only in states with restricted contraceptive access (the association was not significant in states with good contraceptive access): Predicted probabilities ranged from 0.161 (95% CI = 0.106, 0.216) at the lowest rates of binge drinking by men to 0.251 (95% CI = 0.187, 0.316) at the highest rates of binge drinking by men in states with restricted contraceptive access and from 0.178 (95% CI = 0.125, 0.231) at the lowest rates of binge drinking by men to 0.195 (95% CI = 0.136, 0.255) at the highest rates of binge drinking by men in states with good contraceptive access. The interaction is depicted in Figure 1 (left panel), which shows increasing rates of second-hand harms from alcohol as rates of men's binge drinking increase, but only in states without good contraceptive access (top line, dashed).

Table 2. Interactive associations of states' male binge drinking rates and contraceptive access with any second-hand harm from others' drinking [1].

Predictor Variables	Full Sample (N = 7792) OR (95% CI)	Men (n = 3156) OR (95% CI)	Women (n = 4636) OR (95% CI)
Male	0.93 (0.80, 1.08)	-	-
Unmarried	1.36 (1.06, 1.74) *	1.71 (1.26, 2.31) ***	1.13 (0.87, 1.48)
Race/Ethnicity [2]			
Black	1.06 (0.85, 1.31)	1.06 (0.70, 1.59)	1.03 (0.78, 1.37)
Hispanic	0.87 (0.71, 1.05)	0.96 (0.62, 1.49)	0.74 (0.53, 1.03) †
Other/Missing	1.40 (0.99, 2.00) †	1.69 (1.06, 2.69) *	1.21 (0.71, 2.07)
Less than College Degree	1.08 (0.86, 1.36)	1.20 (0.84, 1.69)	1.02 (0.74, 1.39)
Income [3]			
Up to $20,000	1.75 (1.26, 2.43) **	1.42 (0.90, 2.26)	2.05 (1.37, 3.08) ***
$20,000–$60,000	1.41 (1.04, 1.93) *	1.28 (0.76, 2.15)	1.55 (1.06, 2.27) *
$60,001–$100,000	1.11 (0.81, 1.52)	1.21 (0.75, 1.94)	0.96 (0.62, 1.48)
Missing Income	0.99 (0.74, 1.33)	1.09 (0.62, 1.95)	0.90 (0.57, 1.41)
Age	0.98 (0.97, 0.98) ***	0.98 (0.97, 0.99) ***	0.97 (0.96, 0.98) ***
Drinking Status [4]			
Drinker, Does not Exceed Guidelines	1.14 (0.90, 1.45)	0.96 (0.64, 1.44)	1.26 (0.92, 1.74)
At-risk Drinker, Exceeds Guidelines	2.32 (1.89, 2.84) ***	2.14 (1.51, 3.03)	2.53 (1.86, 3.44) ***
State Median Income	1.06 (0.17, 6.65)	0.92 (0.05, 16.82)	1.97 (0.88, 1.17)
State Male Binge Drinking Rate	1.11 (1.01, 1.23) *	1.07 (0.93, 1.24)	1.12 (1.02, 1.22) *
State Female Binge Drinking Rate	1.02 (0.86, 1.22)	1.00 (0.79, 1.25)	1.01 (0.88, 1.17)
Contraceptive Access [5]	0.90 (0.65, 1.24)	0.84 (0.49, 1.43)	0.99 (0.73, 1.32)
Male Binge * Contraceptive Access [6]	0.92 (0.85, 0.99) *	-	0.91 (0.85, 0.97) **
Constant	0.34 (0.12, 0.96) *	0.23 (0.03, 1.60)	0.29 (0.12, 0.69) **

Note: *** $p < 0.001$ ** $p < 0.01$ * $p < 0.05$ † $p < 0.10$; [1] Harm from Others' Drinking = Reported one or more of 8 second-hand harms in the past year; [2] Reference = White; [3] Reference = $100,001+; [4] Reference = Non-drinker; [5] Contraceptive access = The state offered or required insurance coverage of contraception and/or low-income access to family planning, versus neither; [6] Main effects model reported for men because interaction was not significant, $p > 0.10$.

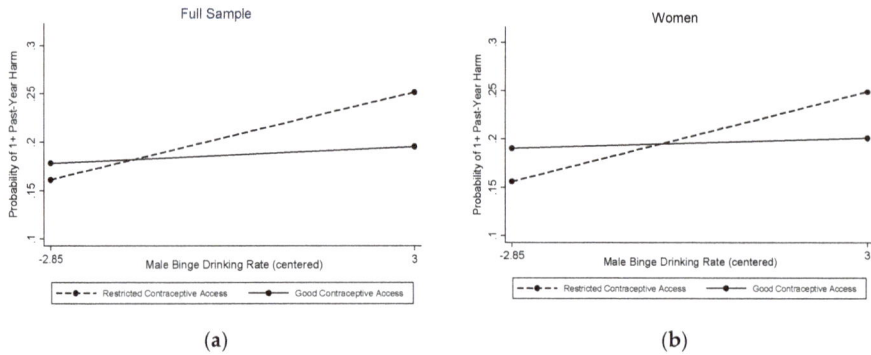

Figure 1. Interaction between male binge drinking rate and contraceptive access in relation to any second-hand harm from alcohol in the past year: (**a**) in the full sample (left panel); and (**b**) for women (right panel).

The stratified models used to test Hypothesis 3 (Table 2 and Figure 1, right panel) revealed this pattern was unique to harms reported by women (OR = 0.91 for interaction and OR = 1.12 for the male binge drinking rate; Wald chi-square (df = 17) = 291.07, $p < 0.001$), with predicted probabilities of experiencing one or more harm due to someone else's drinking ranging from 0.156 (95% CI = 0.113, 0.199) at the lowest rates of binge drinking by men to 0.249 (95% CI = 0.189, 0.309) at the highest rates of binge drinking by men in states with restricted contraceptive access and from 0.190 (95% CI = 0.149, 0.232) at the lowest rates of binge drinking by men to 0.200 (95% CI = 0.149, 0.253) at the highest rates of binge drinking by men in states with good contraceptive access. The interaction was not statistically significant for men, so it was dropped from the model. In the main effects model for men (Table 2), none of the state-level variables were significantly associated with past-year harms from someone else's drinking.

3.2.2. Past-Year Stranger-Perpetrated Harm

A similar pattern of results was found in the full sample when considering stranger-perpetrated harms. Both contraceptive access (OR = 0.89; Wald chi-square (df = 18) = 327.57, $p < 0.001$; Table 3) and abortion rights (OR = 0.90; Wald chi-square (df = 18) = 310.89, $p < 0.001$; Table 4) evidenced significant interactions with the male binge-drinking rate.

As shown in Table 3 and Figure 2, in states with restricted contraceptive access (the reference group), the male binge drinking rate was associated with significantly greater odds of harms from drinking strangers (OR = 1.17). The marginal predicted probabilities showed a significant association of states' male binge drinking rates with past-year harm due to a stranger's drinking only in states with restricted contraceptive access (the association was not significant in states with good contraceptive access): Predicted probabilities ranged from 0.067 (95% CI = 0.031, 0.103) at the lowest rates of binge drinking by men to 0.143 (95% CI = 0.096, 0.190) at the highest rates of binge drinking by men in states with restricted contraceptive access and from 0.070 (95% CI = 0.044, 0.096) at the lowest rates of binge drinking by men to 0.082 (95% CI = 0.051, 0.113) at the highest rates of binge drinking by men in states with good contraceptive access. In the stratified models, the interaction between contraceptive access and men's binge drinking rates was not significant for either men or women, and in the main effect models (Table 3), none of the state-level variables were associated with harm from drinking strangers for either men or women.

Table 3. Interactive associations of male binge drinking rates and contraceptive access with harm from drinking strangers.

Predictor Variables	Full Sample (N = 7792) OR (95% CI)	Men (n = 3156) OR (95% CI)	Women (n = 4636) OR (95% CI)
Male	1.37 (1.07, 1.74) *	-	-
Unmarried	1.34 (1.03, 1.75) *	1.52 (0.96, 2.40) †	1.31 (0.92, 1.87)
Race/Ethnicity [1]			
Black	1.08 (0.74, 1.57)	1.19 (0.67, 2.11)	0.92 (0.57, 1.47)
Hispanic	0.90 (0.66, 1.21)	0.86 (0.51, 1.46)	0.82 (0.44, 1.51)
Other/Missing	1.64 (1.11, 2.42) *	2.49 (1.43, 4.33) **	0.97 (0.48, 1.97)
Less than College Degree	0.90 (0.64, 1.26)	1.21 (0.74, 1.98)	0.67 (0.43, 1.05) †
Income [2]			
Up to $20,000	1.34 (0.85, 2.11)	0.84 (0.43, 1.63)	1.89 (0.91, 3.96) †
$20,000–$60,000	1.23 (0.75, 2.04)	1.21 (0.60, 2.44)	1.19 (0.65, 2.16)
$60,001–$100,000	0.97 (0.64, 1.48)	1.04 (0.53, 2.04)	0.82 (0.38, 1.77)
Missing Income	1.01 (0.61, 1.67)	1.08 (0.52, 2.22)	0.88 (0.36, 2.14)
Age	0.97 (0.97, 0.98) ***	0.99 (0.97, 1.00) *	0.96 (0.95, 0.97) ***
Drinking Status [3]			
Drinker, Does not Exceed Guidelines	0.95 (0.70, 1.29)	0.89 (0.55, 1.43)	0.92 (0.53, 1.61)
At-risk Drinker, Exceeds Guidelines	1.85 (1.41, 2.44) ***	1.80 (1.11, 2.93) *	1.82 (1.06, 3.12) *
State Median Income	1.02 (0.15, 7.11)	0.48 (0.02, 12.16)	1.72 (0.74, 1.18)
State Male Binge Drinking Rate	1.17 (1.04, 1.31) *	1.08 (0.94, 1.25)	1.13 (0.95, 1.36)
State Female Binge Drinking Rate	1.02 (0.85, 1.22)	1.02 (0.80, 1.28)	0.93 (0.74, 1.18)
Contraceptive Access [4]	0.74 (0.48, 1.14)	0.84 (0.38, 1.87)	0.68 (0.35, 1.34)
Male Binge * Contraceptive Access [5]	0.89 (0.81, 0.97) *	-	-
Constant	1.73 (0.44, 0.67) *	0.13 (0.01, 1.32) †	0.32 (0.06, 1.76)

Note: *** $p < 0.001$ ** $p < 0.01$ * $p < 0.05$ † $p < 0.10$; [1] Reference = White; [2] Reference = $100,001+; [3] Reference = Non-drinker; [4] Contraceptive access = The state offered or required insurance coverage of contraception and/or low-income access to family planning, versus neither; [5] Main effects model reported for gender-stratified analyses because interactions were not significant, $p > 0.10$.

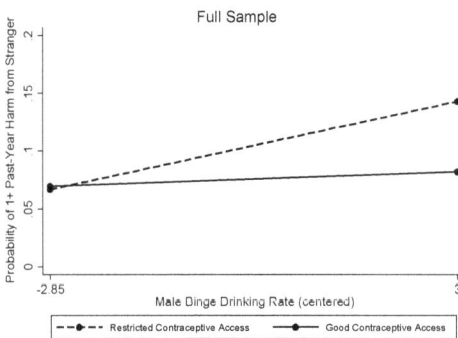

Figure 2. Interaction between male binge drinking rate and contraceptive access in relation to stranger-perpetrated harm in the full sample.

The interaction pattern was consistent when using the indicator of abortion rights. As shown in Table 4 and Figure 3, in states with restricted abortion access (the reference group), the male binge drinking rate was associated with significantly greater odds of harms from drinking strangers (OR = 1.14). The marginal predicted probabilities showed a significant association of states' male binge drinking rates with past-year harm due to a stranger's drinking only in states with restricted abortion access (the association was not significant in states with good abortion access): Predicted probabilities ranged from 0.067 (95% CI = 0.038, 0.095) at the lowest rates of binge drinking by men to 0.131 (95% CI = 0.088, 0.173) at the highest rates of binge drinking by men in states with restricted abortion access and from 0.068 (95% CI = 0.043, 0.093) at the lowest rates of binge drinking by men to 0.077 (95% CI = 0.043, 0.111) at the highest rates of binge drinking by men in states with good abortion access. In the stratified models, the interaction between abortion rights and male binge drinking rates was not significant for men, but it approached significance for women (OR = 0.88; Wald chi-square (df = 17) = 158.01, $p < 0.001$; Table 4).

Table 4. Interactive associations of male binge drinking rates and abortion rights with harm from drinking strangers.

Predictor Variables	Full Sample (N = 7792) OR (95% CI)	Men (n = 3156) OR (95% CI)	Women (n = 4636) OR (95% CI)
Male	1.36 (1.07, 1.74) *	-	-
Unmarried	1.34 (1.03, 1.74) *	1.52 (0.96, 2.41) †	1.31 (0.92, 1.86)
Race/Ethnicity [1]			
Black	1.08 (0.74, 1.56)	1.18 (0.67, 2.08)	0.90 (0.56, 1.44)
Hispanic	0.90 (0.66, 1.22)	0.87 (0.51, 1.48)	0.81 (0.44, 1.49)
Other/Missing	1.63 (1.11, 2.41) *	2.50 (1.44, 4.35) **	0.97 (0.47, 1.97)
Less than College Degree	0.90 (0.64, 1.26)	1.21 (0.74, 1.97)	0.67 (0.43, 1.05) †
Income [2]			
Up to $20,000	1.34 (0.85, 2.11)	0.84 (0.43, 1.63)	1.90 (0.90, 3.99) †
$20,000–$60,000	1.23 (0.75, 2.03)	1.21 (0.60, 2.42)	1.19 (0.65, 2.16)
$60,001–$100,000	0.97 (0.64, 1.48)	1.04 (0.53, 2.03)	0.81 (0.37, 1.76)
Missing Income	1.01 (0.61, 1.67)	1.08 (0.52, 2.22)	0.89 (0.36, 2.16)
Age	0.97 (0.97, 0.98) ***	0.99 (0.97, 1.00) *	0.96 (0.95, 0.97) ***
Drinking Status [3]			
Drinker, Does not Exceed Guidelines	0.95 (0.70, 1.29)	0.89 (0.55, 1.42)	0.91 (0.52, 1.59)
At-risk Drinker, Exceeds Guidelines	1.85 (1.40, 2.43) ***	1.80 (1.11, 2.92) *	1.81 (1.05, 3.11) *
State Median Income	1.68 (0.26, 11.02)	1.63 (0.07, 37.35)	2.87 (0.39, 20.94)
State Male Binge Drinking Rate	1.14 (1.02, 1.29) *	1.06 (0.92, 1.23)	1.18 (0.95, 1.48)
State Female Binge Drinking Rate	1.02 (0.85, 1.22)	1.07 (0.83, 1.38)	0.96 (0.74, 1.25)
Abortion Rights	0.74 (0.49, 1.12)	0.64 (0.30, 1.37)	0.81 (0.46, 1.42)
Male Binge * Abortion Rights [4]	0.90 (0.82, 0.98) *	-	0.88 (0.76, 1.01) †
Constant	0.12 (0.04, 0.40) ***	0.07 (0.01, 0.51) **	0.21 (0.54, 0.84) *

Note: *** $p < 0.001$ ** $p < 0.01$ * $p < 0.05$ † $p < 0.10$; [1] Reference = White; [2] Reference = $100,001+; [3] Reference = Non-drinker; [4] Main effects model reported for men because interaction was not significant, $p > 0.10$.

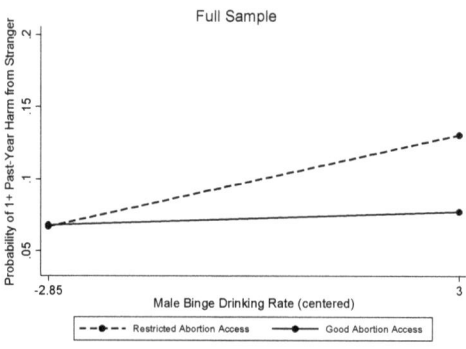

Figure 3. Interaction between the male binge drinking rate and abortion rights in relation to stranger-perpetrated harm in the full sample.

3.2.3. Past-Year Spouse- or Partner-Perpetrated Harm

A different pattern of results emerged for spouse/partner-perpetrated harms. Only economic equality evidenced a significant interaction with the male binge-drinking rate (OR = 1.18; Wald chi-square (df = 18) = 166.53, $p < 0.001$; Table 5). The interaction is depicted in Figure 4 (left panel), which shows a diverging pattern, with higher rates of male binge drinking associated with only slightly higher rates of spouse/partner harm in states with economic equality (solid line) and somewhat decreasing rates of spouse/partner harm in states without economic equality (dashed line).

Table 5. Interactive associations of male binge drinking rates and economic equality with harm from drinking spouse/partner.

Predictor Variables	Full Sample (N = 7792) OR (95% CI)	Men (n = 3156) OR (95% CI)	Women (n = 4636) OR (95% CI)
Male	0.42 (0.26, 0.68) ***	-	-
Unmarried	0.87 (0.56, 1.34)	1.02 (0.38, 2.69)	0.84 (0.50, 1.42)
Race/Ethnicity [1]			
Black	0.96 (0.52, 1.79)	1.49 (0.57, 3.88)	0.80 (0.39, 1.65)
Hispanic	0.78 (0.45, 1.35)	1.38 (0.44, 4.34)	0.66 (0.34, 1.30)
Other/Missing	1.71 (0.87, 3.39)	3.02 (0.90, 10.15) †	1.40 (0.61, 3.23)
Less than College Degree	1.50 (0.98, 2.31) †	1.29 (0.52, 3.20)	1.53 (0.96, 2.44) †
Income [2]			
Up to $20,000	1.81 (0.94, 3.45) †	1.90 (0.71, 5.07)	1.87 (0.76, 4.61)
$20,000–$60,000	1.20 (0.67, 2.17)	0.66 (0.20, 2.24)	1.60 (0.69, 3.68)
$60,001–$100,000	0.95 (0.49, 1.85)	0.80 (0.38, 1.69)	0.98 (0.41, 2.34)
Missing Income	0.58 (0.25, 1.38)	0.77 (1.17, 3.53)	0.49 (0.18, 1.31)
Age	0.98 (0.97, 0.99) ***	1.00 (0.98, 1.01)	0.97 (0.96, 0.98) ***
Drinking Status [3]			
Drinker, Does not Exceed Guidelines	1.51 (0.88, 2.58)	1.64 (0.53, 5.06)	1.39 (0.67, 2.88)
At-risk Drinker, Exceeds Guidelines	2.23 (1.37, 3.65) **	2.68 (1.04, 6.88) *	2.13 (1.06, 4.27) *
State Median Income	2.96 (0.07, 117.38)	7.06 (0.06, 781.29)	5.16 (0.05, 540.02)
State Male Binge Drinking Rate	0.90 (0.76, 1.07)	0.90 (0.71, 1.14)	0.93 (0.74, 1.16)
State Female Binge Drinking Rate	0.90 (0.67, 1.20)	1.02 (0.68, 1.50)	0.85 (0.61, 1.19)
Economic Equality	1.88 (0.97, 3.63) †	1.39 (0.62, 3.12)	1.83 (0.70, 4.80)
Male Binge * Economic Equality [4]	1.18 (1.00, 1.39) *	-	1.25 (1.02, 1.54) *
Constant	0.02 (0.00, 0.12) ***	0.00 (0.00, 0.03) ***	0.01 (0.00, 0.16) **

Note: *** $p < 0.001$ ** $p < 0.01$ * $p < 0.05$ † $p < 0.10$; [1] Reference = White; [2] Reference = $100,001+; [3] Reference = Non-drinker; [4] Main effects model reported for men because interaction was not significant, $p > 0.10$.

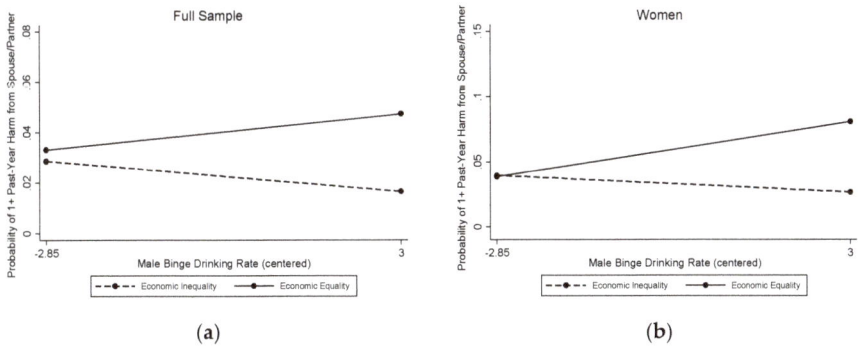

Figure 4. Interaction between male binge drinking rate and economic equality in relation to spouse-perpetrated harms (**a**) in the full sample (left panel); and (**b**) for women (right panel).

The marginal predicted probabilities suggested that states' male binge drinking rates were not significantly associated with past-year harm due to a partner's drinking in either group of states, however: Predicted probabilities ranged from 0.029 (95% CI = 0.015, 0.043) at the lowest rates of binge drinking by men to 0.016 (95% CI = 0.002, 0.031) at the highest rates of binge drinking by men in states without economic equality and from 0.033 (95% CI = 0.013, 0.054) at the lowest rates of binge drinking by men to 0.047 (95% CI = 0.017, 0.078) at the highest rates of binge drinking by men in states with economic equality. The stratified models revealed that this pattern was unique to harms reported by women (OR = 1.25; Wald chi-square (df = 17) = 79.34, $p < 0.001$; Table 5 and Figure 4, right panel), although the marginal predicted probabilities suggested that states' male binge drinking rates were not significantly associated with women's reports of past-year harm due to a partner's drinking in either group of states: Predicted probabilities ranged from 0.039 (95% CI = 0.017, 0.062) at the lowest rates of binge drinking by men to 0.026 (95% CI = -0.004, 0.057) at the highest rates of binge drinking by men in states without economic equality and from 0.038 (95% CI = 0.011, 0.066) at the lowest rates of binge drinking by men to 0.081 (95% CI = 0.023, 0.138) at the highest rates of binge drinking by men in states with economic equality. The interaction was not statistically significant for men. In the main effects model for men (Table 5), none of the state-level variables were significantly associated with past-year harm due to a spouse or partner's drinking.

4. Discussion

In this US study, with the exception of an association between male binge drinking and harms perpetrated by drinking strangers, we did not see any strong independent associations of either gender equality (Hypothesis 1a) or state-level drinking culture (Hypothesis 1b) with second-hand harms from alcohol. Our findings on Hypothesis 1a thus did not replicate prior studies showing an association between gender equality and reduced violence [8,30,31], suggesting the relationship between gender equality and alcohol-related harms is more complex than what can be captured by a main effect model. As hypothesized, we did find evidence that the combination of low gender equality (indexed here by indicators of restricted reproductive rights, including limited contraceptive access and curtailed abortion rights) and high levels of binge drinking by men was associated with increased odds of second-hand harms (Hypothesis 2). This relationship was seen in overall models and it was suggested in results for women, but not seen in results for men (Hypothesis 3). This moderation pattern held for an overall indicator of any second-hand harm in the past year, as well as for an indicator of harm attributed to drinking strangers. Thus, in this nationally-representative US sample, reproductive rights for women appear to buffer against the negative impacts of male binge drinking on others in the community, particularly on women. Future research should seek to replicate our findings, teasing out different types of alcohol-related harms at varying levels of severity, and to examine mechanisms through which these protective effects may occur, such as through changing social norms around violence or allowing women to not be tethered to violent men or to families or communities with high levels of violence.

When we examined alcohol-related harms perpetrated by intimate partners (spouses or boyfriends/ girlfriends), a different interaction pattern emerged. There were somewhat elevated rates of spouse/partner harm in states with economic equality but high levels of male binge drinking, but somewhat lower rates of spouse/partner harm in states without economic equality but high rates of male binge drinking. It may be that there is a backlash against women in these higher-equality, heavy-drinking states [8]. There also may be a tendency for people (women, in particular) in lower-equality, less-heavy-drinking states to label a partner's drinking behavior as problematic, thus resulting in an increased reporting of harms in these contexts. Further, women in environments with greater gender equality may be more likely to divulge alcohol-related harms perpetrated by a partner or spouse. These possibilities should be examined in detail in longitudinal studies that could assess changes in gender equality and changes in second-hand harms from alcohol, as well as in qualitative studies that could describe the social construction of second-hand harms in regions with lower rates of binge drinking or higher economic equality.

We provide new evidence under Hypothesis 1b that a state-level drinking culture characterized by greater binge drinking by men is associated with second-hand harms from drinking strangers. Our findings are similar to prior research, showing that high levels of binge drinking on college campuses were related to reports of second-hand harms experienced by residents of nearby neighborhoods [38]. However, female drinking culture was not associated with second-hand alcohol harms, independently nor in tandem with measures of gender equality. This was not surprising given the contexts in which women drink in the US and other countries, with women tending to drink less often in public settings such as bars than men [32]. Drinking in public settings is associated with higher volume consumption and more opportunities for harms, both due to someone's own drinking and from the drinking of people around them [50,51]. A future study could incorporate the drinking contexts in which these second-hand harms occur to examine differences across levels of gender equality. Furthermore, western drinking cultures generally endorse a normative view of high alcohol consumption among men, whereas women tend to be socialized otherwise [52,53]. However, in many age groups (with the exception of adolescents and young adults), heavy drinking among women in the US is steadily increasing [54] to meet rates comparable to those of men's. Shifting drinking cultures may precede greater occurrences of second-hand harms from alcohol, with women's drinking contributing more to these harms as women's drinking cultures continue to evolve. Intersection of heavy drinking by women with lower levels of gender equality also may put women at greater risk of alcohol-related harm.

To our knowledge, this is one of the first US studies on the topic of state-level gender equality, drinking cultures and alcohol's harm to others. Although we had the benefit of a large, nationally-representative sample of adult respondents, our data were cross-sectional, and causality cannot be implied. Although it is possible that reductions in the second-hand effects of alcohol could precede changes in gender equality, it is less likely that changes in these harms would reduce binge drinking by men or prompt legislators to enact laws and policies protecting women's reproductive rights. Thus, it seems reasonable to assume the outcomes studied here may have been at least partially a result of the policy context and drinking culture of the respondents' state of residence. Stronger causal models would enhance the evidence base on this topic.

Another study limitation is that there may be other important effect modifiers that we did not take into account, such as a respondent's level of education [12] or work status [55], which have been shown to interact with gender equality in studies of drinking behavior. An additional consideration is that some of the US states with the lowest gender equality (such as Idaho, South Dakota and Utah) are also relatively sparsely populated, and may be under-represented in general population samples such as ours.

Further, the indicators of gender equality are not independent, and isolation of their effects may be impossible. For example, four states scored low on all three measures of gender equality, and fourteen states scored low on two of the three measures. Future work may benefit from the utilization of summary scores that better describe the status of women on multiple dimensions. Finally, additional work is needed to disentangle the effects of gender equality, drinking cultures and attitudes toward violence (and particularly violence to women) on alcohol's second-hand harms, as these may be related in complex ways [56]. Future work also should examine overall cultures of violence, using indicators such as levels of violence toward women or state laws on domestic violence and sexual assault, in relation to second-hand harms from alcohol.

5. Conclusions

Findings from a large, population-representative study of US adults suggest detrimental effects of high rates of male binge drinking may be exacerbated by gender inequality, with this effect being particularly harmful for women. As reproductive rights decrease in U.S. states [57], policy makers in states with high levels of binge drinking should be aware that changes in reproductive rights might increase second-hand harms from alcohol experienced by women in these states.

Author Contributions: Conceptualization, K.J.K.-J., C.C.T., W.K.C. & S.C.M.R.; formal analysis, K.J.K.-J. & C.C.T.; data curation, W.K.C.; writing—original draft preparation, K.J.K.-J., C.C.T. & S.C.M.R.; writing—review and editing, W.K.C. & T.K.G.; funding acquisition, T.K.G. & K.J.K.-J.

Funding: This research was funded by the U.S. National Institutes of Health's National Institute on Alcohol Abuse and Alcoholism (NIAAA) grant numbers P50AA005595 (W. Kerr, PI), R01AA022791 (T. Greenfield and K. Karriker-Jaffe, Multiple PIs) and R01AA023870 (T. Greenfield, S. Wilsnack and K. Bloomfield, Multiple PIs).

Acknowledgments: The authors would like to thank biostatistician Libo Li for consulting on analyses.

Conflicts of Interest: The authors declare no conflict of interest. The funders had no role in the design of the study; in the collection, analyses, or interpretation of data; in the writing of the manuscript; or in the decision to publish the results.

References

1. Sen, G.; Ostlin, P. Gender inequity in health: Why it exists and how we can change it. *Glob. Public Health* **2008**, *3* (Suppl. 1), 1–12. [CrossRef]
2. King, T.L.; Kavanagh, A.M.; Scovelle, A.J.; Milner, A. Associations between gender equality and health: A systematic review. *Health Promot. Int.* **2018**. [CrossRef] [PubMed]
3. Borrell, C.; Palencia, L.; Muntaner, C.; Urquia, M.; Malmusi, D.; O'Campo, P. Influence of macrosocial policies on women's health and gender inequalities in health. *Epidemiol. Rev.* **2014**, *36*, 31–48. [CrossRef] [PubMed]
4. Kawachi, I.; Kennedy, B.P.; Gupta, V.; Prothrow-Stith, D. Women's status and the health of women and men: A view from the States. *Soc. Sci. Med.* **1999**, *48*, 21–32. [CrossRef]
5. Homan, P. Political gender inequality and infant mortality in the United States, 1990–2012. *Soc. Sci. Med.* **2017**, *182*, 127–135. [CrossRef] [PubMed]
6. Koenen, K.C.; Lincoln, A.; Appleton, A. Women's status and child well-being: A state-level analysis. *Soc. Sci. Med.* **2006**, *63*, 2999–3012. [CrossRef]
7. Kavanagh, S.A.; Shelley, J.M.; Stevenson, C. Does gender inequity increase men's mortality risk in the United States? A multilevel analysis of data from the National Longitudinal Mortality Study. *SSM Popul. Health* **2017**, *3*, 358–365. [CrossRef]
8. Roberts, S.C.M. What can alcohol researchers learn from research about the relationship between macro-level gender equality and violence against women? *Alcohol Alcohol.* **2011**, *46*, 95–104. [CrossRef]
9. Schwab, K.; Samans, R.; Zahidi, S.; Leopold, T.A.; Ratcheva, V.; Hausmann, R.; Tyson, L.D. *The Global Gender Gap Report 2017*; World Economic Forum: Geneva, Switzerland, 2017; p. 349. Available online: https://www.weforum.org/reports/the-global-gender-gap-report-2017 (accessed on 7 May 2018).
10. United Nations Development Programme Gender Inequality Index. Available online: Http://hdr.undp.org/en/content/gender-inequality-index-gii (accessed on 5 July 2018).
11. Institute for Women's Policy Research. *Status of Women in the States*; Institute for Women's Policy Research: Washington, DC, USA, 2018; p. 7. Available online: Https://iwpr.org/publications/status-of-women-fact-sheet-2018/ (accessed on 7 May 2018).
12. Roberts, S.C.M. Macro-level gender equality and alcohol consumption: A multi-level analysis across U.S. states. *Soc. Sci. Med.* **2012**, *75*, 60–68. [CrossRef]
13. Petticrew, M.; Shemilt, I.; Lorenc, T.; Marteau, T.M.; Melendez-Torres, G.J.; O'Mara-Eves, A.; Stautz, K.; Thomas, J. Alcohol advertising and public health: Systems perspectives versus narrow perspectives. *J. Epidemiol. Community Health* **2017**, *71*, 308–312. [CrossRef]
14. Emslie, C.; Hunt, K.; Lyons, A. Transformation and time-out: The role of alcohol in identity construction among Scottish women in early midlife. *Int. J. Drug Policy* **2015**, *26*, 437–445. [CrossRef] [PubMed]
15. Kuntsche, E.; Kuntsche, S.; Knibbe, R.; Simons-Morton, B.; Farhat, T.; Hublet, A.; Bendtsen, P.; Godeau, E.; Demetrovics, Z. Cultural and gender convergence in adolescent drunkenness: Evidence from 23 European and North American countries. *Arch. Pediatr. Adolesc. Med.* **2011**, *165*, 152–158. [CrossRef] [PubMed]
16. Wilsnack, R.W.; Wilsnack, S.C.; Gmel, G.; Kantor, L.W. Gender differences in binge drinking: Prevalence, predictors, and consequences. *Alcohol Res.* **2018**, *39*, 1–20.

17. Giesbrecht, N.; Cukier, S.; Steeves, D. (Eds.) Collateral damage from alcohol: Implications of 'second-hand effects of drinking' for populations and health priorities. *Addiction* **2010**, *105*, 1323–1325. [CrossRef]
18. Room, R.; Ferris, J.; Laslett, A.-M.; Livingston, M.; Mugavin, J.; Wilkinson, C. The drinker's effect on the social environment: A conceptual framework for studying alcohol's harm to others. *Int. J. Environ. Res. Public Health* **2010**, *7*, 1855–1871. [CrossRef]
19. Karriker-Jaffe, K.J.; Greenfield, T.K.; Kaplan, L.M. Distress and alcohol-related harms from intimates, friends and strangers. *J. Subst. Use* **2017**, *22*, 434–441. [CrossRef]
20. Greenfield, T.K.; Ye, Y.; Kerr, W.; Bond, J.; Rehm, J.; Giesbrecht, N. Externalities from alcohol consumption in the 2005 US National Alcohol Survey: Implications for policy. *Int. J. Environ. Res. Public Health* **2009**, *6*, 3205–3224. [CrossRef]
21. Laslett, A.-M.; Catalano, P.; Chikritzhs, T.; Dale, C.; Doran, C.; Ferris, J.; Jainullabudeen, T.; Livingston, M.; Matthews, S.; Mugavin, J.; et al. *The Range and Magnitude of Alcohol's Harm to Others*; AER Centre for Alcohol Policy Research, Turning Point Alcohol and Drug Centre, Eastern Health: Fitzroy, Australia, 2010; p. 214. Available online: http://www.webcitation.org/5wB6fDhnQ (accessed on 1 February 2011).
22. Wilsnack, R.W.; Kristjanson, A.F.; Wilsnack, S.C.; Bloomfield, K.; Grittner, U.; Crosby, R.D. The harms that drinkers cause: Regional variations within countries. *Int. J. Alcohol Drug Res.* **2018**, *7*, 30–36. [CrossRef]
23. Room, R.; Callinan, S.; Greenfield, T.K.; Rekve, D.; Waleewong, O.; Stanesby, O.; Thamarangsi, T.; Benegal, V.; Casswell, S.; Florenzano, R.; et al. The social location of harm from others' drinking in ten societies. *Addiction* **2019**, *114*, 425–433. [CrossRef]
24. Karriker-Jaffe, K.J.; Greenfield, T.K. Gender differences in associations of neighbourhood disadvantage with alcohol's harms to others: A cross-sectional study from the USA. *Drug Alcohol Rev.* **2014**, *33*, 296–303. [CrossRef]
25. Nayak, M.B.; Patterson, D.; Wilsnack, S.C.; Karriker-Jaffe, K.J.; Greenfield, T.K. Alcohol's secondhand harms in the United States.: New data on prevalence and risk factors. *J. Stud. Alcohol Drugs* **2019**, *80*, 273–281. [CrossRef] [PubMed]
26. Ferris, J.A.; Laslett, A.-M.; Livingston, M.; Room, R.; Wilkinson, C. The impacts of others' drinking on mental health. *Med. J. Aust.* **2011**, *195* (Suppl. 3), 22–26. [CrossRef]
27. Karriker-Jaffe, K.J.; Li, L.; Greenfield, T.K. Estimating mental health impacts of alcohol's harms from other drinkers: Using propensity scoring methods with national cross-sectional data from the United States. *Addiction* **2018**, *113*, 1826–1839. [CrossRef] [PubMed]
28. Casswell, S.; You, R.Q.; Huckle, T. Alcohol's harm to others: Reduced wellbeing and health status for those with heavy drinkers in their lives. *Addiction* **2011**, *106*, 1087–1094. [CrossRef]
29. Greenfield, T.K.; Karriker-Jaffe, K.J.; Kerr, W.C.; Ye, Y.; Kaplan, L.M. Those harmed by others' drinking in the US population are more depressed and distressed. *Drug Alcohol Rev.* **2016**, *35*, 22–29. [CrossRef] [PubMed]
30. Yllö, K. The status of women, marital equality and violence against wives: A contextual analysis. *J. Fam. Issues* **1984**, *5*, 307–320. [CrossRef]
31. Lei, M.K.; Simons, R.L.; Simons, L.G.; Edmond, M.B. Gender equality and violent behavior: How neighborhood gender equality influences the gender gap in violence. *Violence Vict.* **2014**, *29*, 89–108. [CrossRef]
32. Bond, J.C.; Roberts, S.C.M.; Greenfield, T.K.; Korcha, R.; Ye, Y.; Nayak, M.B. Gender differences in public and private drinking contexts: A multi-level GENACIS analysis. *Int. J. Environ. Res. Public Health* **2010**, *7*, 2136–2160. [CrossRef]
33. Roberts, S.C.M.; Bond, J.; Korcha, R.; Greenfield, T.K. Genderedness of bar drinking culture and alcohol-related harms: A multi-country study. *Int. J. Ment. Health Addict.* **2013**, *11*, 50–63. [CrossRef]
34. Room, R. Intoxication and bad behaviour: Understanding cultural differences in the link. *Soc. Sci. Med.* **2001**, *53*, 189–198. [CrossRef]
35. Kerr, W.C. Categorizing US state drinking practices and consumption trends. *Int. J. Environ. Res. Public Health* **2010**, *7*, 269–283. [CrossRef] [PubMed]
36. Naimi, T.S.; Brewer, R.D.; Mokdad, A.; Denny, C.; Serdula, M.K.; Marks, J.S. Binge drinking among U.S. adults. *JAMA* **2003**, *289*, 70–75. [CrossRef] [PubMed]
37. Nelson, T.F.; Naimi, T.S.; Brewer, R.D.; Wechsler, H. The state sets the rate: The relationship among state-specific college binge drinking, state binge drinking rates, and selected state alcohol control policies. *Am. J. Public Health* **2005**, *95*, 441–446. [CrossRef] [PubMed]

38. Wechsler, H.; Lee, J.E.; Hall, J.; Wagenaar, A.C.; Lee, H. Secondhand effects of student alcohol use reported by neighbors of colleges: The role of alcohol outlets. *Soc. Sci. Med.* **2002**, *55*, 425–435. [CrossRef]
39. Stanesby, O.; Callinan, S.; Graham, K.; Wilson, I.M.; Greenfield, T.K.; Wilsnack, S.; Hettige, S.; Hanh, H.; Ibanga, A.; Siengsounthone, L.; et al. Harm from known others' drinking by relationship proximity to the harmful drinker and gender: A meta-analysis across 10 countries. *Alcohol. Clin. Exp. Res.* **2018**, *42*, 1693–1703. [CrossRef] [PubMed]
40. Kaplan, L.M.; Nayak, M.B.; Greenfield, T.K.; Karriker-Jaffe, K.J. Alcohol's harm to children: Findings from the 2015 United States National Alcohol's Harm to Others Survey. *J. Pediatr.* **2017**, *184*, 186–192. [CrossRef]
41. Greenfield, T.K.; Karriker-Jaffe, K.J.; Giesbrecht, N.; Kerr, W.C.; Ye, Y.; Bond, J. Second-hand drinking may increase support for alcohol policies: New results from the 2010 National Alcohol Survey. *Drug Alcohol Rev.* **2014**, *33*, 259–267. [CrossRef]
42. Eliany, M.; Giesbrecht, N.; Nelson, M.; Wellman, B.; Wortley, S. *Alcohol and Other Drug Use by Canadians: A National Alcohol and Other Drugs Survey (1989) Technical Report*; The Unit: Ottawa, ON, Canada, 1992; p. 450.
43. World Health Organization. *Harm to Others from Drinking: A WHO/Thai Health International Collaborative Research Project. Master Research Protocol*; WHO: Geneva, Switzerland, 2012; p. 22.
44. NARAL Pro-Choice America. *Who Decides? The Status of Women's Reproductive Rights in the United States*; NARAL: Washington, DC, USA, 2015; Available online: Https://www.prochoiceamerica.org/wp-content/uploads/2017/04/2015-Who-Decides.pdf (accessed on 7 May 2018).
45. Roberts, S.C.M.; Biggs, M.A.; Chibber, K.S.; Gould, H.; Rocca, C.H.; Foster, D.G. Risk of violence from the man involved in the pregnancy after receiving or being denied an abortion. *BMC Med.* **2014**, *12*, 144. [CrossRef]
46. Institute for Women's Policy Research Status of Women in the States: Download the Data. Available online: Https://statusofwomendata.org/explore-the-data/download-the-data/ (accessed on 21 June 2017).
47. Centers for Disease Control and Prevention. *Behavioral Risk Factor Surveillance System Survey Data and Documentation*; Centers for Disease Control and Prevention: Atlanta, GA, USA, 2013.
48. U.S. Census Bureau. *2011–2015 American Community Survey. Data Profiles*; U.S. Census Bureau: Washington, DC, USA, 2015. Available online: http://www.webcitation.org/6tv0XSKlm (accessed on 2 October 2017).
49. StataCorp. *Stata Statistical Software: Release 15*; StataCorp LLC: College Station, TX, USA, 2017.
50. Rossow, I.; Hauge, R. Who pays for the drinking? Characteristics of the extent and distribution of social harms from others' drinking. *Addiction* **2004**, *99*, 1094–1102. [CrossRef]
51. Seid, A.K.; Grittner, U.; Greenfield, T.K.; Bloomfield, K. To cause harm and to be harmed by others: New perspectives on alcohol's harms to others. *Subst. Abuse* **2015**, *9* (Suppl. 2), 13–22. [CrossRef]
52. Atkinson, A.M.; Kirton, A.W.; Sumnall, H.R. The gendering of alcohol in consumer magazines: An analysis of male and female targeted publications. *J. Gend. Stud.* **2012**, *21*, 365–386. [CrossRef]
53. Peralta, R.L. Raced and gendered reactions to the deviance of drunkenness: A sociological analysis of race and gender disparities in alcohol use. *Contemp. Drug Probl.* **2010**, *37*, 381–415. [CrossRef]
54. Keyes, K.M.; Jager, J.; Mal-Sarkar, T.; Patrick, M.E.; Rutherford, C.; Hasin, D. Is There a Recent Epidemic of Women's Drinking? A Critical Review of National Studies. *Alcohol. Clin. Exp. Res.* **2019**, *43*, 1344–1359. [CrossRef] [PubMed]
55. Kuntsche, S.; Knibbe, R.A.; Kuntsche, E.; Gmel, G. Housewife or working mum—Each to her own? The relevance of societal factors in the association between social roles and alcohol use among mothers in 16 industrialized countries. *Addiction* **2011**, *106*, 1925–1932. [CrossRef] [PubMed]
56. Flood, M.; Pease, B. Factors influencing attitudes to violence against women. *Trauma Violence Abuse* **2009**, *10*, 125–142. [CrossRef]
57. Reingold, R.B.; Gostin, L.O. State Abortion Restrictions and the New Supreme Court: Women's Access to Reproductive Health Services. *JAMA* **2019**, *322*, 21–22. [CrossRef]

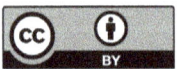

© 2019 by the authors. Licensee MDPI, Basel, Switzerland. This article is an open access article distributed under the terms and conditions of the Creative Commons Attribution (CC BY) license (http://creativecommons.org/licenses/by/4.0/).

MDPI
St. Alban-Anlage 66
4052 Basel
Switzerland
Tel. +41 61 683 77 34
Fax +41 61 302 89 18
www.mdpi.com

International Journal of Environmental Research and Public Health Editorial Office
E-mail: ijerph@mdpi.com
www.mdpi.com/journal/ijerph

www.ingramcontent.com/pod-product-compliance
Lightning Source LLC
LaVergne TN
LVHW070506100526
838202LV00014B/1796